Health Care Practices among the Ao Nagas

Socio-Cultural Study of Nagaland

Pranjal Boruah

CONCEPT PUBLISHING COMPANY PVT. LTD.

NEW DELHI-110059

ISBN-13 : 978-81-8069-845-3

First Published 2012

Published and Printed by

Concept
Since 1974

Concept Publishing Company Pvt. Ltd.
A/15-16, Commercial Block, Mohan Garden
New Delhi-110059 (India)
T: 25351460, 25351794, *F*: 091-11-25357109
E: publishing@conceptpub.com, W: www.conceptpub.com
Editorial Office: H-13, Bali Nagar, New Delhi-110 015, India.

Cataloging in Publication Data--*Courtesy:* D.K. Agencies (P) Ltd. <docinfo@dkagencies.com>

Boruah, Pranjal, 1982-
Health care practices among the Ao Nagas : socio-cultural study of Nagaland /Pranja Boruah.
p. cm.
Originally presented as the author's thesis (Ph. D.)—Dibrugarh University, 2008.
Includes bibliographical references (p.) and index.
ISBN 9788180698453

1. Naga (South Asian people)—India—Nagaland—Social life and customs. 2. Naga (South Asian people)—India—Nagaland—Economic conditions. 3. Naga (South Asian people)—Health and hygiene—India—Nagaland. 4. Ao language. I. Title.

DDC 305.800954165 23

FOREWORD

Health care study in any community is significant from various angles. As a holistic approach it not only reflects the traditional health care system that exists in a community but also provides an idea about the availability of modern medicare system among the tribal communities living in different geographical and environmental situations. The health, nutrition and medico-genetic problems of diverse tribal groups inhabiting widely varying geo-climatic conditions present a formidable challenge for effective health care system. Studies on health problems as well as the health behaviours of different tribal communities from anthropological point of view, therefore, not only contribute to the development of the medical anthropology but also assist the planners and medical practitioners in contemplating appropriate medicare systems that will be acceptable to the common people.

The present work is one of such studies undertaken by Dr. Pranjal Boruah among the Ao Naga of Mokokchung district, Nagaland—one of the dominant tribe of the region. The study of this nature is urgently needed as we have hardly any information about the population in this field.

The present outcome reflects that with the acceptance of Christianity, development occurs in the socio-religious and economic dimension of Ao Nagas no doubt but they still need special attention in the sphere of health care practices. Modern medicare system is not accessible in their area for which Aos still have to subscribe their traditional medicare system. On the basis of micro-level study, the author tries to focus the felt need of the people and is of opinion that efforts should be made by the Government for easy accessibility of modern medical facilities to all sections of Indian population. It is expected that education may be considered as a significant media towards achieving the desired result in the health care practices.

The book may provide interesting material to the scholars both in India and abroad in the field of Health Culture Studies, Medical Anthropology, Sociology of Health and Family Welfare and Planning. It will be of good use to the population planners in modifying the population welfare programmes for this region and for this tribal community in particular. I wish Pranjal Boruah a great success in his life.

I. Barua 23.11.2010

Prof. (Dr.) I. Barua
Department of Anthropology
Dibrugarh University, Dibrugarh

PREFACE

Micro-level studies concerning Socio-Cultural Dimension of Health Care Practices are very limited particularly among the Naga communities in Nagaland. Hence, the present study was undertaken among the Ao Naga tribe of Nagaland with the hope that the outcome of such an in-depth study may reveal the insight which may help population planners to draw a developmental strategy for this population in particular.

The present work has been the outcome of constant guidance, help, support, views, shared experiences and ideas contributed by many persons.

At the very outset, I would like to express my profound indebtedness to my supervisor Dr. I. Barua, Professor, in the Department of Anthropology, Dibrugarh University, for her painstaking guidance, valuable advice, relevant suggestions and constructive criticism in carrying out this work. It was solely because of her scholarly and efficient guidance, support and constant encouragement that I could undertake and carry-out this work. Without her selfless dedicated service and efficient guidance I would not have been able to complete this project successfully.

I would like to record a special note of appreciation for the assistance rendered by Prof. R.K. Kar by providing me with some important literatures relevant to the topic as well as his valuable suggestion and encouragement in the entire course of the project. I am greatly indebted to Dr. H. Goswami, Professor, in the Department of Economics and Dr. B.K. Baruah, Professor, in the Department of Assamese, Dibrugarh University, for their help and suggestions.

It is a pleasure to thank Dr. R.K. Borkotoki (F.R.C.O.G., London) retired Professor of Department of Obstetrics and Gynaecology, Assam Medical College, Dibrugarh and for the pains he took, in spite of his busy schedule, in going through the whole thesis and making valuable suggestions for improving the presentation of the data.

I am indebted to Director, The Eastern Regional Centre, Indian Council of Social Science Research (I.C.S.S.R.), Kolkata for sanctioning a financial grant; and thereby enabling me to pursue the relevant library consultations in different Universities and institutions of the country. I am thankful to the Librarians and other staff members of National Library, Calcutta University Central Library, Anthropology Department Library, Jadavpur University Library, Asiatic Society Library, Anthropological Survey of India Library and Centre for Social Science Studies Library, for allowing me to use their libraries to search relevant literatures. I am also thankful to the Librarians and staff members of Omeo Kumar Das Institute of Social Change and Development (Guwahati) and Tribal Research Institute (Guwahati) for allowing me to use their libraries.

I am also indebted to Dr. A. K. Borah (Trustee) for providing me the financial grant for research work from the J.K. Chowdhury Charitable and Educational Trust.

I am grateful to Manika Baruah, Assistant Librarian, Dibrugarh University Central Library, for her encouragement and support throughout the course of my studies. My sincere thanks are due to all the other staff members of Dibrugarh University Library who helped me by extending their kind co-operation during entire period of my study in the Library.

My special thanks go to my brother-in-law, Mr. Biju Hatikakoti for his co-operation in every step of my fieldwork and without his help I would not have been able to carry-out this work. Here, I would like to mention the name of Mr. Atul Hatikakoti and his family members who extended all possible help during this period.

At this juncture, I would like to express my deep sense of gratitude to all the people of Lirmen, Yajang-A and Yajang-B villages who helped me by extending their kind co-operation during the entire period of the fieldwork. Here, I would like to mention the name of Mr. B. Shilu Walling, I. Tali Jamir, T.C. Jamir who extended all possible help during this period.

I am grateful to Achangla Longcher for her help and support. I am also thankful to Mr. Temsu Wati Ao, District Information Officer, for giving me useful information on the district.

With a sense of profound love and respect, I must express my indebtedness to my parents, without whose encouragement I would have never completed my work; specially my father, who always encouraged me to go for higher studies, and the present Ph.D. thesis is in fact the result of his persuasion and inspiration.

I would fail in my duty if I do not express my indebtedness to my two sisters Progoti and Prostuti for their constant help and encouragement in every step of my work.

I must record my sense of appreciation for I.C.S.S.R., New Delhi for the financial assistance for conducting my doctoral work and Concept Publishing Company Pvt. Ltd., New Delhi for having readily consented to take the responsibility of publishing the work without which the work would have remained the knowledge of only a few.

Last but not the least my special thank is due to Manash Baruah for his helping hand in every step of my work. I am thankful to all my relatives, friends and well-wishers who helped me in one way or the other; and have contributed either directly or indirectly to achieve my goal.

Pranjal Boruah

CONTENTS

LIST OF FIGURES AND MAPS

Figures

Maps

LIST OF TABLES

LIST OF COLOURED PHOTOGRAPHS

1

INTRODUCTION

Health of an individual as well as the community is largely influenced by social and cultural factors which are deeply interwoven with the social fabric of life. These factors have wide variation from one community to another and also within the community itself.

Health and hygiene are a set of biological needs that are common to all human beings. In a community it is directly related to the interaction between socio-cultural life and environment. The socio-economic status of a community has tremendous impact on morbidity pattern, which is largely dependent on social customs, cultural beliefs and health seeking behaviour.

Social, economic and cultural inequality is detrimental to health of any society. Tribal society in this context provides unique opportunity to study socio-cultural dimension of health as the tribal people have distinguished themselves by their unique social, cultural, economical and ethnic identity. The health status of the tribals is mostly affected by insufficient diet, lack of personal hygiene practices, living conditions, non-availability of potable water, socio-cultural practices and inappropriate health care services. Thus, it is apparent that socio-cultural perspectives invariably affect the health care practices and it is, therefore, necessary to understand the community in its socio-cultural context before any health programme is implemented or evaluated.

The cultural structure of a particular society regarding

perception, preference, evaluation and satisfaction shows the pattern of health care. Thus, it becomes imperative to find out personal hygiene, food habits and nutritional status in relation to its culture. The cultural setting of a society influences directly or indirectly people's understanding of the problems of diseases, its treatment, prevention and the pattern of health care. A person's attitudes, daily routine, decisions regarding health maintenance, food habits and food serving practices are reflective of efforts on his or her part to maintain or restore himself or herself to his or her normal state. Even when we know how to prevent some illness or to seek medical care for cure of various diseases, the utilization of such services will depend on the notion people have of health and illness and actions they take in the event of sickness which depends on their understanding of the etiology of a disease. Thus, the attitude of the members towards disease, health, food and eating habits form the matrix of health pattern (Nagla, 2006).

The culture of a community determines also its health culture. Culture generally refers to patterns of human activity and the symbolic structure that give such activity significance. Different definitions of 'Culture' reflect different theoretical bases for understanding, or criteria for evaluating, human activity. In general, the term culture denotes the whole product of an individual, group or society of intelligent beings. It includes technology, art, science, as well as moral systems and the characteristic behaviour and habits of the selected intelligent entities. In particular, it has specific more detailed meanings in different domain of human activities.

Anthropologists most commonly use the term 'culture' to refer to the universal human capacity to classify, codify and communicate their experiences symbolically. This capacity has long been taken as a defining feature of the humans. It can also be said that culture is the way people live in accordance to belief, language, history or the way they dress.

According to Dube (1996), "Culture refers to all those parts of the Universe that have been created by humankind. Beliefs, ideas and attitudes, religious, social and economic organization, material culture, science and technology are all parts of the complex network that is our culture".

Culture refers to the relationship that we develop with nature, society and the supernatural world. It denotes all historically created designs for living that we inculcate and learn. These designs are transmitted from generation to generation, although they are constantly being modified by pressures from within the culture and from outside (Dube, 1996).

Culture maintains the biological functioning of the human organism by providing for the needs of food, drink, warmth, shelter, sexual gratification and reproduction, affection and encouragement. It is through culture that we develop a conception of self, society and God. Culture provides us a system of meaning and motivation. Through culture, we set our goals and obtain the outlets for creative expression. It is also responsible for the maintenance of internal and external security. In its more dynamic aspects, culture provides for adaptation and adjustment to the changing natural, social and psychological environments (Dube, 1996).

Interaction with outside world opens a community or a society to a theoretically unlimited range of available raw materials, finished goods, technical knowledge and ideas. Furthermore it brings about cultural change in a society (Wells, 1980). Culture is the characteristic way of life inspired by fundamental values in which a people live. It is the sum total of the values expressed through art, religion, literature, social institutions and behaviour the ever acts of individuals and mass action inspired by collective urges. The dress we wear, the factories we set up or the dams we build are only a part of the civilization, the material equipment of life which tends to increase in complexity with scientific progress. But essentially culture has little to do with material equipment of life (Kumar, 2003).

The health of a community is also affected/influenced by its culture. The socio-cultural and economic variables of health are interrelated and interdependent. Every culture, irrespective of its simplicity and complexity has its own notion regarding health and health seeking behaviour, and this is often referred to as 'Health culture'. It is an integral component of the overall culture of the community. The health of any community, particularly of a tribal community, by and large, is a function of the interaction between socio-cultural and socio-biological practices, the genetic attributes and the environmental conditions. The widely varying prevalent health practices, use of indigenous herbal drugs, taboos and superstitions are also responsible for determining the health behaviour and health status of tribal groups (Kar and Gogoi, 1995).

Culture determines to a large extent not only the type and frequency of disease/illness but also the way people perceive, explain and treat diseases as well as the manner in which they respond to the delivery of modern medicine. Thus, culture is an invariable determining factor of a community's understanding of health and illness (Kannuri, 2005).

Environmental control is the ability of members of a particular cultural group to plan activities that control nature or direct environmental factors. Included in this concept are the complex systems of traditional health and illness beliefs, the practice of folk medicine, and the use of traditional healers. This particular cultural phenomenon plays an extremely important role in the way clients respond to health-related experience, including the ways in which they define health and illness and seek and use health care resources and social supports (Spector, 1996).

The social environment in which people grow up and live plays an essential role in their cultural development and identification. Children learn their culture's responses to life events from the family and its ethno religious group. This socialization process is an inherent part of heritage-cultural, religious and ethnic background. Social organization refers to the family unit (nuclear, single parent, or extended family) and the social group organizations (religious or ethnic) with which clients and families may identify. Countless social barriers, such as unemployment, underemployment, homelessness, lack of health insurance, and poverty, can also prevent people from entering the health care system (Spector, 1996).

Social scientists have been actively engaged in empirically examining the social factors which contribute significantly in promoting good health and controlling diseases. Their persistent efforts to understand health from social perspective have firmly rooted social scientists in addressing larger issues related to causes and cures of health problems. In this context, Dalal and Ray (2005) opines four sectors that cover most of the areas and disciplines of social sciences. These four sectors are: socio-economic concomitants of health, health services and systems, health care practices and health attitudes and perceptions. This sectoral model of health is presented below (Fig.1.1).

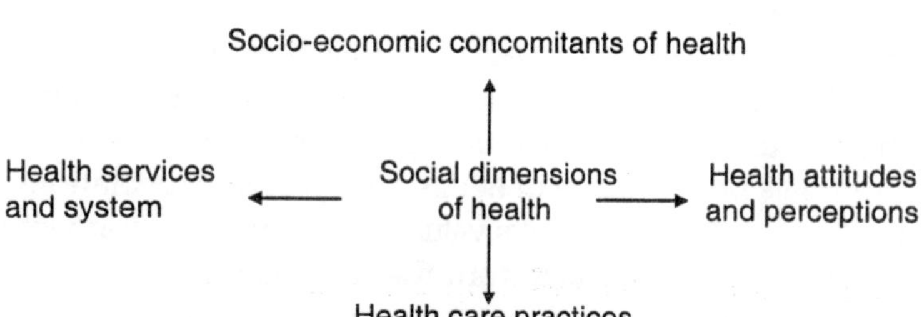

Fig.1.1 : Sectoral Model of Health

Source : Dalal and Roy; 2005.

Socio-economic concomitants of health: Socio-economic conditions of the people determine their health status in terms of longevity, infant mortality and morbidity. People lows on socio-economic ladder are not only more vulnerable to infection and respiratory diseases but also have lower access to health services. In general, people below poverty line, children, women, aged and displaced ones suffer more from health problems than other strata of the society.

Health systems and services: Health systems have existed ever since people made systematic attempts to protect their health and treat diseases. Throughout the world, the traditional practices based on herbal cures and/or spiritual counselling and providing both curative and preventive care, have existed for thousands of years, and even today have survived despite the dominance of modern medicine. The modern health systems, aiming to cater to the needs of a large mass of population, existed barely a century ago. In many countries, the existence of hospitals has a larger history than the organised health system. With the onset of industrial revolution, there occurred a transformation in the lives of the people, especially in relation to health and health systems.

Most of the information available on health system refers to the provision of investment in health services, i.e. health care, including curative, preventive and palliative interventions, whether directed to individuals or population. People come into direct contact with a health system as patients attended by the health care providers. It matters very much how the system treats people's health needs, meets their expectations, treats them with dignity, pays value to their time and anxiety and how it raises revenues from them, including how much protection it offers them from financial risk. Again, in order for an individual to utilize a service, they must believe that the service will benefit their health. Some studies have focused on the perceptions and motivations to use health services reveal that care is often inadequate and ineffective. Moreover, location of services and transportation problems in accessing services can be a barrier to the utilization of health facilities. Sometimes, corruption in public health services creates aversion among the care seekers.

Health care practices: Health behaviour is a kind of

social behaviour and as such, affects and gets affected by various socio-cultural parameters. For example, understanding of a disease is not a medical issue but is largely dependent on the shared knowledge of a particular community. Traditions, social practices and role relationship—all contribute to our dealings with health and illnesses. The sick role behaviour largely depends on how a community expects its sick members to behave. These social aspects of health form basis for informal systems of health care.

Medical anthropologist, Arthur Kleinman has classified health care practices into three sectors: popular, folk and professional. These three sectors not only differ in terms of their explanations of illness but also in the treatment regimen and the mode of social interaction. The popular sector refers to those informal health practices that primarily rely on familial and social network knowledge to deal with diseases. Home-made remedies, knowledgeable people who can be consulted, visiting spiritual centres are all parts of the popular sector. These practices are the outgrowth of shared experiences and transfer of knowledge from one generation to the other. According to Kleinman, 95 per cent of the health problems in a society are taken care of by this popular sector. The folk sector is rather a more organised system of dealing with health and illness. These are the informal systems, which have evolved over a very long period of time, and are integrated within the community life. The folk sector comprises herbal medicine, shamans and traditional healers and time-tested indigenous medicines. These folk treatments have survived for centuries because they share the belief systems of the community and are consistent with the social and religious practices. Kakar has evidenced that, what are considered as primitive and superstitious practices have their rationality rooted in a coherent worldview and in efficiency in dealing with a wide range of health problems. Even, in this scientific age, the popularity of these folk practices has not declined. The third sector, i.e. professional sector, refers to organised professional systems, like medical system, acupuncture and *Ayurveda*, which have a formal system of practising. These systems are based on well laid-out theoretical basis, system of education and professional bodies and code of conduct. Such professional systems compete for public patronage and their co-existence is characterized by suspicion and underlying tension.

Health perceptions and attitudes: In this sectoral approach health is understood from the people's perspective. It views a person as embedded in a socio-cultural context, in which he or she imbibes certain belief system. These socio-cultural beliefs would determine the way a patient evaluates and gives meaning to his/her sickness. Kleinman has made a distinction in his research between disease and illness. Whereas disease is an organic malfunctioning as diagnosed by a medical practitioner, illness is a subjective construction of the experience of a disease by the patient. It is patient's own interpretation and perception of the disease, which is greatly influenced by the culture to which the patient belongs.

Human health and quality of life are strongly influenced by the environment. Both environmental and genetic factors, however, are involved in the production of disease, while genetic factors usually give rise to congenital diseases and environmental factors to acquired ones, there is often an interplay between the two (Swarap, 1992). The Government of India was a signatory to the *Alma Ata* Declaration, and the South East Asian Health Charter with WHO for achieving the goal of "Health for All by 2000" (Sharma, 2005).

Health and disease are very often considered to be the polar words (Kar, 1997). To many people, good health means simply that they have no obvious illness or physical problems. But some people who are depressed, lack vitality and say they are 'not feeling well', cannot be shown to have any specific illness. For this reason, the World Health Organization defines health as, 'a state of complete physical, mental and social well-being and not merely the absence of disease and infirmity' (cited in Coleman and Cressey, 1987). It is clear that health involves social and psychological conditions as well as biological ones. Health, thus, connotes an efficient functioning of the body and the mind as well as, a capacity to participate in social activities and being able to discriminate and abide by the moral principles. It takes a holistic perspective in which nutritional status, immunity from diseases, better quality of social and family life, peace and contentment are important. Thus, good health is taken as synonymous to general well-being of a person.

The definition of good health varies between notions and even between different classes within the same notion. There is overwhelming evidence that poor people have more health problems than those who are better off. The effects of poverty are obvious in the over populated agricultural nations.

A state of disease on the other hand, is a condition of the organism that seriously obtrudes against these adaptive requirements; and causes partial or complete disablement; and physical or behavioural dysfunction. But these are necessarily relative terms and especially so when they are applied to the human being. Webster defines disease as a "discomfort, a condition in which bodily health is seriously attacked, deranged, impaired, a departure from a state of health, an alternation of human body interrupting the performance of vital functions" (cited in Mehta, 1977).

It, however, becomes apparent that while disease is considered to be a diagnosed and defined concept of a particular type of illness or infirmity of body, health is a holistic view. In other words, it is as much a social as a biological issue. As a social issue, it depends on a society's technology and distribution of resources. Culture shapes the concepts of health as well as responses to illness.

The marked variation in health from nation to nation and from society to society provides a strong evidence of the link between health and society. Historical pattern too confirms this connection. Thus, Kar (1997) observes that health is not only the result of interaction between an individual's hereditary contribution with his or her natural and cultural environment, but it is also largely determined by the biological and cultural adaptation and evolution of the society and the population. Health and diseases are measures of the effectiveness with which a human group has adapted to the environment. It is thus apparent that the standard of health and well-being varies with the environment, which of course varies enormously among population, or even their sub-groups.

Thus, social and cultural elements as a whole do influence the health of a community both positively and negatively. The various cultural do's and don'ts, especially in food and drinking habits, pregnancy, child birth practices, etc., will have a direct impact on the health.

On the whole, Health and Disease are related to biological and cultural resources of a community in a specific environment. That is why concept of health and disease though biological, are often culturally comprehended as these have been connected with variation in socio-cultural circumstances and habit patterns.

Of late, it has been realized by both social scientists and medical practitioners that there is a close relationship between health problems on the one hand, and socio-cultural and economic factors on the other hand. Thus, Kar (1993) observes that health is not the exclusive domain of medical sciences. It needs a co-ordination between social scientists and medical practitioners to deal effectively with both prevention and cure of disease. Health cannot be given to people, nor can it be bought or sold as a commodity. It invariably calls for people's active participation.

The social and cultural aspects of maintenance of health and etiology of disease are infecting deeply rooted in medical history. Again, beliefs and practices constitute a major element in every culture. Therefore, it is very important to gain an understanding of the people's lives; and to identify different communities' health needs. Likewise, the socio-cultural matrix of health and disease in relation to a particular society must be properly understood for inflicting any change of concept for the purpose of the implementation of any developmental programme. It is assumed that the socio-cultural phenomena are by and large very important factor that acts as either promoter or barrier for accepting modern practices.

Thus, man's medical history can only be understood through an analysis of the socio-cultural milieu. It is necessary to know the community structure, their social and cultural pattern, attitude towards health, their beliefs and health practices etc., before introducing any health programme on any population. Anthropological studies have shown that every known human society has developed a concept regarding health and disease and also the methods of cropping with them. They practise some form of preventive or curative medicine according to their own concept of the cause. Medical science is directly involved with the study of health condition, disease and its treatment. But an interdisciplinary approach is more essential for the improvement of health and biological qualities of mankind. In recent years the need to study human population by interdisciplinary approaches has been increasingly realized. In the implementation of public health programme communities' acceptance and participation is very essential. Here a joint effort of the medical sciences and social and behavioural sciences is necessary. Anthropology can play a greater role in this regard as it tries to understand human groups from both biological and cultural point of view (Das, 1997).

In anthropology, an emphasis is always placed on the group and on the study of human being within the framework of culture. Culture, in the simplest words may be defined as a set of beliefs and behaviours, shared by a group of people. Culture provides people with a way of perceiving the world at large and with the ways in which a person should be treated when ill. It is the culture that determines why people suffer from certain disease and what type of treatments need to be followed; and so on and so forth.

Thus, the anthropologist has to find out the underlying socio-cultural, economic and other factors that relate to the health and health-seeking behaviour of a community.

The tribal communities of India constitute a sizeable portion of the total population of a country. They have distinctive problems because of their special kind of placement in difficult areas and circumstances in which they live. These groups inhabit widely varying ecological and geo-climatic conditions in different concentrations throughout the country. The health of tribal depends on various interacting factors. The health problems of tribal's stem from a double burden—the burden of health problems associated with low income (poverty), mal (or under) nutrition, poor sanitation and underdevelopment and other burden placed upon them by ecological/ environmental changes (Tyagi, 1997). NFHS-II (IIPS, 1995) has revealed that Scheduled Tribes (STs) are lagging behind in social development. All indicators of mortality and morbidity show that STs have not benefited from development as much as others. Among the tribes death rates is general and maternal mortality rates in particular are very high (Sharma, 2005).

Health is man's natural condition, therefore, it is always a major concern of the community development and problems of health are the problems of national importance. It is well-known fact that health and disease are interrelated and their concept varies from culture to culture and people to people, especially in tribal and other backward communities, because their concept of health and health seeking behaviour is a part of their culture. Health status and health seeking behaviour of different tribal and backward groups are influenced by their entire way of life like culture, including social and economic condition, nutrition, living condition, housing, education, food habits, taboo and superstition, socio-religious beliefs and practices, use of indigenous medicare system, income, communication and transportation, ecology, demography, socio-biological practices, genetic attributes and health services etc. (Yadav and Sharma, 2002).

Thus, all these above mentioned characteristics of the tribal societies, not only have an observable reflection on their overall health status, but also add to the people's reluctance and resistance to accept the available modern medicare services. The prevalence of low economy, illiteracy, hostile environment etc., and decline in their traditional curative knowledge of diseases make it more important to study their health problems.

However, living condition, poverty, illiteracy and ignorance etc. also contribute towards their enhanced fertility, mortality and morbidity, the very important parameters in assessing the health status of a community. It thus becomes apparent that to understand the health scenario of a community, particularly a simple one; it is necessary to have a total knowledge of the society and its culture, especially the health culture.

The Problem

The foregoing discussion thus makes it apparent that it is the culture which consists of the acquired or cultivated behaviour and thoughts of individuals within a society, as well as of the intellectual, artistic and social ideals and institutions which the members of the society profess and to which they strive to conform. In other words, culture has dynamism. It grows and this growth is attained by culture processes. Culture processes and culture change go together.

Again health of a community is also affected/influenced by its culture. Culture provides people with a way of perceiving the world at large and with the ways in which a person should be treated when ill. It is the culture that determines why people suffer from certain disease and what type of treatment needs to be followed; and so on and so forth. The socio-cultural elements as a whole do influence the health of a community both positively and negatively. The socio-cultural and economic variables of health are interrelated and interdependent and every culture, irrespective of its simplicity and complexity has its own notion regarding health and health seeking behaviour.

Thus, health of an individual and community is largely influenced by social and cultural factors which are deeply interwoven with the social fabric of life. These factors have wide variation from one community to another and within the community itself. It is, therefore, necessary to understand the community in its socio-cultural context before any health programme is implemented or evaluated.

Though the rapid advances in the field of medical science in the last century have helped in reducing mortality, the morbidity has significantly increased. There are more people suffering from various diseases today than ever in the past. Pollution, poverty, lifestyle, food habit, social and personal stresses and many other factors have contributed to this sense, health and social development cannot be separated from each other, and social sciences research is of much significant in health care planning.

The health problems need special attention in the context of tribal communities in India because of their settlements in difficult areas and circumstances. The health, nutrition and medico-genetic problems of diverse tribal groups inhabiting widely varying geo-climatic conditions present a formidable challenge for effective health care delivery. Similarly, the common beliefs, customs and practices connected with health and disease are intimately connected with the treatment of disease.

Despite gradual expansion of modern education and increasing contact with the outside world, very often it is observed that the social, economic and cultural factors poise as barrier in availing of modern medicare facilities.

Studies on health problems as well as the health behaviours of different tribal communities from anthropological point of view, therefore, not only contribute to the development of the sub-discipline (i.e. medical anthropology) but also assist the planners and medical practitioners in contemplating appropriate medicare systems that will be acceptable to the target beneficiaries.

Since the health care practices of a community are also prescribed its deep-rooted tradition. like beliefs, customs, practices, literacy and prevailing health care facilities, therefore, studies on socio-cultural correlated of the tribe will help to understand their health seeking behaviour which in turn will be helpful to plan interventions to improve their health status.

Keeping all these facts, observations and views in mind; and also in view of the fact that studies on health problems among the tribal in Nagaland, particularly among the Ao Nagas are very scanty, the present study is proposed to be carried out among the Ao Nagas under rural setting in Nagaland, to examine their socio-cultural life and to understand the socio-cultural dimension of health as well as the nature and extent of the interaction between their traditional health care practices and the modern medicare system.

In order to have a detailed holistic understanding of the problem, it has been decided to make the study an intensive one. For that purpose, it is proposed to carry out the study in three homogeneous Ao Naga villages (micro-field), namely Lirmen, Yajang-A and Yajang-B under rural setting in Mokokchung district, where they are numerically a dominant group.

Review of Literature

The following pages have been devoted to have a brief review of some of the available and accessible relevant literatures.

To start with we may mention about the important work carried out by Horam (1977) among the Tangkhul Nagas of Manipur to bring to lighi their socio-cultural life. His study highlights the social organisation, village administration, head hunting, festivals, songs and dances and social change that had been taken place due to Christianity.

Das Gupta's ethnographic study (1984) on the War Khasis of Meghalaya embraces almost every facet of the tribe's life and culture, describing the characteristic War Khasi village, home, agriculture, livestock, tools, dress, ornaments, vocations, domestic chores, hunting pursuit armory, means of travel, recreations, pastimes, family, clan, marriage, divorce, kinship, rules of inheritance, social practices, beliefs, myths, superstitions, funeral rites and a lot more.

Tangmi (2002) did his doctoral dissertation on ethnographic study among the Thangal (Koirao) tribe of Manipur. His study also brings to focus the socio-economic, political and religious life of the Thangals and their changing aspects after Christianity.

Chutia (1984) did her doctoral dissertation on continuity and change among the Chaudangs of Assam. Her work highlights the ethnicity and social stratification of the Chaudangs of Assam and also religion and festivals, economic profile etc.

Ahmed (1995) in his doctoral dissertation carried out in-depth study on socio-economic changes among the Kaibartas of Barak valley, Assam. In his work he discussed about the family, religion, economy, material culture, community life and the changing scene among the Kaibartas.

Roy (2002) worked among the Garos. In his work he traces the successive development and changes of the Garo Hill people down the ages, from the ancient times to the present decade. He traced the social origin and evolution of the peoples of the Garo Hills district in Meghalaya, from the ancient Vedic time to the modern period. He also makes an attempt to evaluate the impact of Christian missionaries and the role they played in transforming the social profile of the Garo people.

Singh (1985) did his doctoral dissertation on changing orientation of Mongsang tribe of Manipur. His in-depth study highlights the domestic life, economy, religion and its socio-economic implications, village government and politics, emergent identity orientation etc.

Dutta (1990) carried out a research on socio-cultural life of the Singphos of Arunachal Pradesh. His study also highlights the social, political, religious and domestic life of the Singphos.

An elaborate work was done by Bhagabati (1991), on the social formation of the Tangsa tribe of Arunachal Pradesh. His study highlights the social change and the dynamic identity orientation among the Tangsa tribe.

Barua and Bharali (2001) carried out a project on socio-religious life of the Deoris of Assam. Their study brings to light that the life and culture of Deoris are strongly religious oriented and religion, as a matter of fact, is a very dominant force and its manifestations are revealed in almost all aspects of Deoris social structure

Rongmei and Kapoor (2005) carried out a study on the Zeliangrong tribe of Manipur. Their study brings to light all the cultural customs, traditions, living system, occupation, marriage system and physical features of Zeliangrong.

Saikia (2003) carried out a study on religion of the Angami Nagas in Nagaland. The study brings to light about the past and present religion of the Angamis and the impact of religion on the socio-economic and cultural life in transition from tradition to modernity.

Bairathi, (1991) studied the tribal problems with special emphasis on the inter-play of culture, economy and health care practices of the Saharias of Rajasthan.

Majumdar (1933), Vidyarthi (1963) and Chaudhuri (1986) observed that socio-cultural and religious beliefs and practices are associated with the health care practices among some primitive and tribal societies in India.

Barua and Phukan (1998) carried out a study on the Sonowal Kacharis of Assam. Their study highlights the socio-religious aspects in relation to health and well-being of the Sonowal Kacharis and the various beliefs and practices and restrictions associated with health.

Pandey *et al.* (2000) worked on fertility behaviour of Gond tribe of Jabalpur district of Madhya Pradesh. In this work, they analyzed how fertility is affected by the social, cultural and economic factors, such as the socially considered appropriate age of female marriage culturally controlled cohabitation activities, economic and educational factors that govern or affect the marriage ceremony.

Bhagwat and Chirmulay (1997) worked on the traditional remedies followed for certain illness, perceived causes and the associated beliefs in a rural area of Karnataka. Their work also brings to focus that despite the popularity of modern medicine in the area, the traditional medical system persists and is mainly related to the belief system of the society.

Dalal and Roy's (2005) edited book *Social Dimensions of Health* is the outcome of articles presented in the National Seminar on Social Dimension of Health organised by Centre for Behavioural and Cognitive Sciences, University of Allahabad.

Maheo (2004) carried out a demographic anthropological study on the Mao Naga tribe of Manipur. Her study highlighted the general demographic profile of the population; reproductive profile of women; knowledge, attitudes and practices of birth control measures; mortality; mother and child health status and health care practices.

Patel (1985) studied among the Khond tribals and Tibetan refugees. His study highlighted the problems and inter-relationship between undernourishment, social environment and work-output.

Pokarana (1994) carried out his project titled 'Social Beliefs, Cultural Practices in Health and Disease' in two villages in Jaipur, Rajasthan. He made an effort to understand the health conditions, health problems, health beliefs and health practices, traditional health care institutions, faith healers, sickness and role network, modern medical care and its impact, environmental sanitation and personal hygienic conditions and role of voluntary organizations in health care system in rural setting.

Nagla (2006) carried out a study on attitudes and beliefs towards medicine and medical care systems and organizations in two different settings, i.e. urban and rural settings in Haryana.

Duarah and Pathak (1997) studied the health care practices among the Nishis of Arunachal Pradesh. Their study highlighted the overall hygiene and food among the people, their morbidity pattern and treatment by using local medicinal herbs. The study also brings to light about the trend of development of using modern medicinal treatment.

Bhadra and Tirkey (1997) carried out a comparative study to find out the situations of acceptance and non-acceptance of modern medical system among some tribal workers of tea plantation and scheduled caste peasants.

Mandal (1997) studied the social and cultural dimensions of mother and children health in a Muslim village in West Bengal. His study also brings to light that there is a general ignorance and unawareness of modern health care system for mother and child. Their health is a socially controlled factor and the reasons of negative attitudes towards modern health care system are mainly social and cultural. The study also reveals that the mother and child not only experiences morbidity and mortality but also are affected by malnutrition, poor health care, lack of proper treatment.

Roy *et al.* (1997) studied the health status of Kharia and Mankria women of Orissa. Their study reveals that the Kharia and Mankria females are undernourished and the reason for such condition is not only for malnutrition and poverty but also for lack of proper medical facilities.

Kar and Barua (1997) studied the morbidity and health behaviour among the migrant Munda Tea labourers in Upper

Assam. Their study brings to light that socio-economic factors such as lack of education, superstition, ignorance about the nutritional value of diet, insufficient per capita income along with unhygienic living conditions, poor environmental sanitation and unsanitary habits etc. are responsible for high frequency of these diseases among the people. The people believe that diseases are inflicted through three agencies, i.e. natural, human and supernatural and to cure these diseases they approach the traditional medicine man both herbal and magico-religious.

Dwivedi and Sharma (2005) carried out a study on utilization of health and family welfare services among the Baigas of Samnapur in Madhya Pradesh. In the study he brings to light that Baigas have little interest in modern system of medicine and have a strong faith in their traditional system of medicines and other magico-religious activities performed by village folk healer.

Yadav and Sharma (2002), studied health culture and assessed the health seeking behaviour among the Semi Nomadic Lohar Godiyas of Madhya Pradesh.

Das (2003) carried out a study on ethnomedicinal practices among the Karbis of Goria Ghuli of Sonapur, Assam. His study also brings to light the female health problems.

Sharma and Ali (2005) studied the Kaibartas society and economy and the occupational changes noticed among them due to the impact of urbanization.

Dzuvichu (2005) studied the health problems of the aged Angami Nagas of Nagaland. His study brings to light that majority of aged suffer from one or a combination of ailments and the medical facilities available for the aged are inadequate and many aged are compelled to seek help from private practitioners in spite of their poor economic status.

Verma (2002) carried out a study on Antenatal care and Birth related practices among the Baigas of Madhya Pradesh.

Prasad and Nagraj (2001) conducted a study on a rural community of Andhra Pradesh to examine socio-demographic correlates of place of delivery and person conducting the delivery and look at possible interventions.

Tiwari and Sharma (2001) carried out a study on multireligious population in Sagar city of Madhya Pradesh to assess the influence of socio-demographic and environmental factors on the incidence of cases of maternal malaria.

Pandey *et al.* (2001) carried out a study on the Pando Tribe of Madhya Pradesh. His study brings to light how studies on socio-cultural correlates of the tribe will help to understand their health seeking behaviour which in turn will be helpful to plan interventions to improve their health status.

Kar and Gogoi (1995) carried out a study on appraisal of some aspects of health culture of the Noctes of Arunachal Pradesh. Their study highlights the living conditions, personal hygiene, sanitation, food habits, concepts of health, disease and treatment etc. that prevail among the people.

Thakre (1995) carried out a study to analyse the family, marriage and inheritance system in the social, economic and religious set-up of the Bhills by focusing on marriage age, bride price, family planning, adultery, divorce, remarriage and other related issues.

Ajala *et al.* (2005) carried out a study to examine the accessibility to health care facilities in the rural areas of Osun state and its implication for sustainable development was highlighted.

Nanda and Stephenson (2001) carried out a project in Orissa to evaluate the infant mortality rate taking into account socio-economic and household environmental factors. Their study highlighted the correlation between infant mortality rate and poverty in Orissa, with focus on the impact of household conditions, for which the 'Household Environment Index' is taken as a measure.

Mojumder (2006) carried out a study in an interdisciplinary framework to investigate how pattern of utilization of care is affected by different socio-economic, demographic and other relevant factors in the rural and urban areas of Cooch Behar and Jalpaiguri district of North Bengal.

Maiti *et al.* (2005) studied on health care and health condition among the tribal women in comparison to the non-tribal women in the newly formed state of Jharkhand. Their study also highlights the antenatal, delivery and postnatal characteristics of tribal and non-tribal women, delivery and post-partum care, contraceptive use and problems and nutritional status and identifies many lacunae.

Medhi and Paul (2004) carried out a study on health and hygiene of the Nahs of Arunachal Pradesh. Their study brings to light that due to bad communication system, the people live principally with their traditional health care practices under the given ecological condition. The study also highlights how the impinging modern medicine system adjusts and reacts with the traditional one in Nah heritage.

Biswas and Kapoor (2005) carried out a study on health status and health seeking behaviour on Saharia tribe of Madhya Pradesh. Their study highlights that due to inhabit in remote area, they are totally isolated from advanced society and entangled in socio-economically backward situation while achieving low extent of literacy rate. They are highly constrained to respect to their socio-cultural orthodox. Health seeking behaviour focuses that most of the Saharia bear very weak health status, sustain sickness of their early age and old age, suffer from various diseases and tolerate some of the sickness for long time. Consultations with the doctors for their sickness are usually depended on their socio-cultural temperament. Initially they prefer the treatment under their traditional healer. The study also highlights the people's comments against the unhealthy role of their local hospital.

Rajaratnam *et al.* (1997), in their study among the Malto tribes in Bihar, attempts to highlight the maternal and child health practices and nutritional status of mothers and their children. Their study reveals that the health care practices of the Malto tribe is poor.

Sharmeen and Sharmeen (2005) carried out a study on traditional health practices of Munda women in Naogaon district, Assam. The study brings to light about the position and status of a Munda woman in her social, cultural and economic domain within the community. It also emphasizes on the belief system, cultural practices and dietary restrictions related to the period during pregnancy, lactation and in the rest of her life. This also recognizes the heavy work burden, and vicious cycle of malnutrition that is attributed through different socio-cultural practices that apparently lead towards drastic physiological and gynaecological disease. It also highlights the health seeking behaviour and the nature and access to reproductive health care system.

Medhi and Hasan (2003) carried out his study about the ethno-medicine system of the Garos of Assam. Their study reveals that they practice ethno-medicine extensively and intensively.

Joshi (1992) carried out his study in a Nagaland village on concept of health, illness and their relationship with social structure. He also discussed about the ethno medicine of Nagaland.

Babu (1998) conducted his study in the Madugula Mandal of Andhra Pradesh and discussed about how differential health care is employed at various stages of any illness. The study also reveals that the socio-cultural beliefs, education, economy etc., influence the health scenario of the people.

Barua (1994) in her Ph.D. project carried out an in-depth study on the socio-cultural dimension of health practices among the migrant Mundas working in tea plantations of Assam. The study reveals that their socio-cultural and magico-religious beliefs and practices till date, dominate the overall attitude towards health care system.

Singh (2000) did his doctoral dissertation on health culture among the Mishings. His study also brings to focus that their socio-religious beliefs and practices dominate their day-to-day life including the health behaviour of the community. Despite the urban influence, they show preference to their traditional medicare system.

Bora (2001) did her doctoral dissertation on child care and development among the Mishings. The study reveals the socio-cultural and magico-religious beliefs associated with the reproductive health.

Dutta (2002) did her doctoral dissertation on health status and health seeking behaviour among the tea labourers. The study reveals about the concept of health, disease and treatment among the people and socio-cultural and magico religious beliefs associated with health.

Konwar (2001) did her Ph.D. dissertation on reproductive health of Ahom women in Upper Assam. The study reveals the reproductive health of women folk living in both rural and urban settings.

Objectives of the Study

The objectives of the present study are —

(1) To describe the socio-cultural life of the Ao Nagas.
(2) To trace the health care practices and how the socio-cultural life influences the health care practices of the Ao Nagas.

The following parameters are considered to deal with the above-mentioned objectives :

(i) Some relevant socio-demographic aspects: (a) Type, composition and size of the families, (b) level of education by age and sex of the individuals' and (c) economic background of the people.

(ii) To examine the nature of changes in the concept of health, disease and treatment and the causes of disease under the new socio-cultural system.

(iii) To understand the overall living condition, personal hygiene and environmental sanitation that is prevalent among the people *vis-à-vis* their health scenario.

(iv) To collect information about the food habit of the people including food timing, food taboos and the possible distribution of the proximate principles etc.

(v) Access to modern medical services as well as traditional medical services (i.e. available health resources).

(vi) To collect the morbidity history.

(vii) Concept of health, disease (ailment), etiology (disease causation) and traditional beliefs, customs and practices with regard to treatment (curative measures).

(viii) To get an idea about the traditional preventive, curative and promotive health care practices that is prevalent among the people.

(ix) To identify the factors that contributes towards acceptance/non-acceptance of modern health care practices.

(x) To examine people's view towards both traditional and modern medicare system and the level and the extent of interaction between the two.

(xi) To understand the mother and child health care practices and the changing trends.

Methodology

The most important aspect of any scientific study is its methods, without which the investigation or the experiment will not be fruitful. Methodology is referred to as the procedures, rules, techniques and the stages of conducting experiment and gathering of the mass of data.

The basic themes of different disciplines may be the same but the methodologies are generally different. Anthropological study of any group of people is a holistic one that tries to understand the community's culture from an ethnic perspective. This is due to the tradition of this discipline that anthropologists observe the human beings and their activities staying with them. Thus in anthropological context, methodology refers to the overall systematic approach to the problems of fieldwork-based research and to the broad scientific principles in the light of which the anthropologist approaches his task (Bhagabati, 1991).

Social and cultural anthropologists study the people, their society and culture living among them and participating in their day-to-day activities and performances. Thus, it is possible for the researcher to find out the deeply rooted and hiding principles, practices, activities and behaviours of the study group. It also helps the researcher to establish a very good rapport with the people which is a prerequisite in an anthropological fieldwork. With the establishment of a good rapport, the people in course of time accept the researcher as an insider and thereby extend their maximum co-operation to generate the requisite amount of reliable data from the field.

As noted earlier, the present study has been carried out among the Ao Nagas, one of the major tribes of Nagaland.

The main considerations for selecting the Ao Nagas for the present study are:

(i) They are one of the numerically dominant tribe in the Mokokchung district in Nagaland.

(ii) No such intensive study has till date been carried out among them.

The purpose of the study is to bring out the socio-cultural life of the Ao Nagas under the impact of Christianity and to examine health care practices and the role of health care providers among the people. It has also been emphasised to understand the people's beliefs, practices, customs and the manners in which their ways of life influence their health behaviour and their concepts and views on health, disease and treatment etc. In the study, it is also intended to understand the degree and extent of interaction between the traditional and the modern health care systems and to identify the factors that contribute towards acceptance/non-acceptance of modern health care practices.

With regard to the present study, in the beginning, I visited few Ao Naga villages in Mokokchung district in Nagaland. However, explorations were made as to the prospective convenience with regard to easy accessibility in terms of transport and communication and anticipated co-operation in terms of availability of formal permission etc., from the village authority. Considering all these factors it was finally decided to carry out the intensive investigation among the Ao Nagas under Japokong range in Mokokchung district, Nagaland. To have a total understanding of the problem, three Ao Naga villages having differential accesses to modern health services were selected as the micro-field for the purpose of the study. Thus, the present study on socio-cultural life and health care practices of the Ao Nagas is methodologically a study of a three homogeneously living Ao Naga villages.

During the field investigation various techniques have been applied simultaneously depending on the nature of the data that were to be generated. All efforts have been made to collect both primary and secondary data and also both quantitative and qualitative data. Secondary data have been collected from the available sources (published literatures). During the agricultural season, the villagers by and large, were not available during the day time. Thus, the data were collected either in the evening or by meeting and talking to them in the agricultural field during the day time. However, on Sunday everyone remains at home and on that day everyone co-operate in generating the data for the present work. Thus, the fieldwork timings had to be adjusted according to the convenience of the people.

The methods and techniques that have been employed in generating the data from the field are as follows:

(i) Household census schedule.

(ii) Interview; individual and group, structured and unstructured.

(iii) Observation.

(iv) Collection of concrete case histories and life histories.

(v) Informal discussion.

At first, with the help of household survey schedule, all the households in the study area were censused to get some basic data on age and sex, literacy, marital status, occupation, family composition etc. At the same time relevant qualitative data regarding morbidity and mortality, women's reproductive health were also generated with the help of pre-formulated relevant interview schedule by conducting door-to-door survey. Specific informants have been selected, in keeping with the requirements the specific enquiry. Thus for example, data on village administration have been collected from the village council members and chairman of the village council. Information on Church organisation, have been collected from the Church authority. To get an idea about their traditional socio-religious and economic life, the elderly persons have been interviewed. Regarding educational institutions, data have been collected from the school teachers. To get information on the district, the District Information Officer has been interviewed.

Data on morbidity and mortality history have been collected from the heads of the families and housewives, as well as from traditional and medical practitioners. Information on prevailing disease and availability of modern medical facilities as well as people's attitude towards modern medicare system, have been collected from the modern medical practitioners as well as the elderly and some knowledgeable persons.

To get an idea about their traditional medicare system, the traditional healers have been interviewed. Likewise, to have an idea about the people's attitude towards both the systems (modern and traditional) data have been collected from a cross section of the people as well as the medicine man and so on and so forth.

Data on traditional beliefs, taboos, values and practices have been collected more from the elderly persons. On the other hand, data on reproductive performance and child care and various beliefs and taboos related with these have been collected from married woman respondents. Data on public health and modern family planning facilities have been collected from the health attendants.

Information on food habit has been gathered through observation and interviews. The details of the housing condition, environmental sanitation and personal hygiene have been collected mainly through prolonged personal observation during the entire period of the field investigation. To collect data on beliefs and practices with regard to health, disease, pregnancy and birth; accessibility to modern medical and traditional systems; and preventive, promotive and curative health practices, prevalent among them; structured and unstructured interviews have been conducted.

In this process the required mass of data have been generated from the field to bring into light an empirical picture of their present socio-cultural life including living condition, food habit, fertility, morbidity, mortality and other relevant facts, directly or indirectly associated with the overall health scenario.

The quantitative data have been analyzed using the simple

statistical tools and techniques and have been presented in statistical tables. Qualitative data have been also properly analyzed and systematized for detailed presentation distributed in a number of chapters. Whenever necessary, data obtained from one informant have been cross-checked from other sources. To make the dissertation more holistic and readable the relevant figures, photographs and maps also have been incorporated.

Presentation of Data

The entire mass of data generated from the field as well as collected from other sources have after proper organization, analysis and interpretation been arranged systematically and presented conveniently in eight different chapters in the dissertation.

In *Chapter One (Introduction)* an attempt has been made to introduce the problem as well as its relevance. A brief review of the relevant and accessible literatures has also been attempted here. The broad objectives of the investigation have also been laid out in the chapter. Further, the chapter deals with the overall methodology including, the mode of presentation of the analyzed and organized data on the dissertation.

Chapter Two (The Ao Nagas), is devoted to provide a brief historical note on the Nagas including the origin of the word Naga, their migration, racial affinity, geographical distribution, language and cultural commonalities and way of life. A brief ethnographic account of the Ao Nagas including their origin, migration and distribution etc. has also been presented in the chapter.

Chapter Three (The Setting), provides a brief introduction with proper geographical perspective to the micro field (the land as well as the people) where the present intensive investigation has been carried out.

Chapter Four (Social Life) is devoted to incorporate a discussion on the social life of the Ao Nagas under investigation. A detailed discussion about the family, educational attainment, clan, marriage, inheritance of property and village administration has been attempted in this chapter.

In *Chapter Five (Religious Life)*, a detailed description has been made on religious life of the people under investigation. The chapter incorporates some discussion on the traditional religion and Christianity among the Ao Nagas, Church organization and impact of Christianity on the life of the Ao Nagas.

Chapter Six (Economic Life), deals with the economic life of the people under investigation. The prevailing food habit of the people has also briefly been introduced in this chapter. A detailed description about the overall living condition of the people including housing condition, personal hygiene and environmental sanitation have also been attempted in this chapter.

In *Chapter Seven (Health Scenario Among The People)*, an idea about the available and accessible health care facilities in and around the micro-field have been attempted. A discussion has also been made on the nature and extent of utilization of the different health care systems by the people. Some morbidity and mortality scenario of the people has also been discussed. The chapter also incorporates some discussion on mother and child health care and the nature of interaction between the traditional and modern health care systems among the people under investigation.

The *Eighth Chapter (Summary and Conclusion)* is the last chapter in the dissertation. It is devoted to summarize the entire work and highlight the salient findings of the study. Some relevant concluding remarks have also been incorporated here and there.

2

THE Ao NAGAS

The Term Naga

The term 'Naga' applies to all the people living in compact area between the Brahmaputra river and the Chindwin river, i.e. in between 93° -96° longitude and 24° - 27° latitude (Shimray, 1985). 'Naga' is a generic term that comprises various tribes with different but more or less allied cultures.

The origin of the word 'Naga' is obscure. There are different theories regarding the origin of the word 'Naga'. Tajenjuba (Ao Naga) has opined that the name 'Naga' originated from the Kachari language. According to him, the Nagas were known to the Kacharies as 'NAHNGRA', meaning warrior or fighter. The earnest contra version of this term in Assamese became NHUGA and from NHUGA, the Anglicized form became NAGA (cited in Shimray, 1985: 39).

According to Horam the name 'Naga' originated from Tangkhul Naga language—NAOKHOKA, meaning a very brave child. According to him, in course of time, NAOKHOKA was known as NAOKHA. When Naokha people came into contact with the Ahoms of Assam, the Ahoms called them NOGA in their own peculiar way and thus the word Naga came into being (cited in Shimray, 1985 : 40).

Few other scholars explained it as a derivative of nag meaning 'snake'. The etymology of naga or noga may be explained in another way. Sanskrit 'naga' means 'hill' and naga with the suffix—a, which means 'definiteness' or 'the dwellers', or 'live in' indicates the hill dwellers (Boruah, 1993: 1).

To quote Mills, "Naga is the corruption of Assamese 'Nanga' (pronounced as NOGA) probably meaning, mountaineer from Sanskrit 'Nog' a mountain or inaccessible place" (cited in Shimray, 1985: 40).

Gait, Peal and Helcombe have opined that the word Naga is derived from Sanskrit word 'NOK' or 'NOG' meaning people or folk (cited in Shimray, 1985: 41).

Mills, an authority on the Nagas, wrote, "It is generally assumed in a vague sort of way that these tribes which were spoken of as Nagas have something in common with each other which distinguished them from many other tribes found in Assam and entitles them to be regarded as a racial unit in themselves" (cited in Shimray, 1985).

According to Rowney the word 'Naga' means a serpent (cited in Elwin, 1969). Among the Burmese the word 'Naka' means people with pierced ears (Horam, 1975).

Phizo, the most popular Naga leader, maintained that Burmese word 'Naka' was the origin of the word Naga. In Burmese 'Na' means ear and 'Ka' means pierced—one whose ears are pierced or those who bears earrings. The Naga people in olden days used to pierce their ears for putting flowers and creepers, as they were lovers of natural beauty. Hence the term Naga is closely related to the Burmese word 'Naka' (cited in Singh, 2004).

According to Elwin (1961), the derivation of the word 'Naga' is obscure and they are as Indo-Mongoloid folk living in the North-Eastern Hills of India. According to him, the derivative form of the word 'Naga' is 'Nok' which means 'people'.

According to Peal, the true term of this word is not Naga, but Noga, from a root nog, nok, meaning "people" (cited in Smith, 1857).

According to Butler, the term Naga is derived from the Bengali word nangta, or the Hindustani word nanga, meaning 'naked', 'crude', 'barbarous' (cited in Smith, 1857).

Ptolemy writes of them as 'Nagalog' which means the realm of the 'Naked'. However, Phemberton, in the Report on the Eastern Frontier of British India, in describing the Western Naga tribes mentioned that the Kabuis who then resided on the several ranges of hills between Manipur and Cachar were known in Bengal by the term 'Naga' (cited in Shimmi, 1988: 46).

According to Sen (1987: 20), "The term 'Naga' has been given by the neighbouring plain people of Assam. A view is that the word Naga was derived from the Sanskrit word 'Nagna' which means naked. In the remote past, the Nagas were known by their scanty of clothes. They used to cover, at that time, their private parts with a loin cloth and practically they were naked and nude. Another view says that throughout India the words 'Naga Sannyasi' are applied to the naked mendicants. As the naked Sannyasi is called Naga so also the naked people of this area are called from the remote past as Naga. They did not have their any original generic term for the whole of their race".

Origin and Migration and Racial Affinity

The origin of the Nagas is a vexed question. Nagaland exhibits racial inter-mixtures in a great range: it forms a meeting centre of the Himalayan, Burmese, Japanese, Thai, Malaysian, Philippinian, Polynesian, Indonesian and Melanesian cultures (Bareh, 1970).

While discussing about early Naga migration, Jamir and Lanunungsang (2005) wrote, "There are many theories on the origin and early migration of Nagas. It is evidently clear that many Mongolian races now living in the North Eastern India in Himalayan region have migrated from China and South

East Asia. During the ancient Indo-China relation, the Chinese visitors came to India following the Yunan river bank through the present Myanmar. It is believed that the Nagas also came through such route during the end of B.C. and in the beginning of A.D. According to recent research findings, Nagas have migrated from South East Asia through the present North West Myanmar following different directions and places. It is to be noted that the migration of the Naga tribes did not take pace in one wave only."

The different legends and stories though varied and dissimilar in detail have, however, one thing in common, that the Nagas have come from the eastern part of the world (Horam, 1975).

Sema (1986) opined that the Naga tribe now living in Nagaland, Assam, Arunachal Pradesh and Manipur have migrated to these places through Burma.

According to Jamir and Lanunungsung (2005), "It is believed that the first Naga groups who landed in the present homeland are said to be Maos, Angamis, Chakesangs, Sumis, Rengmas, Rongmais and Lothas. They migrated somewhere from West China, Indo-China, Malaya, Burma, Thailand, Indonesia and Philippines. The second groups are said to be the Aos, Changs, Khiamniungan, Sangtams, Tikirs and Thangkhuls. It is believed that they came crossing the Thangdut-Chindwin Rivers. The Aos might have come across the present Thangkul, Mao and Chakesang country *via* Tuensang-Wokha-Zunheboto districts. The third group consists of the Konyaks and Phoms. They came through North-East Myanmar."

Butler writes, "The Nagas are a fine, stalwart, cheerful, bright and light colourful race" (cited in Shimray, 1985). Nagas may be classified as Tibeto-Burman group of Mongoloid people (Ghosh, 1982).

The Nagas are one of the Mongolian racial groups found in Assam, Meghalaya, Tripura, Mizoram, Manipur, Arunachal Pradesh, Burma, Bangladesh, Bhutan, Sikkim, Nepal, Tibet, the fringe of the U.P., Himachal Pradesh and Kashmir of the Himalayan tracts (Yonuo, 1974).

To quote Elwin, "They are a fine people, of whom their country is proud, strong and self-reliant with the free and independent outlook characteristic of highlanders everywhere, good to look at with an unerring instinct for colour and design, friendly and cheerful with a keen sense of humour, gifted with splendid dances and a love of song" (cited in Shimray, 1985).

Generally, the Nagas bear the Mongolian physical features and cultural traits. They have a broad head, complexion light, dark light and golden brown but black too with a yellowish tinge, hair black, straight, coarse, vigorous, wavy and negrito frizzy in some cases, with scanty hair on face, stature short or below average in the standard way, nose fine to broad, face characteristically flat, eyelids often oblique (Yonuo, 1974).

The Nagas belong to Tibeto-Burman group of Indo-Mongoloid people. They are medium to above medium stature, Mesocephalic head, Euryprosophic round face, broad high cheek bones, flat platyrrhine nose, brownish yellow skin, narrow Mongoloid eyes with black eye colour, Epicanthic fold is remarkably absent in the eyes. The hairs are often straight, Leiotrichy but wavy and woolly hairs are, however, rarely found among them. They are strong and sturdy. The Naga tribes have the affinities with the tribes of South-East Asian countries. They belong to Indo-Mongoloid family of race (Sen, 1987).

Geographical Distribution

The Nagas, comprising about 40 odd tribes are found in North East India and North West Myanmar. In India, the Nagas are concentrated in four States—Nagaland, Manipur, Assam and Arunachal Pradesh which constitute about 2/3 of Naga population of about 4 million. In Myanmar, the Nagas are concentrated in the Somrah Tract bordering India which comes under two administrative units, viz., Kachin State and Sagaing Sub-division.

Nagaland State as the name bears is dominated by the Nagas. The Naga tribes found in this State are—Ao, Angami, Sema, Konyak, Lotha, Chakhesang, Rengma, Pochuri, Sangtam, Yimchunger, Khiamnungan, Phom and Zeliangrong (Zeme, Liangmei and Rongmei). Apart from these, there are also some Naga tribes settled in Nagaland State, namely Tangkhul, Mao, etc.

The Angami Nagas are concentrated in Kohima district and some parts of Dimapur (a newly created district as of later 1997 and erstwhile sub-division of Kohima district) while Mokokchung district is said to be the abode of the Aos. The Semas are mainly concentrated in Zunheboto and Dimapur districts and fringes of Tuensang district. The Lothas and the Konyaks dominate Okha and Mon districts respectively. Phek district is said to be the homeland of the Chakhesangs and Pochuris. The Rengmas are mainly concentrated in the Tseminyu sub-division in Kohima district. Tuensang district is dominated by the Yimclumgers, Khiamnungans, Phoms and Sangtams (the Sangtams are also concentrated in Phek district). The Zeliangrongs are mainly concentrated in Peren sub-division (of Kohima district) and Dimapur district. The Tangkhuls and Maos among others, are also settled in Dimapur and Kohima.

In Manipur, the Nagas dominate in four districts, namely Ukhrul, Senapati, Tamenglong and Chandel. Ukhrul district is dominated by the Tangkhuls, even so is Tamenglong district by the Zeliangrongs. Tamenglong is also the home of the Kharam Nagas. The Maos, Poumais, Marams, and Thangals are concentrated in Senapati district. In Chandel district, 8 Naga tribes are found, namely Maring, Anal, Lamkang, Moyon, Monsang, Chote, Chiru and Tarao. Koirengs, Chirus and Chotes are sparsely distributed in Chandel, Bishnupur and Senapati districts.

In Arunachal Pradesh, three Naga tribes have been identified. They are Tangsha, Wancho and Nocte. They are concentrated in Tirap and Changlang districts of Arunachal Pradesh.

In Assam, two Naga tribes are found, namely Zeliangrongs (Zeme, Rongmei) and Rengma.

In Myanmar, the Naga tribes found are: Konyak, Tangkhul, Phom, Yimchunger, Moyon, Pangsha, Hemi, Hkalak, Tsaplo, Htangan, Lainung, Shangpuri, Pangaw, Pyangoo and Rangpan (cited in Vashum, 2000: 10).

According to Boruah (1993: 2), "the major groups of Naga tribes in Nagaland are—Konyak, Ao, Sema, Lotha, Angami, Chakechang, Phom, Rengma, Chang, Sangtam, Yimchunger, Khenmungam, Kuki and Zelang and other minor groups. Comparatively, Konyaks are more numerous than the Aos. Each of them has their own tongues which vary widely from one language to another."

Hutton has divided the Naga communities into four main divisions : (i) The southern Naga consisting of Kacha Naga and Kabui and the Naga tribes of Manipur (Tangkhal, etc.); (ii) the western Naga consisting of the Angami (including the Memi, Moram and Chakechang sub-tribes), Sema, Rengma and Lotha; (iii) The central Naga; the Tangkhul, Ao, Sangtam, Yachumi (Yimchunger), Chang and Phom; and (iv) The eastern Naga consisting of the Konyak tribes of Tamlu and the area north-east of Dikhu extending along the border of the Sibsagar and Lakhimpur districts to the Patkai range and apparently southwards along that range of the east of the Phom and Chang countries (cited in Singh, 1994).

Language

According to different philologists the languages and dialects of the Nagas belong to the Tibeto-Burman (Yonuo, 1974). The colourful tribes of this region are speaking Tibeto-Burman language in their respective tribal dialects of their own but, 'Nagamese' (Naga + Āssamese), which is much similar to Assamese language, is their common Lingo. In this language some Hindi, English and Nepali words also entered along with some Naga words. Hindi is now spreading very much and taking the place of their common speaking language where Nagamese not yet introduced. They do not have their own script. They are using English script (Sen, 1987).

Grierson has divided the Naga language into five sub-groups as follows:

(a) Western sub-group: It includes Angami, Sema, Rangma, and Kezhama;

(b) Central sub-group: It includes Ao, Lotha, Tengsa, Thukumi and Yachumi;

(c) Eastern sub-group: It includes Angwanku or Tablung Chingmegna or Tamlu, Banpara, Mutonia, Mohongia, Chang or Mojung, Assiringia, Moshang and Shangge;

(d) Naga Bodo sub-groups: It includes Mikir, Kachcha Naga, Kabui and Khoirao; and

(e) Naga Kuki sub-group: It includes Sopvoma or Mao Naga, Maram, Miyangkhang, Kwoireng on Liyang, Luhupa and Luppa and Maring (cited in Boruah, 1993).

According to Boruah (1993), Nagaland has many uncultivated and mutually unintelligible languages, which belong to Assam-Burmese sub-family. These languages or dialects have got no script for their own. According to the Nagas popular belief they had their own script which was originally written on animal skin and ate up by somebody, and thus their script was lost. That traditional story still prevails in their society. They have adopted Roman script to their speeches. The district-wise geographical distributions of the languages mainly are as follows:

(a) Kohima: Angami, Kachari, Kuki, Zemi Liangmei, Rongmei, Rengma, Mao and Kheza.

(b) Mokokchung: Ao (Chongli, Mongsen, Chanki).
(c) Mon: Konyak.
(d) Phek: Pochuri, Chokri.
(e) Tuensang: Phom, Chang, Sangtam, Yimchunger, Khinmungan, Mukwara, Tirkhir, Chin.
(f) Wokha: Lotha.
(g) Zunheboto: Sema.

Cultural Commonalities and Way of Life

According to Vashum (2000:13), "It is rather difficult to bring out common cultural factors of the Nagas, for the simple fact that there is no exactly similar culture among the Naga tribes." In the words of Mills (1922), "It is generally assumed in a vague sort of way that those tribes which are spoken of as Nagas have something in common with each other which distinguishes them from the many other tribes found in Assam and entitles them to be regarded as a racial unit in themselves.... The truth is that if not impossible it is exceedingly difficult to propound any test by which a Naga can be distinguished from other Assam or Burma tribes which are not Nagas."

According to W.C. Smith (1857), the general characteristics of the Naga culture are:

1. Head hunting;
2. Common sleeping houses for the unmarried men, which are taboo to women;
3. Dwelling houses built on posts or piles;
4. Disposal of dead on raised platforms;
5. A sort of trial marriage, or great freedom of intercourse between the sexes before the marriage;
6. Betel chewing;
7. Aversion to milk as an article of diet;

8. Tattooing by pricking;
9. Absence of any powerful political organisation;
10. The double cylinder vertical forge;
11. A large quadrangular or hexagonal shield; and
12. Residence in hilly regions and crude form of agriculture.

The Nagas were a people who, though unaware of the democratic principles of the western civilizations, lived and were governed by democratic principles and practices since time immemorial. Perhaps, the Nagas are a people which have the heritage of one of the oldest democracies of the world. The Nagas lived in villages and each village was a democratic unit of the tribes they represented. Each village was sovereign and self-sufficient in itself. Each village was headed by a council of elders. These leaders represented each clan that existed in the village. They exercised powers not according to the hereditary systems as in the monarchic and feudal systems. They were elected to leadership on the basis of their merit and (potential) efficiency. All disputes in the villages were settled by them. They formed the ultimate authority in maintaining fraternity and protecting peace in their respective villages (Lasuh, 2002:15).

The traditional faith of the Nagas was animism (paganism). They worshipped no idol or creatures. They did not belong to any major religion of the world but like many other tribal of the world they believed in and feared spirits (Lasuh, 2002: 16). Naga religion is described by the sociologists to be animistic which lays emphasis on the existence of the deified manifestations of nature and propitiation of spirits both benevolent and malevolent (Bareh, 1970). In the words of Sen (1987), "In 1901, 96 per cent of the Naga population were animist. But now they are mainly the Christians. Majority of them belonged to American Baptist Mission. There are also Roman Catholic, Pentecostalism, and Assembly of God etc."

For the Nagas, 'head-hunting' was one of the main necessary mechanism for 'defense', 'offence' and regulation of life in a sovereign setting just like the modern warfare. It is also seen as a mechanism for survival itself. In order to maintain and sustain a sovereign entity of village republic and/or monarchy, there is bound to be some mechanism measures and regulations. 'Head-hunting fulfils one of these criteria or requirement of existence and maintenance (Vashum, 2000: 15). Usually, 'head hunting' takes place when any one and/or villager from outside it village state trespasses, hurts, harms, humiliates, and/or mistreats any of citizens/villagers and whoever an individual, a village or sometimes groups of villages try to invade or mischievous with the village/villagers. It is restarted when situation demand. 'Head hunting' was also usually associated with bravery and social recognition for the able head hunters. Head hunters enjoyed great prestige. It inspired wonderful dances. 'Head hunting' was also associated with religious rituals and economic prosperity. They believe that head hunting would result in a better yield of crops. Spread of Christianity gradually decreased the head hunting practice among them and now it is already abolished. There is also government rule to debar from head hunting practice and there is also government rule for serious punishment, if any.

Naga people build their houses high above the ground on long pieces of wooden pillars and there is always a sitting-platform at the back side of the room. Some are crowned the roof with crossed wooden horns; some have gable projecting in the front side roof of the room. The trophies are proudly displayed by them in the front porch.

The Nagas are patrilineal, patrilocal and patrichal. They are generally endogamous and clan exogamy is their fundamental rule for marriage. Bride price is not an essential matter for them. Monogamy is generally practised by them but sometimes polygamy is, however, seen among some rich people of Naga tribes. For that, they construct separate house for each wife because, no wife is willing to live under the same roof when there is more than one wife. Now-a-days there is no restriction to marry outside the tribe. For that inter-tribal marriage has increased. Marriage in the same clan is prohibited but modern educated youth are, however, often not following this customary rule. Polyandry is never allowed. Parallel cousin marriage is strictly prohibited among them. Sexual freedom is found among them. Divorce is also found among them which is very simple as it does not require going to court etc. If the husband divorces his wife for the reason other than barrenness, adultery, sickness of incurable diseases, he is to pay some fine depending on the seriousness of the case. This used to settle after discussing by the parties concerned. Divorced wife is allowed to leave her husband by keeping all the children with her husband except the suckling one and for that infant she is to take some amount from her divorced husband to maintain that issue with her.

The Naga also consider more children for their better living. In earlier days the mother generally observed genna after the birth of her child, six days for male baby and five days for female. It, however, varies from tribe to tribe. But now-a-days the Christian does not follow this genna. They have several rituals for death. Most of the Naga tribes bury their dead. During the pre-British days the Nagas used to keep the dead body exposed on a platform for many days, even a month and then throw the bones outside the villages. After death and before burial, generally a feast with rice and beef are given by the family members of the deceased. A genna is observed for ten days after the death. Within the genna period the family members exclude certain foods and not work in their agricultural field. In some tribes, however, there is no restriction of food during the genna period. They erect stone-structure for their respectable and old rich deceased in the burial ground where they burry so that they remember that dead member, generation after generation. Now-a-days the Christians are using coffin to keep the dead body to bury.

The Nagas also have the dormitory system which is known

as 'Morung'. In the words of Vashum (2000:15), "Morung (youth dormitory), is one common and very important socio-cultural and political institution of the Nagas. In the modern sense, the nearest equivalence would be 'educational institution'". "Furer-Haimendorf, while writing about the dormitory system (morung) of the Nagas opines that the morung belongs, together with the logdrum, to the oldest cultural stratum of the Naga Hills. The morung was the centre of warfare in the sense of imparting to its members the required lessons for fighting the enemy and of guarding the village" (Singh, 1994). As the Naga young boys attain puberty, they are trained of the art of warfare and code of conduct, traditional values etc. in the 'morung'. They continue to be in the 'morung' till they get married. The youth in the 'morung are not only provided knowledge and physical training but they were also deployed for various assignments by the village authorities should need arise, especially for general welfare of the village and security purposes. The girls are also given training in such institution ranging from moral codes to handicrafts and to their roles for the welfare of the village. 'Morung' is also used as a place for guarding the village from the enemies and also as recreation club. Now-a-days, the 'morung' system, those who have, are fading away due to education, spread of Christianity and acculturation.

Among the Nagas, the main weapons are spears, bows and arrows, daos, helmets of dyed cane and cane made shields and even country made rifles. They use daos for all multipurpose work. They ornamented their spears and daos with goats hair dyed in red colour. They are good and efficient hunters and they use these weapons to kill the animals. Naga people are also good fishermen with nets, fishing rods, fishing wickers etc. There are community hunting and fishing among them.

The Naga women have a high position in work. They work with their men-folk in the agricultural field and play an important role in agricultural activities. But the married one has almost no right in the property of her father. All the movable and immovable property of dead father is inherited only by the sons and unmarried daughters. The widow also not getting any property of her husband except her own cash and ornaments and clothes, weaving apparatus given to her by her father but not by her husband. But these cannot be taken with her if she desires to live with her parents or remarry. However, the unmarried girls have their rights in their parental property. The share of property of an unmarried sister usually goes to her brother after her death. If a married daughter gets landed property from her father, in an exceptional case, she can be mistress of that till her life and it goes to her sons soon after her death. If she dies without having any son then her father re-inherits that property. In case her father is dead then her brother inherits that property.

The Nagas are mainly jhum cultivators. The staple food is rice which is taken with meat and vegetables or with chillies. They like chillies very much and huge quantity is consumed by all young and old people. They consume all kinds of animals such as rat, dog, cat, snake, monkey, tiger, bear, elephant, mithuns, spiders, crab, beef, pork, chicken, mutton etc. The meat of elephant and roasted dog is their favourite delicacy food. They also eat fresh and dried fish. Indigenous wine was at one time an inseparable asset of the Nagas which was considered something more than the usual item that is taken as nutritious food. But with the coming of Christianity, such consumption of wine has become a thing of the past for the majority of the Nagas. In the past, they dislike drinking milk and milk made items and used to take tea without milk. But now they use to drink milk.

Water scarcity is a major problem in interior villages of Nagaland. Generally, the female members of the house collect water by going down a steep hill for thousand feet or more to fetch water from local pits and ponds and they draw water in their big bamboo tubes. The water of these pits and ponds is the general cause of wide incidences of intestinal diseases.

Respiratory, intestinal, skin diseases, malaria, tuberculosis, pneumonia, dysentery, and small pox are the common diseases found among the Naga people.

Naga people observe several festivals. These festivals are mostly related to seasons or stage of agricultural operations. At that time they observed their particular set of genna. During festival, dance and music take main part. The important festivals of Nagas are: *Sekrenyi* (Angami tribe), *Tsukhenyie* (Chakhesang), *Aoling* (Konyak), *Monyu* (Phom), *Moatsu* and *Tsungremong* (Ao), *Mia* and *Tsokum* (Khiamangan), *Noknyalan* (Chang), *Tuluni* (Sema), *Medemmeo* (Yimchunger), *Mongmong* (Sangtam), *Tsokum* (Khiamngan), *Tokhu Emong* (Lotha), *Ngada* (Rengma), *Nga-ngoi* (Zeliang) etc. Rice beer plays an important role in these festivals as they widely consume it during these festivals. But with the coming of Christianity, change is also found in the traditional way of observing such festivals.

The Ao Nagas

The second biggest tribe in Naga Hills, with a population of over 45,000 is the Ao. The Aos are entirely different from the Angami Nagas and so is their language. Ao Naga villages are situated in Mokokchung sub-division which is now a district with a compact area. About 54 Ao villages are divided over five ranges of hills, namely Ompangkong, Longpangkong, Asutkong, Chankikong and Japvokong (Singh, 1987:40).

According to Sen (1987: 40), "The Ao tribes are inhabited mainly in Mokokchung district. They call themselves Ni-so-meh and Sa-mai-na."

Mills (1926:4) in his book 'The Ao Nagas' opined that "The Aos, who numbered 30,599 at the census of 1921, occupy a portion of the Naga Hills bounded by the Dikhu River on the south-east, the edge of the plains on the north-west, the Konyaks on the north-east and the Semas and Lothas on the south-west."

According to Singh (1994: 70), "The Ao call themselves Aor or 'those who came' crossing over the Dikhu river."

The name Ao means went or went away. It is understood that in prehistoric age before we entered into Nagaland and even after our entry we the Nagas were nomadic tribe and during their wanderings from place to place, once they came to a big river and they had to cross it by means of a bridge made up of cane. So when the bridge was made, a group of them, so to say the first group moved away across the bridge to the other side of the river and landed on the bank. But no sooner had they landed on the bank then they cut down the bridge so that nobody could come to their side. On seeing the treacherous act of the first group in cutting down the bridge behind them, the rest were badly disappointed and as a result they gave an appropriate name Ao to the group which means went or went away, leaving behind the other tribes or groups on the other side of the river. Thus from there the name Ao has been originated and then and there the name Merir also has been originated. Its meaning is hate or dislike. The Merir are a people hated or disliked by Aos because they left them behind. Ever since then we the Aos are calling them by the name of Merir and they are no other than the Sangtams, Changs, Yimchanger, Kongyaks, Phoms, Khaimnugan, etc. Our forefathers had said that the very river stated above is no other than the Dikhu river. But to us who knows, it may be one of the big tributaries of the Irrawaddy like the Chin win river in Burma (Aier, 1990:6).

According to mythology of the Aos, they claim that their ancestors emerged from the stone (Jamir and Lanunungsang, 2005).

Mills (1926:6) opined that "Ao traditions states quite definitely that the ancestors of the tribe came out of the earth at Lungterok (Sixstones), sometimes called Ungterok, lying on the top of a spur on the right bank of the Dikhu just opposite Mokongtsu." According to Aier (1994:6), "We the Aos belong to a major tribe of the Naga nation and it seems we might have come from South-East Asia. Because, racially we belong to Mongoloid Stock".

Horam (1975) opined that the Aos must have come from the south eastern parts of Burma and passed through Manipur upwards to Wokha in the Lotha country which they occupied for a considerable period. From there the Ao ancestors probably went to Naotistime where stand their traditional Six stones or Longtorok or Langthoruk (incidentally in Tangkhul dialect also 'lung' means 'stone' and 'thoruk' means 'six' Naotistime is a day's journey east of Mokokchung. It is from these six stones that the Aos believe they have emerged.

Ao traditions say that they originated from Longtorok (or Longrok) the Six Stones, in Chungliyimti village in Sangtam area which lies directly on the east of Ao area and is some 20 km. from Mokokchung. It is maintained by the Aos that it is at Chungliyimti that Ao society was thoroughly organised and their marriage and other customs were given definite shape (Ghosh, 1982:46).

According to Ghosh (1982:48), "Though the exact route of Ao migration is not known, from various cultural traits left behind it is believed that they came from Burma to Manipur, Manipur to present Chakhesong area, from there to Yimchunger area and from there to Sangtam area where lies Chungliyimti in their northward move. From Chungliyimti they crossed to the present place in the north west of the state of Nagaland."

Singh (1987:40) while discussing about Ao Nagas wrote, "Ungma, the biggest Ao village, Lungkum, the fortrees of Aos, Mokokchung, the headquarters, Chuchuyimlung, the richest and the second biggest Ao village, Impur, the mission station, Changk, the most educated village, Merangkong, Changtongia, Mongenyimiti, Longchang, Khensa, Chungliyimsen, Linamen, Lakhuni and Chuchuyimbang are notable Ao Naga villages."

Physically the Ao is classed almost or as Brachycephals.

The Ao from many aspects exhibit cultural traits of the Thai and Monkhemer and seem to have come from the south-east. The language of the Ao is also classed in the Tibeto-Burman but not in the Siamese Chinese (Shimmi, 1988:34).

Linguistically, the Ao Nagas are divided into three sub-tribes: Chonglee, Chungke and Mong-sen. The common word for marriage, in standard Ao language is *kiyemba*. Clan exogamy remains the most important marriage rule among the Ao and thus marriage within the patriclan is prohibited. Marriage within the matriclan is permitted, if it is not one's own clan. The system of Dowry is not prevalent among them. Divorce among them is very common. Both man and woman are allowed to remarry at any stage.

Nuclear type of families is predominantly found in the Ao community. Kinship obligations shape the interpersonal and inter-group relations. Inheritance is in the male line and in case of absence of sons, only the close agnatic male members inherit the property, particularly the landed property. A daughter cannot inherit landed property.

Succession to different positions in the traditional politico-religious set up has strictly been in the male line. The main clan elders selected through an age set system could form the *putu menden* or the village council. Above these elders, only a senior male member, *ongre*, of the pongen clan, could hold the supreme position. The chief priest and priests are selected from amongst these elders.

Cultivation among Ao is mostly jhum cultivation. Land and forest are the major economic resources for most of the Ao people. The Ao are strictly non-vegetarian. The mithun has traditionally been the significant non-vegetarian food item. The cow, buffalo, pig and large varieties of wild animals and fish are eaten. Rice is the staple food of the Ao. Due to spread of Christianity, tea is more commonly taken now than 'Yi' (Ao wine). Beides, Naga-dal remains an important food item. A large variety of jungle fruits and leafy vegetables are consumed by them. Tubers and roots are also collected from the jungles for self-consumption. Tea without milk is an important drink of the Ao. Alcoholic foreign drinks are also purchased from shops in the urban and semi-urban areas for self-consumption.

Like other tribes, the Ao also observe several rituals during childbirth, marriage and death. In case of birth of a male child, the ritual *kinimong* is observed for six days and in case of a female child, the ritual is observed for five days. Among the Ao and other Naga tribes, a ritual, a festival and a taboo is spoken of as *genna*. Another ritual known as *tenarong-jokba* in Mongsen dialect and *tengrong-atuba* in Chongli dialect is performed, in which the ear hole of the child is done by an elderly man of the clan. The elder person acting as the religious specialist in this *genna*, sacrifices a cock in the name of the Tiaba tribal god *Tiaba*.

The Ao has symbolic value in the process of first rice-feeding. After birth of a child, the mother shall put a little boiled rice into the child's mouth within a few days and with that the ritual of rice feeding is accomplished. The clan elder gives names of ancestors to the child during this ritual. Now-a-days mostly the pastors give Bibalical names to new born kids.

In older days the Ao made special arrangements to physically separate the male and female children and allow them to join their respective dormitories (*morung*) during adolescence. The dormitories of the boys were more structured and functional in nature than the girls' dormitories. The girls' dormitories generally functioned only as sleeping house for girls. The boys were allowed to visit the girls sleeping houses and choose their life partners but the girls were prohibited to enter the boys' dormitories. These dormitory (*morung*) systems are fading away gradually due to education, spread of Christianity and acculturation.

In marriage ceremony, on the marriage day, the priest (*putir*) will bring one cock on behalf of the bridegroom to his house and sacrifice the same to a god with a prayer for a prolonged happy married life. The oldest male member of the bridegroom's clan will participate in a feast to be given at the bride's house on the second day of marriage. In case of death, the eldest clan member of the deceased person will visit the family and perform a simple ceremony. He will kill one cock and mix the liver with rice and place it near the body of the deceased. Male and Female relatives of the deceased are prohibited from going to the jungles or to the fields for six and five days respectively. However, due to acculturation and conversion of Christianity they are now westernized and as a result majority of them have abandoned most of these life-cycle rituals. In almost all lifecycle events, the pastor prays on behalf of the family and gives blessings.

The Ao people have their own dress and ornaments which are distinct from other Naga tribes. Men wear a piece of black cloth round their waist which comes up to the knee. Upon this, a number of long narrow lines of beautiful white coloured linear stripe cloth made of cotton thread is used by them to decorate their front part, from lower part of their abdomen to the knee. Sometimes, a jacket type of cotton made of small cloth they wear to cover their upper part. Upon this, a small red coloured decorated scurf they put on their chest from their right shoulder. They wear short necklace *shipu* made of wild boar tusk and a long sized necklace *shiretzuk*, made of cowrie shells and small glass beads. Sometimes they wear a collar (small sized, black coloured) ribbon. They put *temko*, a headgear, which is black round based made of bear's hair, on which, feathers of hornbill are also fixed. They wear ivory armlets, *kampang*, and wristlet of white cowrie shells. A cleaver or axe (*dao*) is fastened by them in a wooden sheath which they keep behind their body with the help of a cotton string round their waist. The women wear red coloured decorated cloth, from their waist to the knee. A white blouse with sleeves they wear to cover the upper part. Their necklaces are with numerous strings of red and blue coloured cornelian beads and with most beautiful traditional conical objects look very nice. They decorated the upper part of their ear with brass made large sized rings. A feather of hornbill bird is also used by them to decorate the head. They use a brass-made bracelet. The Ao shawl with a decorated stripe in the middle depicting various animals and designs is commonly used by men. Conversion of Christianity and acculturation also influence the way of wearing cloths. Now-a-days people use to wear all kinds of modern dresses.

The Aos have two important festivals, *Moatsu* and *Tsungrem Mong*. *Moatsu* is observed after the sowing is done and the mother earth begins to show the sign of fertility. In the past, they observed it for six days in the month of May and from 1st May. But now they observe it only for a day. They select the suitable day in the first week of May. Aos have another festival called *Tsungrem Mong*. It is celebrated in the eve of the harvest. However, now-a-days the Aos observe this festival only for a day in the first week of August and most of the Christians now abandoned to observe this festival.

3

THE SETTING

The Land

India's North East, a region of mystic splendours and rich cultural heritage. From times immemorial, it has been the meeting point of many communities, faiths and cultures. North East India comprises eight states: Assam, Arunachal Pradesh, Manipur, Meghalaya, Mizoram, Nagaland, Tripura and Sikkim. It shares its international border with five foreign countries, namely—Bangladesh, Bhutan, Burma (Myanmar), China and Nepal.

North East India is located between latitudes 22°N and 29°3′N and longitudes 89°46′E and 97°30′E. The region, covering 255,082 square kilometres of uneven surface, supports a population of 31.4 million (1991), which accounts for 7.7 per cent of the total land surface and 3.72 per cent of the total population of the country.

North East is home to a total of 39,035,582 people (provisional population total, census 2001), which is 3.80 per cent of the country's population. It includes 20,162,752 males and 18,872,830 females with a density of 149 persons per sq. km. The entire region can be geographically divided into two parts: plains and the hills. The majority of those living in the plains of the region are Hindus and Muslims while a substantial proportion of the hill tribes inhabiting the states of Meghalaya, Mizoram and Nagaland are Christians. The region has a high concentration of tribal population. The states of

Arunachal Pradesh, Meghalaya, Mizoram and Nagaland are mostly inhabited by a number of native tribes. Each tribe has its own distinct tradition of art, culture, dance, music and lifestyles. The festivals and celebrations in the North Eastern states of India are a colourful reflection of the people and their lives. Around one-third (1/3) of the total number of the listed tribes for the whole of India are to be found in this region and therefore, the area may be regarded as 'living laboratory' for anthropological research where different theories could be tested and new ideas and thoughts can be formulated and developed.

Nagaland is a paradise-state for social sciences as it is a most fertile field to study Anthropology and Sociology for its colourful cultural traditions, folklore, myths and legends as well as customs of the Naga tribes which carry the traces of their ancient chronicle. The state is situated approximately between 25°11′55″ and 27°2′10″ North Latitude and between 93°02′0″ and 95°17′10″ East Longitude. After Sikkim, this is the second smallest state of India covering an area of 16,579 sq. km. It is almost triangular in shape, lying at about an angle 45 degree. It is one of the North Eastern most state of India, sharing the international border with the adjacent nation Burma on its maximum part of the south-east. Nagaland is bounded by the states of Assam on the west from north-west to south-west and Manipur on the south; Burma on the east and Arunachal Pradesh, the Union Territory (now a state) of India, on the northern part of the eastern border. Geopolitically Nagaland is very much sensitive state as the nation like Burma in the east, China is being close in the north and Bangladesh near to its western borders.

According to 2001 census, its total population is 1,988,636 of which there are 1,041,686 males and 946,950 females. The rate of literacy is 66.59 per cent.

Nagaland has been divided into eight administrative districts, namely Mon, Mokokchung, Wokha, Tuensang, Phek,

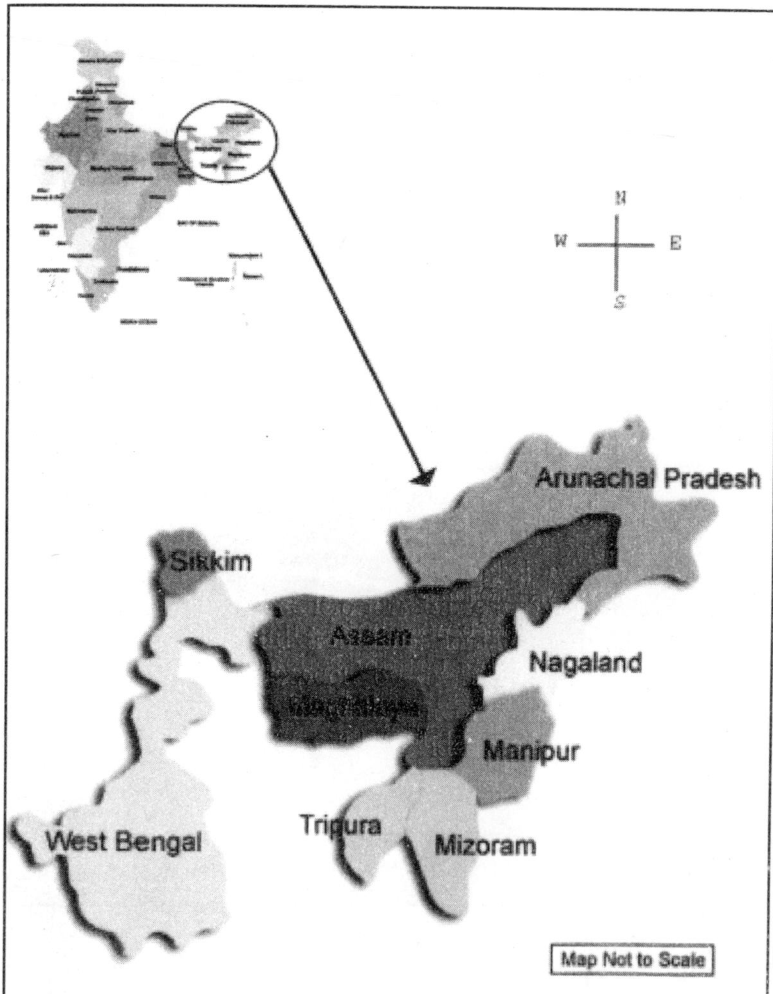

Map 3.1 : Map of North-East India

Zunheboto, Dimapur, Kohima. But recently three more districts have been added, namely Kiphire and Longleng (both formerly under Tuensung district) and Peren (from Kohima district). So, the total number of district is eleven.

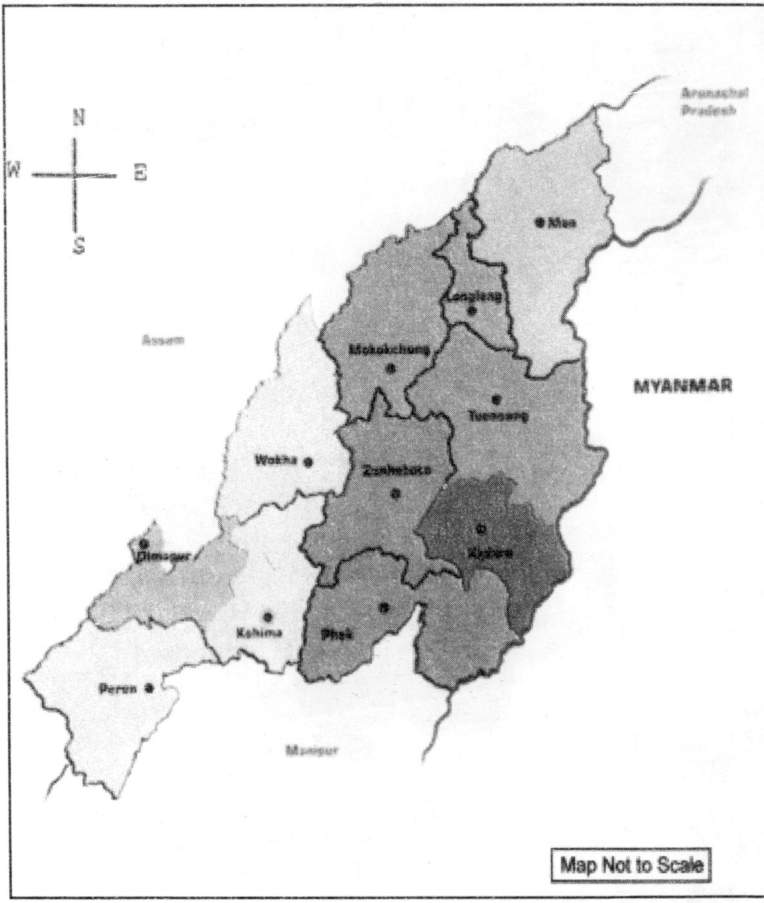

Map 3.2 : Map of Nagaland

Mokokchung District

The micro-field, selected for the purpose of the present investigation falls under the jurisdiction of Mokokchung, one of the eleven districts of Nagaland. The district was formed by decreasing the original Mokokchung district due to reorganization in 1973 to form two more districts along with the present Mokokchung district. The two more districts are Wokha and Zunheboto. Mokokchung district is bounded by Sibsagar district of Assam in the north, Jorhat district of Assam in the west, Zunheboto and Wokha districts of Nagaland in the south and Tuensang district of Nagaland in the east. It lies between 93.53 and 94.53 degrees longitude and 25.56 degrees latitude. The altitude of Mokokchung towns which is the headquarters of this district is 1325.08 metres above the sea level. The area of the district is 1,615 sq. km. The total population is 2,27,230. Rural population is 196,026 and the urban is 31,204. The density of the population is 140 per sq. km. and the literacy rate is 84.27 per cent (prov. census 2001).

Mokokchung district has two sub-divisions: Mongkolomba and Tuli. Mokokchung district has nine administrative town circles. These are Ongpangkong, Kubolong, Mongkolemba, Longchem, Alongkima, Changtongya, Chuchuyimlang, Tuli, Mokokchung sadar.

Physiographically, the district is a hilly area. This district is divided into six distinct hill ranges. These ranges are more or less parallel to each other and run south east direction. These are: Tzurangkong range, Japukong range, Changkikong range, Asetkong range, Longpangkong range, Ongpangkong range. Road communication, in this district is much better than the other districts of Nagaland.

The Aos is the main tribe of this district who inhabited on these hill ranges. The main rivers of this district are: Melak, Dikhu, and Tserang. The Melak flows through the heart of this district touching Tuli on its way to turn towards the Brahmaputra river of Assam. The Dikhu flows in between Mokokchung and Tuensang districts and forming a boundary between these two districts.

The available minerals of this district are oil and gas. There is sericulture farm, pineapple fibre unit, cultivation citronella farm, district industry centre etc. Timber, bamboo, thatch, grass, palm leaves are the main forest products. There are

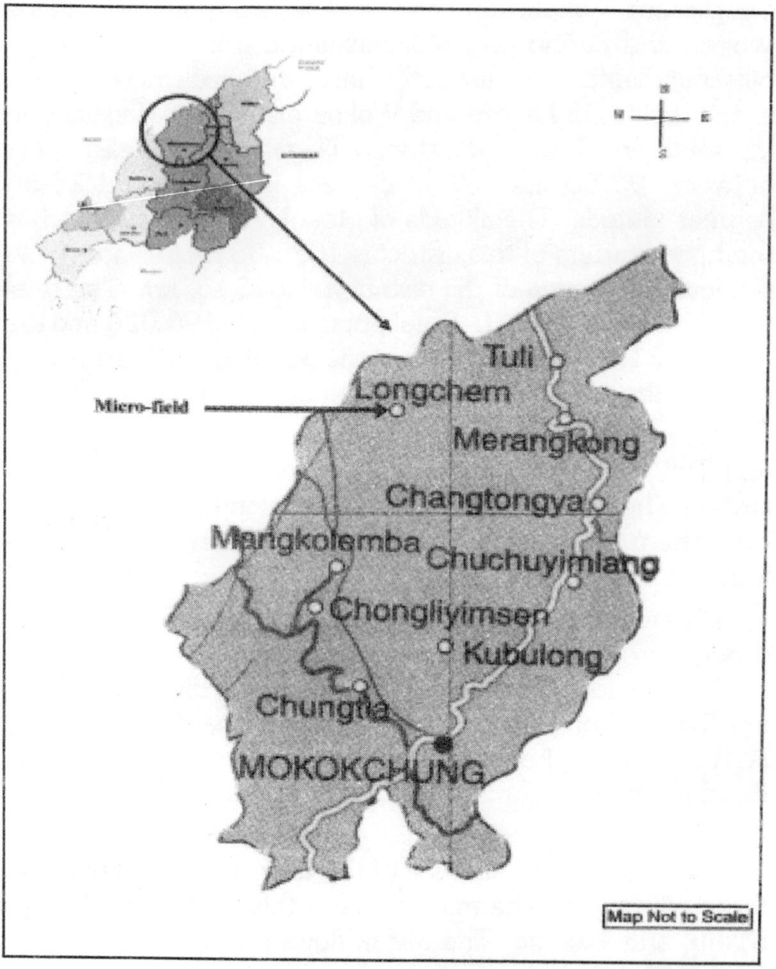

Map 3.3 : Map of Mokokchung District

private forest areas, which are owned either by community or some individuals. In this forest area the customary rights are regulated.

The principal crop is paddy which is cultivated under shifting cultivation. Maize, betel leaf, tapioca, ginger, potato, sugarcane and mustard seed are cultivated under shifting cultivation.

Coal, limestone, cobalt, magnesite, cromite, nickel etc. are available in this district. The important industry, pulp and paper mill is situated at Tuli of this district.

THE MICRO FIELD

As noted earlier, the present study has been conducted among the Ao Nagas in a rural setting under the Mokokchung District in Nagaland, North-East India. The district has two administrative sub-divisions, namely Mangkolemba and Tuli. The present micro-field falls under the jurisdiction of Mangkolemba sub-division having its headquarters at Mokokchung. The villages under study also fall within the service area of EAC Longchem Circle.

The intensive study has been carried out in three homogeneous villages, namely; Lirmen, Yajang-A and Yajang-B. All these three villages are within the jurisdiction of Longchum police station and are located in an identical geographical setting. The villages under study are homogeneously inhabited by the Aos, the tribe under investigation. The people are mainly agriculturalists and live in pile-dwellings. They by and large, have still been retaining their traditions and culture in-spite of the conversion to Christianity and the impact of westernization and education.

Lirmen village

Lirmen village is situated in the Mongkolomba sub-division under Mokokchung district of Nagaland. It is located northern side at a distance of about 100 km. from the district head-quarters. The village falls under the jurisdiction of Longchem police station and under the range Japokong.

The nearest railway station is Mariani (Assam) which stands at a distance of 45 km. from the village. The road transports are available from Longchem to anywhere in the country which is 13 km. far from the Lirmen village.

The village is surrounded by paddy fields, rivers and other villages. On the northern side of the village there is Yajang-A village, on the southern side there is Anokpu village, on the eastern side there is Waromong village and on the western side of the village there is Naginijan T.E.

Regarding the name and history of the village, it has been found that it was before 400 years when seven members came to this place and set under a big amla tree which is in their local term known as *Liri*. Out of these seven members, two were *Longchar*, two *Longkumer*, two *Sangpang* and one *Walling*. As they, after reaching the spot set under the Liri tree the name becomes Lirimen. *Liri* means amla and *men* means sit. Thus, the village was recognised as Lirmen.

Yajang-A village

The village Yajang-A is situated in Mongkolomba sub-division under Mokokchung district of Nagaland. It is located on eastern side at a distance of 105 km. from the district headquarters. The village falls under the jurisdiction of the Lonchum police station and is in the range Japokong.

The nearest railway station is Amguri (Assam) which stands at a distance of nearly 25 km. from the village and Haluwating is the nearest developing town from where road transports are available to anywhere in the country.

The village is surrounded by jhum fields, rivers, hills and other villages. On the northern side of the village there is Assam, on the southern side there is Lirmen, on the eastern side there is Molong and on the western side of the village there is Assam.

The village was formed by the people who were coming from three different places, e.g. Waramong, Molong and Lirmen. In the time of origin there were 30-40 households. The village was established in the year 1882. At the time of establishment of the village, except Molong, the people from Waramong and Lirmen were not Christian. The people from

Molong popularised the Christianity and after that all of them embraced Christianity. In 1885 after 3 years of the establishment of the village the Church was established there. The word Yajang has two meanings *Ya* means this and *Jang* means cross, i.e. away from enemy.

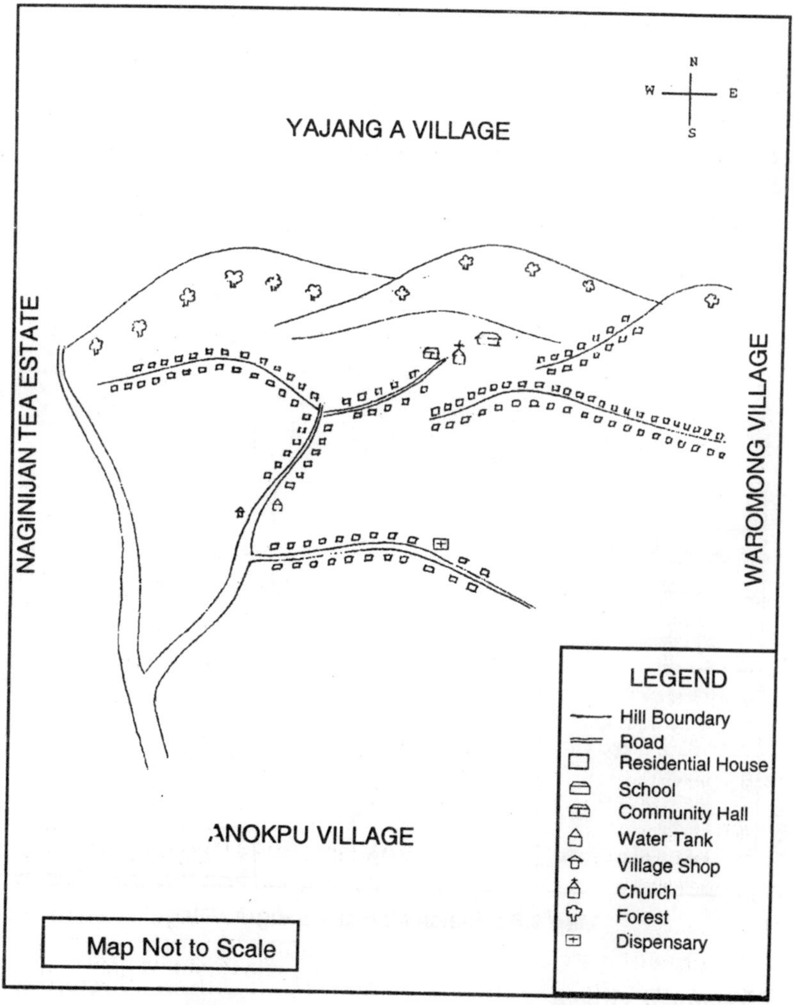

Map 3.4 : Sketch Map of Lirmen Village

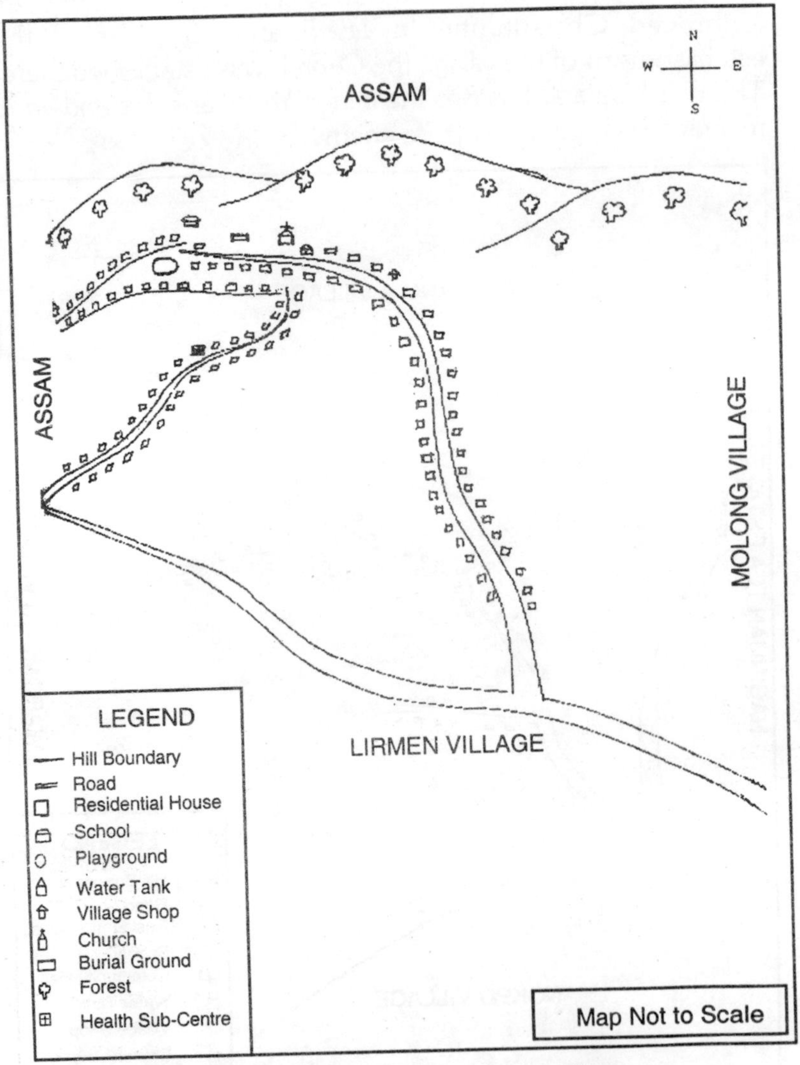

Map 3.5 : Sketch Map of Yajang-A Village

Yajang-B village

The village Yajang-B is situated in Mongkolomba sub-division under Mokokchung district of Nagaland. It is located on western side at a distance of 115 km. from the district headquarters and 10 km. away from the Yajang-A village. The village falls under the jurisdiction of the Longchem police station and is in the range Japukong.

The nearest railway station is Amguri which stands at a distance of nearly 15 km. from the village and Haluwating is the nearest developing town from where road transports are available to anywhere in the country.

The village is surrounded by jhum fields, rivers, hills and other villages. On the northern side of the village there is Yajang C, on the southern side there is Yajang-A village, on the eastern side there is Molong village and on the western side of the village there is Assam.

During the establishment time there were fifty members who came to this place from Yajang-A in the year 1970. The main cause of their migration to this place is the growth of population and lack of land in the village Yajang-A. They also did not go to the Lirmen side, i.e. upward because there is also already a large population. Finally, they came to downward as it was convenient to settle in their jhum land and get settled there. The people of this village Yajang-B is a part of Yajang-A. Village-wise distribution of the households, families and the population in the micro field are presented in Table 3.1.

Table 3.1 shows the distribution of the households, families and the population in the three villages. It will be seen from the table 3.1 that the total population is 1168 (male 53.25% and female 46.74%) that has been distributed in 259 families. With regard to their household dimensions however, it has been observed that each of the families occupies a household independently. That is why we find that 259 families have been accommodated in 259 households.

With regard to the number of family as well as population size, Lirmen seems to be the largest and Yajang-B the smallest village. Lirmen has 130 (50.19%) families with a total population of 624 (53.42%), whereas there are 28 (10.81%)

Table 3.1 : Village-wise distribution of the households, families and the population in the micro field

Sl. No.	Name of Villages	Number of Households (%)	Number of Families (%)	Population (%) Male	Female	Total
1	2	3	4	5	6	7
1.	Lirmen	130 (50.19)	130 (50.19)	333 (28.51)	291 (24.91)	624 (53.42)
2.	Yajang-A	101 (38.99)	101 (38.99)	220 (18.83)	194 (16.60)	414 (35.44)
3.	Yajang-B	28 (10.81)	28 (10.81)	69 (5.90)	61 (5.22)	130 (11.13)
Grand Total (%)		259 (100.00)	259 (100.00)	622 (53.25)	546 (46.74)	1168 (100.00)

families with a total population of 130 (11.13%) in Yajang-B Village. It will also be seen from Table 3.1 that the total number of families in Yajang-A village is 101 (38.99%) and the total population is 414 (35.44%).

Topography

Generally topography varies from range to range. All the three villages under Japokong Range are situated on hill tops. The houses are scattered haphazardly. Some places are steep and rugged, others are thick dark forests and yet others are meadow and plain.

Hydrography

There are two rivers, namely *Tzurang* and *Phuno* flowing from north to east and north to south nearby the Lirmen village.The river *Tzurang* is flowing through the Yajang-A village from east to north of the village. There is a small stream known as *Makumdang* which is flowing through the village

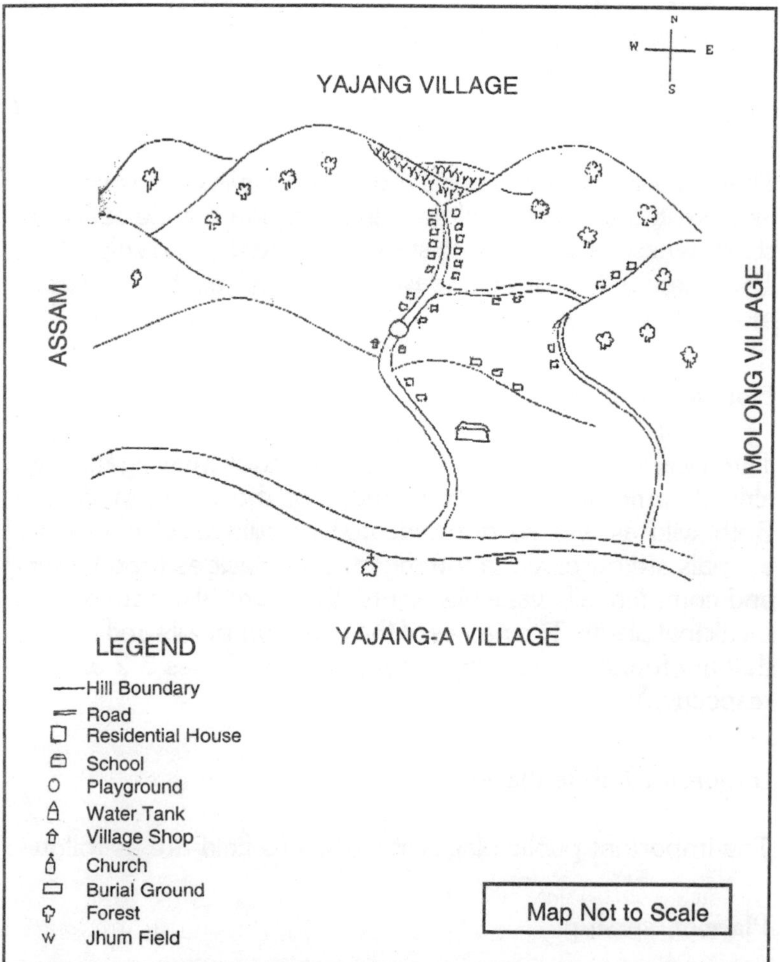

Map 3.6 : Sketch Map of Yajang-A Village

Yajang-B. People use this river water for fishing purposes. There are some Government infrastructural facilities for water such as there are some provision of water tanks. But they are to bring water from these tanks in bamboo pipes. They use this water for all their household purposes. They also store water in bamboo pipes. In rainy seasons they also store the rain water in their own tanks. For agricultural purposes they have to depend upon rain water.

Climate

The climate of the villages is moderate. As Assam is not very far from it, the climate is almost similar to the climate of Assam, characterized by hot and moist summer and dry and cold winter. The autumn and spring seasons are marked by favourable moderate weather.

Flora and Fauna

The flora and fauna of all the villages under investigation are almost same and identical to those of the areas of Assam. Both wild as well as domesticated or cultivated plants and animals are observed in the micro-field. Besides food bearing and commercially valuable plants, there are also found some medicinal plants. The names of the common plants and animals that are found in the villages are provid in Tables 3.2 and 3.3 respectively.

Important Public Places

The important public places in the micro-field are as follows:

Place of worship

The people of the micro field are Christians and Church is the place of worship for them. Each village has one Baptist Church. The names of the Churches are Lirmen Baptist Church which was established in 1931, Yajang-A Baptist Church and was established in 1885 and Yajang-B Baptist Church which was established in 1970. On every Sunday at 10.30 a.m. all the people come to their respective Churches and pray. The priest comes there and teaches them religious lessons.

Table 3.2 : The common flora present in the micro field

Sl. No.	*Local Name*	*English Name*	*Scientific Name*
1	*2*	*3*	*4*
1	Teti	Mango	*Mangifera Indica*
2	Polong	Jack fruit	Atrocarpus heterophylus
3	Luzu (c)/ Liri (m)	Amla	Emblica oficinalis
4	Leshi	Litchi	Litchi chinesis
5	Kozu (c)/ Koi (m)	Betel nut	Areca nut
6	Patio (c)/ Patiwa (m)	Betel leaf	*
7	Modhrem (c)/ Bogre(m)	Guava	Psidium guayava
8	Naring(c)/Chamben(m)	Orange	Citrus reticulata
9	Mamazu (c)/Mamalizang(m)	Papaya	Carica papaya
10	Mongo (c)/Mango(m)	Banana	Musacae species
11	Tinga	Lemon	Citrus species
12	Same	Atlas	*
13	Moji(c)/Motsu(m)	Sugarcane	*
14	Joro	Pineapple	Annanas comosus
15	Menti	Corn	*
16	Mapo (c)/Lao(m)	Pumpkin	Cucurbita moschata
17	Sungmok(c)/Songsing(m)	Ginger	Zingiber officinale
18	Sung sung(c)/Molichila(m)	Naga ginger	*
19	Manu(c)/Ami(m)	Arum	Colocasia species
20	Mersu (c)/Merchi (m)	Chilli	Capsicum annum
21	Bagana	Tomato	Lycopersicum esculentum
22	Sungerlikok (c)/ Pantu (m)	Brinjal	Solanum melongena
23	Aao (c)/Longmi (m)	Bamboo	Bamboosa species
24	Zungi (c)/Majhi (m)	Cucumber	*Cucumis sativus*

c= chongli term, m=mongseng term, *Scientific names could not be made available.

Table 3.3 : The common fauna present in the micro field

Sl. No.	*Local Name*	*English Name*	*Scientific Name*
1	*2*	*3*	*4*
1	Nashi (c)/Mashi (m)	Cow	*
2	NapangAk (c)/Aok (m)	Goat	Hemitragus suidae
3	Azu (c)/Ai (m)	Pig	Scrofa domestica
4	Tanu (c)/Mochi (m)	Dog	Caris familiaris
5	Per (c)/Afu (m)	Cat	Felis domestica
6	Jang (c)/Apang (m)	Snake	Reptila species
7	AnShishang (c)/Thanksu (m)	Buffalo	*
8	Ango (c)/ Anga (m)	Elephant	*
9	Lulng (c)/ Lang (m)	Fowl	*
10	Shisang (c)/ Tangchi (m)	Squirrel	Dremomys lokriah
11	Mesu (c)/ Metsu (m)	Deer	*
12	Angu (c)/ Anga (m)	Fish	Pisces
13	Ninang Mochitsu (c)/ Longnang nagotsu (m)	Honey bee	Apis species

* Scientific names could not be made available.

Educational Institutions

Each of the villages under study has at least one Lower Primary School. In one village there is also a M.E. (Middle Elementary) school. All these schools are provincialised by the Government. There are two schools in Lirmen village. Out of these, one L.P. School named as Government Primary School, Lirmen and another is Government Middle School and was established in the year 1972 but, provincialised in the year 1931. The M.E. School is housed in an Assam type structure made of brick, cement and C.I. Sheet. There are 9 teaching staff (two female and the rest male) in the M.E. School and the total number of student is 54. The building of the L.P. School is also of concrete work with C.I. sheet roof, where six teachers are there. Out of these, two females and four males. All the teachers of both the schools are belonging to the same village and tribe.

There is only one L.P. School provincialised by the Government in 1945 in Yajang-A village. The building is made of bamboo and C.I. sheet. There are five teachers (four males and one female) in the school. The total number of students is 80. All the teachers are belonging to the same village and tribe.

The village Yajang-B, has only one L.P. school. The school was established in the year 1970 but was provincialised in the year 2005. The building is bamboo made and roofed by C.I. sheet. There are three teachers (all male) in the school and are belonging to the same village and tribe. The total number of students is 45.

Playground

All the three villages have playgrounds within the village premises. The young boys and the children play football, cricket and volleyball etc. in these grounds. They also use the playgrounds in festival and Christmas time.

Shops and Market

There are a few shops in the villages under study. The village Lirmen has three shops. The village Yajang-A has 5 shops and the village Yajang-B has one shop. All these shops of the three villages are found in the residence of the owners and the owners are the village people. All these shops deal in both stationery and grocery items. The shops deal in almost all the material necessities of domestic life. Due to very far from the town area, most of the people buy the items of their day to day life from these shops.

The marketing places of the people are the nearly townships. The people of Lirmen village go to Naginijan for marketing, where on every Saturday a market is held which is under Jorhat district, Assam and is 9 km. away from the village. The people of Yajang-A and Yajang-B come to Haluwating the nearest developing town for marketing where two weekly markets are held, one on Tuesday and the other on Friday. All the necessary commodities from cloth to spices are available there. People buy their necessary goods from the market. For any major purchase, as well as for necessary purchases on other days they go to Amguri town, Jorhat, Morioni.

Medical Facility

As regards medical facility, the village Lirmen has one government dispensary with a pharmacist, one nurse and one midwife. The village Yajang-A also has one health sub-centre with one nurse and one midwife. But there is no any dispensary/sub-centre in the village Yajang-B and for that people of this village either go to Yajang-A or Yajang-C village where there is one sub-centre. In case of emergency, the people of these villages go to Haluwating, Jorhat, Amguri, Dimapur, Mokokchung.

Burial Ground

As the people are Christian, they bury their dead ones in their respective burial ground. Each of the village possesses one burial ground. The burial ground of Lirmen village and Yajang-B village is in the road side but the burial ground of Yajang-A village is near the Church.

Community Hall

Both Lirmen and Yajang-A village has one community hall, where all village meetings are held. Sometimes the women also use for their meeting. But the village Yajang-B does not have the community hall and for meeting purpose they use their own houses.

Transport and Communication

As the villages under study are in a rural setting, the transport facility is not good. In the villages, a few families have bicycle and a few families possess scooter and bike. Most of the people use to visit the neighbouring villages and towns on foot. Only those who possess scooter and bike can move with their vehicles to the nearabout villages and towns. When the people want to go to some far places they hire taxi from their nearest town. Besides, Nagaland State Transports (NST) are available from their nearest town. The people of Lirmen village either come to Tzudikong or go to Morioni from where NST are available. Morioni is the nearest railway station for them.

The people of Yajang-A and Yajang-B village come to Haluwating from where NST are available. For them the nearest railway station is Amguri.

There is no postal facility available within these three villages. However, the nearest B.P.O. is Longchem which is 7 k.m. away from the villages. Though there is no provision of land telephone connection but a few families now possess mobile phones. There is no public telephone booth for other residents. For this facility also people are to go to nearest town. However, W.L.L. phone is available in Lirmen village.

The People

As noted earlier, the present study has been carried out among the Ao Nagas under Mokokchung district, in Nagaland. The Aos are one of the dominant tribes of Nagaland and at present their principal settlement is to the Mokokchung district of Nagaland.

A detailed discussion with regard to their origin and history has already been presented in Chapter 2 (The Ao Nagas).

The intensive study has been carried out in three homogeneous villages (Lirmen, Yajang-A and Yajang-B) which is revealed by generating data from the field. The total population is 1168 which is distributed in 259 families.

The people under investigation are short to medium statures, strong built, complexion light, hair is black, straight, course with scanty hair on face, nose fine to broad, and with a flat face which are the characteristic features of Mongoloids.

Linguistically, the Ao Nagas are divided into three sub-tribes: Chonglee, Chungki and Mongsen. The people under investigation are also belonging to two linguistic groups, i.e. Chonglee and Mongsen. The people of Lirmen village speak Mongsen dialect and the people of Yajang-A and Yajang-B village speak Chonglee dialect. But all of them can speech Nagamese and a few of them (the educated one) can speak English and Hindi.

With regard to the religion all people are Christian and they are under the Baptist Church Association.

The Ao people have their own dress and ornaments which are distinct from the other Naga tribes. In the present setting, it has been seen to wear all kinds of modern dresses by the people. They wear their traditional dress and ornaments only during the festival occasion (*Moatsu*) which always starts from 1st May. During the time of this festival, both male and female wear their typical specially designed clothes and ornaments and traditionally dance and engaged themselves with different tunes and melodies followed by drums which have considerable artistic values.

Population Analysis

For the purpose of the present investigation, data have been collected from a sample of 259 families. A brief analysis of the people of the micro-field is attempted below:

Distribution of the Population by Age and Sex

In Table 3.4, the analysis of the total population by age and sex of the micro-field under study has been given. The total population of the villages under study is 1168. Out of this, there are 622 (53.25%) male and 546 (46.74%) female (Table 3.4).

It will be seen from the table that age group 20-24 years contains the largest population (11.81%) in both the sexes. The second largest population is in the age group of 15-19 years (being 11.30%). On the other hand, the least number of people are found in the age-group of 85-89 years (0.17%).

Considering the villages under study independently, it is seen (Table 3.5) that the total population of the village Lirmen is 624 (53.36% male and 46.63% female). The largest population falls in the age group of 20-24 years (being, 12.98%). On the other hand, the least number of people are found in the age group of 85-89 years (0.16%).

In the village Yajang-A (Table 3.6) the total population is 414. Out of this, there are 220 (53.14%) male and 194

Table 3.4 : Distribution of the population of the villages under study by age and sex

Sl. No.	Age group (in years)	Male (%)	Female (%)	Total (%)
1	2	3	4	5
1	0-4	39 (3.33)	44 (3.76)	83 (7.10)
2	5-9	47 (4.02)	40 (3.42)	87 (7.44)
3	10-14	52 (4.45)	53 (4.53)	105 (8.98)
4	15-19	64 (5.47)	68 (5.82)	132 (11.30)
5	20-24	76 (6.50)	62 (5.30)	138 (11.81)
6	25-29	80 (6.84)	49 (4.19)	129 (11.04)
7	30-34	52 (4.45)	41 (3.51)	93 (7.96)
8	35-39	37 (3.16)	31 (2.65)	68 (5.82)
9	40-44	30 (2.56)	35 (2.99)	65 (5.56)
10	45-49	33 (2.82)	26 (2.22)	59 (5.05)
11	50-54	26 (2.22)	32 (2.73)	58 (4.96)
12	55-59	23 (1.96)	24 (2.05)	47 (4.02)
13	60-64	25 (2.14)	15 (1.28)	40 (3.42)
14	65-69	7 (0.59)	8 (0.68)	15 (1.28)
15	70-74	18 (1.54)	12 (1.02)	30 (2.56)
16	75-79	3 (0.25)	4 (0.34)	7 (0.59)
17	80-84	8(0.68)	2 (0.17)	10 (0.85)
18	85-89	2(0.17)	0	2 (0.17)
Grand Total		622(53.25)	546(46.74)	1168(100.00)

Table 3.5 : Distribution of the population of the village Lirmen by age and sex

Sl. No.	Age group (in years)	Male (%)	Female (%)	Total (%)
1	2	3	4	5
1	0-4	11 (1.76)	17 (2.72)	28 (4.48)
2	5-9	19 (3.04)	15 (2.40)	34 (5.44)
3	10-14	24 (3.84)	24 (3.84)	48 (7.69)
4	15-19	40 (6.41)	40 (6.41)	80 (12.82)
5	20-24	45 (7.21)	36 (5.76)	81 (12.98)
6	25-29	43 (6.89)	22 (3.52)	65 (10.41)
7	30-34	30 (4.80)	28 (4.48)	58 (9.29)

(Contd...)

Table 3.5 *(Contd...)*

1	2	3	4	5
8	35-39	21 (3.36)	15 (2.40)	36 (5.76)
9	40-44	18 (2.88)	22 (3.52)	40 (6.41)
10	45-49	16 (2.56)	10 (1.60)	26 (4.16)
11	50-54	16 (2.56)	24 (3.84)	40 (6.41)
12	55-59	13 (2.08)	14 (2.24)	27 (4.32)
13	60-64	17 (2.72)	11 (1.76)	28 (4.48)
14	65-69	3 (0.48)	6 (0.96)	9 (1.44)
15	70-74	12 (1.92)	4 (0.64)	16 (2.56)
16	75-79	2 (0.32)	2 (0.32)	4 (0.64)
17	80-84	2 (0.32)	1 (0.16)	3 (0.48)
18	85-89	1 (0.16)	0	1 (0.16)
Grand Total		333 (53.36)	291 (46.63)	624 (100.00)

Table 3.6 : Distribution of the population of the village Yajang-A by age and sex

Sl. No.	*Age group (in years)*	*Male (%)*	*Female (%)*	*Total (%)*
1	*2*	*3*	*4*	*5*
1	0-4	18 (4.34)	18 (4.34)	36 (8.69)
2	5-9	19 (4.58)	20 (4.83)	39 (9.42)
3	10-14	20 (4.83)	22 (5.31)	42 (10.14)
4	15-19	20 (4.83)	20 (4.83)	40 (9.66)
5	20-24	28 (6.76)	23 (5.55)	51 (12.31)
6	25-29	31 (7.48)	18 (4.34)	49 (11.83)
7	30-34	17 (4.10)	12 (2.89)	28 (6.76)
8	35-39	11 (2.65)	11 (2.65)	23 (5.55)
9	40-44	7 (1.69)	11 (2.65)	18 (4.34)
10	45-49	14 (3.38)	13 (3.14)	27 (6.52)
11	50-54	8 (1.93)	7 (1.69)	15 (3.62)
12	55-59	9 (2.17)	9 (2.17)	18 (4.34)
13	60-64	7 (1.69)	2 (0.48)	9 (2.17)
14	65-69	4 (0.96)	1 (0.24)	5 (1.20)
15	70-74	4 (0.96)	5 (1.20)	9 (2.17)
16	75-79	1 (0.24)	2 (0.48)	3 (0.72)
17	80-84	2 (0.48)	0	2 (0.48)
18	85-89	0	0	0
Grand Total		220 (53.14)	194 (46.85)	414 (100.00)

(46.85%) female. The largest population falls in the age group of 20-24 years (12.31%) and the least number of people are found in the age group of 82-84 years (0.48%).

Similarly, from Table 3.7 it has been observed that the total population of the village Yajang-B is 130 (53.07% male and 46.92% female). The largest population falls in the age group of 0-4 years (being 14.61%). On the other hand, the least number of people are found in the age group of 65-69 years and 85-89 years and is respectively same (0.76%).

Table 3.7 : Distribution of the population of the village Yajang-B by age and sex

Sl. No.	*Age group (in years)*	*Male (%)*	*Female (%)*	*Total (%)*
1	*2*	*3*	*4*	*5*
1	0-4	10 (7.69)	9 (6.42)	19 (14.61)
2	5-9	9 (6.92)	5 (3.84)	14 (10.76)
3	10-14	8 (6.15)	7 (5.38)	15 (11.53)
4	15-19	4 (3.07)	8 (6.15)	12 (9.23)
5	20-24	3 (2.30)	3 (2.30)	6 (4.61)
6	25-29	6 (4.61)	9 (6.92)	15 (11.53)
7	30-34	5 (3.84)	2 (1.53)	7 (5.38)
8	35-39	5 (3.84)	4 (3.07)	9 (6.92)
9	40-44	5 (3.84)	2 (1.53)	7 (5.38)
10	45-49	3 (2.30)	3 (2.30)	6 (4.61)
11	50-54	2 (1.53)	1 (0.76)	3 (2.30)
12	55-59	1 (0.76)	1 (0.76)	2 (1.53)
13	60-64	1 (0.76)	2 (1.53)	3 (2.30)
14	65-69	0	1 (0.76)	1 (0.76)
15	70-74	2 (1.53)	3 (2.30)	5 (3.84)
16	75-79	0	0	0
17	80-84	4 (3.07)	1 (0.76)	5 (3.84)
18	85-89	1 (0.76)	0	1 (0.76)
Grand Total		69 (53.07)	61 (46.92)	130 (100.00)

4

SOCIAL LIFE

Social life is the essence of human life. It grows out of constant patterning of social interactions and relationships that take place within some institutionalized grouping among human beings.

Man is a social animal by nature and necessity. He has to meet his basic needs like food, shelter and social needs like companionship, recreation, religious activities, games etc. He thus forms groups or associations with the help of other men and builds up certain institutions (e.g. marriage and family etc.), with the help of those groups, which help him to satisfy his needs. To quote Firth (1961:41), "All community life involves methods of grouping and grading people for an effective carrying out of the various types of activities demanded by the common existence."

In this context, it may be emphasised that family is considered to be the most important element in social life, as it forms the first sphere in which individuals combine. It is the fundamental social institution that fulfils various needs of human being in his life.

Therefore, in order to have an understanding of the social life of the Ao Nagas under investigation, the discussion has conveniently been confined to their family life and marital alliances. Education, being an important variable of social life, information regarding educational attainment of the people has also been included here. Brief discussions have also been incorporated on their clan system, inheritance system and village administration.

Family

The family is the most important primary group in a society. It is the most basic of all social groupings. As an institution it is the most permanent and the most pervasive of all social institutions.

Murdock (1965: 1) defines family as "A social group characterized by common residence, economic co-operation and reproduction. It includes adults of both sexes, at least two of whom maintain a socially approved sexual relationship and one or more children, own or adopted, of the sexually cohabiting adults."

According to Robert H. Lowie, "A family is a group based on marital relations, rights and duties of parenthood, common habitation and reciprocal relations between parents and children" (cited in Jha, 1994: 89).

In most of the societies, the establishment of a family is based on marriage, which unites a man and a woman having social sanction to live together with the purpose of establishing a family. Thus, "the family in this sense is based on marriage, which is defined as a union between a man and a woman such that children born by the woman are recognized as the legitimate offspring of both the parents" (Notes and Queries in Anthropology, 1971: 1).

Many scholars perceive the family as the cornerstone of society. As a carrier and mediator of culture its role in socialization and personality development is very well recognized. Goldstein has truly narrated it as "More than a legal entity or a social institution. It is the cradle into which the future is born and the nursery in which the new democratic social order is being fashioned. The family is related to the past through traditions but is also related to the future through social responsibility and trust" (Thakre, 1995).

The family as the standard social unit has been found in one form or another at almost all levels of cultural development. The form and basis of familial groupings have varied from time to time and from place to place. Different types of families have been observed in different societies and at different points of time and space. But as a basic social group, family existed in all societies at all times.

For the purpose of the present discussion the term family has been operationally and synonymously used with the term household. A family then includes all the members dwelling under the same roof and sharing common food from same hearth.

Being the basic and primary unit of socialization, in the following pages, it is proposed to have an overall idea about the family life of the people under investigation.

To start with, let us first have an understanding of the operational meaning of some of the concepts used in the discussion on familial organisation.

Nuclear or Elementary Family

It refers to a family, which is composed of husband, wife and their unmarried children. Family without having children or/ and having one or two unmarried dependents have also been included in this category.

Extended or Joint Family

The term extended family denotes the family where extension to an elementary family has taken place by marriage, either horizontally or vertically. In horizontally extended family, more than one brother lives together with their respective families. And, in vertically extended family patrilineal extension takes place on the basis of parent-child relationship and generally it extends up to three generations.

Broken Family

When a family consists of either the parents with unmarried children or of the siblings, or a group that has lost or lack one or more relationship to constitute an elementary family, it has been termed as a broken family.

In every kind of family, generally the eldest member is regarded as the head of the family; and he/she is usually an earning member. In a joint family, however, sometimes the head may not be an earning member. A widow becomes the head of the family after the passing away of her husband leaving the children imrnature.

The head of the family takes dominant role in the management of the institution. The other members, however, take active role in running the day-to-day affairs while taking major decisions, the members generally discuss amongst themselves. But, the final decision is taken or is to be approved by the head.

Among the Ao too, family is considered to be the smallest social unit comprising a married man and wife with one or more children. The Ao families live in houses called *ki (chongli)/ aki (mongsen)*. The term *kibong (chongli)* or *kiong (mongsen)* means the family and the members of the family, whereas *kinunger (chongli)* or *kiyaa (mongsen)* refers to relatives. The form of Ao family is patriarchal and patrilineal in nature, so the head of the family is father or an elder male individual and the major shares of property go to the sons rather than the daughters. He is the owner and administrator of the family property and right. He is the main bread earner of the family although he is assisted by his wife and children. Children have no specific responsibility during their childhood. But as they grow up they assume specific responsibilities on the basis of sex. Mostly, they are dependent. Elder children, however, assist their parents in taking care of their younger siblings. The head of the family (male) represents the family in case of village court and other village level collective activities. In some cases, like loss of father, during childhood, mother takes the administrative role in the family. In the absence of father, the grown up eldest son assumes the role of his father although constant consultation with his mother is made.

The married couples have greater preference for male children rather than female as they are going to represent the family or clan for generations to come and also for the property right as traditionally, inheritance among the Ao was through male line. Most of the females are housewives and assistants to their husbands besides their duties of nourishing their young one and household management.

Type and Composition

The Ao mostly live in small families as they follow nuclear family. After the marriage, the newly married couple lives separately in a new house constructed by the husband. Therefore, the nuclear family is the main type that prevails among the Aos, other types which show characteristics of joint and extended family types are very rare.

An analysis of the type and composition of the Ao families under investigation has been presented in Tables 4.1, 4.2, 4.3 and 4.4.

It will be seen from Table 4.1 that majority of the families is of nuclear type. There are 217 (83.78%) nuclear families as against 4 (1.54%) extended and 38 (14.67%) broken ones.

With regard to the composition, the table reveals that the maximum number of nuclear families (71.04%) have husband, wife and unmarried children as the inmates. In case of extended families, it is dominated by husband, wife, married son, son's wife and children (1.54%).

To have a comparative idea, village-wise distributions of the family type and composition have been presented in the Tables 4.2, 4.3 and 4.4.

Table 4.1 : Distribution of the families of the under study villages according to type and composition

Sl. No.	*Type*	*Composition*	*No. of families (%)*
1	*2*	*3*	*4*
1.	Nuclear Family	Husband and wife	24(9.26)
		Husband, wife with unmarried children	184(71.04)
		Husband, wife, unmarried children and husband's unmarried brother and sister	1(0.38)
		Husband, wife and unmarried children and husband's unmarried sister.	1(0.38)
		Husband, wife and husband's widow mother	1(0.38)
		Husband, wife and unmarried children and husband's widow mother and unmarried brother and sister	1(0.38)
		Husband, wife, and unmarried children and husband, widow mother	3(1.15)
		Husband, wife, and unmarried children and husband's widower father	1(0.38)
		Parents in law with widow daughter-in-law and her children unmarried	1 (0.38)
	Sub-Total		217(83.78)
2.	Joint or Extended Family	Parents with married son and unmarried children	4(1.54)
	Sub-Total		4(1.54)
3.	Broken Family	Widower and unmarried children	8(3.08)
		Widow and unmarried children	15(5.79)
		Unmarried siblings	9(3.47)
		Only widower	3(1.15)
		Widow with unmarried son	2(0.77)
		Widow with unmarried brother	1(0.38)
	Sub-Total		38(14.67)
	Grand Total		259(100.00)

Table 4.2 : Distribution of the families of the village Lirmen according to type and composition

Sl. No.	*Type*	*Composition*	*No. of families (%)*
1	*2*	*3*	*4*
1.	Nuclear Family	Husband and wife	7(5.38)
		Husband, wife with unmarried children	97(74.61)
		Husband, wife, unmarried children and husband's unmarried brother and sister	1(0.76)
		Husband, wife and unmarried children and husband's unmarried sister.	1(0.76)
		Husband, wife and husband's widow mother	1(0.76)
		Husband, wife and unmarried children and husband's widow mother and unmarried brother and sister	1(0.76)
		Husband, wife, and unmarried children and husband, widow mother	1(0.76)
		Husband, wife, and unmarried children and husband's widower father	0(0.00)
		Parents in law with widow daughter-in-law and her children unmarried	1 (0.76)
	Sub-Total		110(84.61)
2.	Joint or Extended Family	Parents with married son and unmarried children	2(1.53)
	Sub-Total		2(1.53)
3.	Broken Family	Widower and unmarried children	6(4.61)
		Widow and unmarried children	11 (8.46)
		Unmarried siblings	1(0.76)
		Only widower	0(0.00)
		Widow with unmarried son	0(0.00)
		Widow with unmarried brother	0(0.00)
	Sub-Total		10(13.84)
	Grand Total		130(100.00)

Table 4.3 : Distribution of the families of the village Yajang-A according to type and composition

Sl. No.	*Type*	*Composition*	*No. of families (%)*
1	*2*	*3*	*4*
1.	Nuclear Family	Husband and wife	13(12.87)
		Husband, wife with unmarried children	69(68.31)
		Husband, wife, unmarried children and husband's unmarried brother and sister	0(0.00)
		Husband, wife and unmarried children and husband's unmarried sister.	0(0.00)
		Husband, wife and husband's widow mother	0(0.00)
		Husband, wife and unmarried children and husband's widow mother and unmarried brother and sister	0(0.00)
		Husband, wife, and unmarried children and husband, widow mother	1(0.99)
		Husband, wife, and unmarried children and husband's widower father	0(0.00)
		Parents in law with widow daughter-in-law and her children unmarried	0(0.00)
	Sub-Total		83(82.17)
2.	Joint or Extended Family	Parents with married son and unmarried children	0(0.00)
	Sub-Total		0(0.00)
3.	Broken Family	Widower and unmarried children	1(0.99)
		Widow and unmarried children	4 (3.96)
		Unmarried siblings	7(6.93)
		Only widower	3(2.97)
		Widow with unmarried son	2(1.98)
		Widow with unmarried brother	1(0.99)
	Sub-Total		18(17.82)
	Grand Total		101(100.00)

Table 4.4 : Distribution of the families of the village Yajang-B according to type and composition

Sl. No.	*Type*	*Composition*	*No. of families (%)*
1	*2*	*3*	*4*
1.	Nuclear Family	Husband and wife	4(14.28)
		Husband, wife with unmarried children	18(64.28)
		Husband, wife, unmarried children and husband's unmarried brother and sister	0(0.00)
		Husband, wife and unmarried children and husband's unmarried sister.	0(0.00)
		Husband, wife and husband's widow mother	0(0.00)
		Husband, wife and unmarried children and husband's widow mother and unmarried brother and sister	0(0.00)
		Husband, wife, and unmarried children and husband, widow mother	1(3.57)
		Husband, wife, and unmarried children and husband's widower father	1(3.57)
		Parents in law with widow daughter-in-law and her children unmarried	0(0.00)
	Sub-Total		24(85.71)
2.	Joint or Extended Family	Parents with married son and unmarried children	2(7.14)
	Sub-Total		2(7.14)
3.	Broken Family	Widower and unmarried children	1(3.57)
		Widow and unmarried children	0(0.00)
		Unmarried siblings	1(3.57)
		Only widower	0(0.00)
		Widow with unmarried son	0(0.00)
		Widow with unmarried brother	0(0.00)
	Sub-Total		2(7.14)
	Grand Total		28(100.00)

A cursory glance of Tables 4.2, 4.3 and 4.4 will show that the general trend of distribution of the major nuclear type of family is by and large identical.

Size of the Family

For the understanding of size of the family under investigation, the family size has conveniently been divided into 5 categories. These are single (1 individual), small (2-3 individuals), medium (4-6 individuals), large (7-9 individuals) and very large (10 and above it, individuals). Distribution of the families according to size has been presented in Table 4.5. It will be seen from the table that maximum number of families (159; 61.38%) fall in the medium category. It is followed by small (62; 2.39%) and large (32; 12.35%) categories. Very large families are not found among the people. The average size of a family has been found to consist of around 4.50 individuals.

Table 4.5 : Distribution of the families of the villages under study according to size

Sl. No.	*Categories of families*	*Size (No. of individuals)*	*No. of families (%)*
1	*2*	*3*	*4*
1	Single number	1	6 (2.31)
2	Small	2 – 3	62 (2.39)
3	Medium	4 – 6	159 (61.38)
4	Large	7 – 9	32 (12.35)
5	Very large	10 and above	0
	Grand Total (%)		259 (100.00)

Tables (4.6, 4.7 and 4.8) show the independent distribution of the families of the three study villages according to size. The tables show that the general trend of distribution of different sizes is by and large similar. The average size however, is slightly more (4.8) in the Lirmen village as compared to that in Yajang-A village (4.0) and Yajang-B village (4.6).

Table 4.6 : Distribution of the families of the village Lirmen according to size

Sl. No.	*Categories of families*	*Size (No. of individuals)*	*No. of families (%)*
1	*2*	*3*	*4*
1	Single number	1	1(0.76)
2	Small	2 – 3	24(18.46)
3	Medium	4 – 6	85(65.38)
4	Large	7 – 9	20(15.38)
5	Very large	10 and above	0
	Grand Total (%)		130 (100.00)

Table 4.7 : Distribution of the families of the village Yajang-A according to size

Sl. No.	*Categories of families*	*Size (No. of individuals)*	*No. of families (%)*
1	*2*	*3*	*4*
1	Single number	1	5(4.95)
2	Small	2 – 3	29(28.71)
3	Medium	4 – 6	62(61.38)
4	Large	7 – 9	5(4.95)
5	Very large	10 and above	0
	Grand Total (%)		101 (100.00)

Table 4.8 : Distribution of the families of the village Yajang-B according to size

Sl. No.	*Categories of families*	*Size (No. of individuals)*	*No. of families (%)*
1	*2*	*3*	*4*
1	Single number	1	0
2	Small	2 – 3	9(32.14)
3	Medium	4 – 6	12(42.85)
4	Large	7 – 9	7(25.00)
5	Very large	10 and above	0
	Grand Total (%)		28 (100.00)

Family Life

Family is the most basic social group and of primary importance in the socialization of the young. In this respect, the family is supposed to be the most effective agent in the transmission of the social heritage.

The quality and content of the family life do play a very important role in shaping the prospect of education in particular and the overall social health in general of the members of the younger generation in a cultural group.

Every association of people; it may be a state, nation or a tribe; has its own distinctive culture; its mode of living and world view, which are developed as a response to the peculiar circumstances of the environment; natural as well as ideological. The family is the agency through which the members of the growing generations are made familiar with the existing traditions. The purpose is once again, two-folds. By teaching the individual what situations to anticipate, how to behave and what behaviour to expect, by giving him/her the gifts of language and other traits which integrate him/her within his/her cultural ethos, the family provides a personal satisfaction. It also facilitates adjustment with the people and groups outside the family circle.

Keeping all these facts in mind, in the following pages, an attempt has been made to have an overall understanding about the family life of the people under investigation.

A. Daily Life

The daily activities of the people vary from season to season and from person to person, depending on the nature of the job requirements. However, the flow of life is by and large, the same throughout the year.

The people usually lead a busy daily routine of work. As the people are mostly *jhum* cultivators, most of the inhabitants belonging to both sexes except the old persons and children are engaged in their *jhum* field for the entire year. Generally, the people stir themselves to life before the sunrise. Women folk get up from the bed earlier than the men folk. They clean their teeth, wash face and go to their pit latrine for attending to nature's call. After then, they sweep their houses and courtyards. After all these are over, they do not take bath and go directly to kitchen for preparing morning meal for their respective families. During this time the men folk get up and those who possess cattle at first bring them out of the shed, give them fresh feeder and water and milk them. The cattle are then driven out for grazing in the grazing field. Those who do not have cattle either help in some domestic work or look after the kitchen garden or do some light repairing work in the fencing or so. In the meantime, the children also wake up and all of them take tea either black/white. Sometimes milk is given to the children.

The children then sit down to study or play outside. By this time the woman members get busy in the preparation of morning meal. The menu for morning meal is not much varying from the evening. The items in their menu include rice, sauce and dry fish and boiled vegetables. If available, meat is also added to their menu. They occasionally sometimes take the pulse. They are fond of bamboo shoot and chilli and they take it often in their items.

Before 7.30 a.m. they complete their breakfast. Then both men and women go out to their respective *jhum* field and they carry the required amount of tiffin from the prepared morning meal with them to have in the lunch time.

The children those who go to schools get ready at 7.30 a.m. after taking meal. Some take bath before going to school and some take bath after coming back from school. Majority of the children do not go to school and play about the whole day barring the time when they eat or feel too tired to play.

Some boys and girls generally look after their infant and

toddler brothers and sisters during day time in the absence of their parents. The adult daughters do the household work and also help mothers in preparing food. The unemployed young boys help their fathers in domestic works and in the *jhum* field. Some of them go out in search of job on daily wage basis. Sometimes they spend their time by hunting in the forest.

Elderly people who are too old to work in the agricultural field, work on some basketry (for domestic use only), fencing or in the kitchen garden, or simply sit down and wait for the day to pass. Generally, the men folk if sometimes do not go to the *jhum* field they get busy with work on basketry, repairing of their house and some other occasional tasks like bamboo work etc. The women folk also sometimes do not go to their *jhum* field and engage themselves in domestic works and other relevant activities.

Usually, the people work in the *jhum* field up to 4.30 p.m. and after then they leave their field and come back to their respective home. In the returning time from the field they carry betel leaf, various roots and shoots, broomstick, firewood etc. with their baskets. Usually they sell the betel leaves on the way.

After reaching home both men and women take bath. After taking bath the womenfolk get busy in the preparation of night meal. Mothers having adult daughters need not do it themselves. The daughters do it either entirely by themselves or help their mothers in household works.

The men folk generally spend the evening by gossiping with the neighbours. Some of them go to fetch water in bamboo pipes. Usually both men and women and the children (if needed) also fetch water in bamboo pipes as required. Occasional shopping in the nearby shops is also done in the evening by the men folk. Some members of the men folk in the evening stay at home to feed the cattle and to do a little bit household work.

Just when the sun sets the women folk pray to god and

then prepare the night meal. The students generally sit with their books. After having the night meal, which is usually finished by around 8 p.m. they go to sleep.

On Sunday, the people do not have any definite routine work. They do not go to the *jhum* field and no one work on that day. Just after completing the usual morning works all the family members get ready to go to the Church to pray. The Church time is from 10 a.m. and by this time all the people complete their bath and morning meal. At 11 a.m. the Church is over and all the people come out gossiping with each other. The village council members sit in their respective place and hold their meetings on that day as they do not get free time to discuss about village matter except on Sunday. The women folk also hold their meeting on that day. Some people visit to their friends/relatives in the nearby villages and some go to the nearest town to purchase their necessary items.

Usually, the council members are very busy on Sunday and they spent their time on that day by holding meetings. The young boys and girls have their youth activities in the Church from 2 p.m. to 3 p.m. on Sunday. In the evening time the young boys spend the time by playing cricket and volleyball.

The daily routine of activities of the people discussed above thus, make it apparent that the women folk remain relatively busier as compared to their men counterpart. They do not get much leisure in the midst of their multifarious pre-occupation. From early morning till night women generally remain busy with their work at home as well as in *jhum* field in addition to the child bearing and child rearing exercises.

B. Intra-Family Relationship

Even though emotions and feelings are the main bases of family life, it is not completely devoid of reasons. A sense of responsibility among its members in relation to each other is an aspect, which is more rational and reasoned than emotional and instinctive. The feeling of personal responsibility towards one another is very important to ensure the smooth working of familial grouping and consequently of society as a whole and therefore, we find society stepping into ensure it through customs and mores (Majumdar and Madan, 1967: 61).

The relationship prevailing among the inmates of a family in the studied group has been presented in brief in the following pages.

(a) *Husband and Wife*

The main occupation of an Ao being agriculture he requires a helping hand in the field. For this purpose, the easiest way to obtain such help is to get married. After the marriage, the wife becomes the mistress of the household and stays with her husband under his guardianship and protection.

The relationship between husband and wife is very cordial and open. Normally, the husband is older than the wife and the wife is always loyal and obedient to the husband. The wife talks to her husband freely and shares their feelings.

The husband and wife have equal responsibilities in the welfare of the family and the upbringing of the children. The children born of their wedlock also help the parents in the field when they grow up. The wife becomes the real helpmate of her husband in all the domestic affairs. She does not only day-to-day household chores but also helps her counterpart in the field. As they develop sound relationship and mutual understanding, she follows her husband in every respect of life throughout their lives. Though there is a broad division of labour in the household activities; and most of the works are allotted to the females, in case of necessity both of them work together.

Both husband and wife spend their earnings in smooth running of the family. It may, however, be noted here that as a tradition, the major decisions in the family are generally taken by the husband. The wife, however, is consulted by the husband in the practice.

Most of the free time seems to be spent by husband and wife in household activities and in the midst of their friends circle. A couple very rarely goes out together for recreation or visiting others.

The relationship between husband and wife is characterized by love and affection along with due respect and responsibilities towards each other.

(b) Relationship between Other Members of the Family

Although a nuclear family result out of the establishment of an independent household by a married son, it has been observed that in many cases the agnates carry on their economic activities in the agricultural field in collaboration and participate in common ceremonies and rituals in their natal family. In most of the important matters of the natal family, a son always takes interest. A brother also helps his brother in crisis.

The mother is the centre of the family. The infant and the mother establish an intimate emotional tie with each other soon after the baby's birth. Usually, both the parents establish love ties with their children but use these ties of emotional dependency to force the children towards attaining gradual independence. In other words the parental roles combine authority and intimacy.

As the adolescent moves into adulthood, an offspring constantly threatens the authority of the parents by the simple process of maturation. The son and daughter are to be given to marriage, usually arranged by parents. But now-a-days selection of a spouse by the adult himself is also not infrequent. The daughter, even after marriage keeps contact with the parents. The sons become junior friends of the father after marriage and they help their father in every aspect even though live separately. Relationship between a daughter-in-law and the parents-in-law is comparable to that between daughter and parents with a certain degree of reservation in frequent interaction, which again is more rigid with the father-in-law. In the old age, the parents are generally looked after by their sons and daughter-in-law.

With regard to the relationship among the siblings, it has been found to be very friendly and affectionate. The elder siblings are generally given some respect by the younger ones and they also claim certain degree of authority over the others. In the absence of parents, they look after younger ones in all spheres as demanded by the situation.

Finally, with regard to the relationship among the member in a joint family (though rare), it has been found that though there are occasions of minor outbursts, the relation between the various members is more or less cordial and happy. The head of the household, with the assistance of the contribution of other earning members, manages and controls the family. He is respected and obeyed by the junior members of the family.

Family Rituals

Among the Aos no any family level ritual is found except the rituals associated with the individual lifecycle. There are three rituals, associated with the individual lifecycle. These are birth, marriage and death rituals. Every family performs these rituals.

In the following pages an attempt has been made to provide an idea about these three rituals.

Birth Ritual

Among the people, the birth ritual is very simple. On the birth-day of the new born, the family members and attended persons pray to God for giving the baby and then all of them together have a feast with chicken or pig meat whatever available.

On the third day from birth of new born, they observe the naming ceremony (*tenung ajaba* in chongli and *tening chuba* in mongsen) of the new born. On that day, they invite their clan members from both father and mother sides. The eldest clan member generally takes the major role in this ceremony. Presence of Pastor of the Church on that day is also essential and therefore, they also invite the Pastor on that day and he offers a prayer of blessing in favour of the newly born child. The eldest persons give a few name and they call with these name to the baby. Out of these names they give that particular name which is seen to be accepted by the baby. If the newly born is girl, then they also pierce the ears on that day by an elderly man and give red thread to wear in the ear holes. This is known as *tenarong atuba* in chongli and *terarong tuba* in mongsen. After naming, ceremony, all the people invited are entertained with a feast. Depending on their economic condition they also invite the neighbouring people on that day. This naming ceremony is observed by the people for their every issue.

Marriage

As the people are Christian by religion, the most socially accepted marriage is the Christian marriage in the Church. According to their rules of marriage, no marriage can be possible within the same clan. Thus, marriage within the patriclan is prohibited. The Pastor conducts the marriage ceremony on that appointed day in the Church. At the end of the marriage solemnization in the Church, all the village people and invited guests come to the bridegroom's house to have the wedding feast.

Death

Under the Christian religion, the people of the villages have the custom of burying the dead bodies. There is a common burial ground in every village which is known in their dialect as *leptza* in mongsen and *leper* in chongli. When someone dies in a family, the Church authority is informed first and then the

Church bell is rung continuously. This bell is different from the usual bell of the Church and by hearing the sound of the bell all the villagers come to know that someone have died. Then all the villagers come to that particular house to mourn the death. The people pray for the departed soul and the clan members of the deceased person offer them tea, biscuits, betel-nut etc. with great affection and hospitality. On that day they also arrange a feast for all the people and each person is offered a packet (*chiten*) of few pieces of meat of pig/cow and rice.

In the meantime, the carpenter (of the village) takes the measurement of the dead body to make a coffin. Some villagers with the appropriate measurement goes to the burial ground and dig out the ground for the burial. After preparing the coffin it is carried to that house and dead body is put inside it. The Pastor chants some hymes and after that the dead body is carried to the burial ground, i.e. the funeral rites follow. If there is something to say about the deceased person, they complete it before the funeral rite start. If someone dies in the night, they do not go to the burial ground in night and wait for the morning. All the villagers abstain from doing any work on that day.

Educational Attainment

Education as a part of human life is as old as civilization and has become an important field of social research. Education makes a man social, aware of modern science and technology and enables him to apply the same in practice.

Education has been considered to be the most important instrument of change be it social, economic, political (Lynden and Khonglah, 2004).

According to Bairathi (1991), education is an important media for bringing about change in any society. By educating people, their economic and social development can be promoted and backward sections of the society can be brought close to advanced communities.

Education has been conceived as one of the most powerful instruments for socio-economic uplift and for bringing about socio-economic transformation on an egalitarian line (Sinha, 1996).

Thus, education has always been considered to be a very important dimension of any agenda for development programme in a society.

Educational attainment of the people by age and sex has been shown in Tables 4.9, 4.10, 4.11 and 4.12.

It will be seen from Table 4.9 that around 8.98 per cent (men 4.36%, women 4.62%) of the people is illiterate. This however includes the children (approximately 7.00%) who are too young to study. Among the literates, 2.22 per cent have read up to preprimary level, 11.81 per cent have read up to primary level. There are 68.92 per cent of the people who have read up to class X. The table further reveals that the majority section of the people (58%) with formal education belongs to the age between 5 years to 34 years. This is probably indicative of the fact that education is gaining momentum in the younger generation.

People with post-secondary level education though not many in number, the scenario in this regard is not very discouraging. There are 25 (2.14%) matriculates, 34 (2.91%) intermediates, 30 (2.56%) graduates and 5 (0.42%) post-graduates. It may however, be noted here that women, as compared to men are relatively less educated in the population.

With regard to the state of affairs in this regard in the three villages independently (Tables 4.10, 4.11 and 4.12), it will be seen that education has made a better inroad in the Lirmen village, at least numerically.

Clan

Clan is an exogamous group which comes next to the family. According to Lewis, "Membership in a clan depends on kinship

Table No.4.9 : Distribution of the population of the villages under study by age, sex and level of education

Sl. No.	Age Group (in years)	Illiterate			Literate											
					Pre-primary			Primary			Secondary			H.S.L.C.		
		Male (%)	Female (%)	Total (%)	Male (%)	Female (%)	Total (%)	Male (%)	Female (%)	Total (%)	Male (%)	Female (%)	Total (%)	Male (%)	Female (%)	Total (%)
1	2	3	4	5	6	7	8	9	10	11	12	13	14	15	16	17
1	0 – 4	36 (3.08)	38 (3.25)	74 (6.33)	3 (0.25)	5 (0.42)	8 (0.68)	0	0	0	0	0	0	0	0	0
2	5 – 9	4 (0.34)	3 (0.25)	7 (0.59)	9 (0.77)	9 (0.77)	18 (1.54)	34 (2.91)	29 (2.48)	63 (5.39)	0	0	0	0	0	0
3	10 – 14	1 (0.08)	0	1 (0.08)	0	0	0	19 (1.62)	16 (1.36)	35 (2.99)	32 (2.73)	37 (3.16)	69 (5.90)	0	0	0
4	15 – 19	0	0	0	0	0	0	0	5 (0.42)	5 (0.42)	61 (5.22)	61 (5.22)	122 (10.44)	1 (0.08)	1 (0.08)	2 (0.17)
5	20 – 24	0	0	0	0	0	0	4 (0.34)	4 (0.34)	8 (0.68)	55 (4.70)	51 (4.36)	106 (9.07)	6 (0.51)	2 (0.17)	8 (0.68)
6	25 – 29	0	2 (0.17)	2 (0.17)	0	0	0	1 (0.08)	1 (0.08)	2 (0.17)	64 (5.47)	38 (3.25)	102 (8.73)	1 (0.08)	1 (0.08)	2 (0.17)
7	30 – 34	1 (0.08)	0	1 (0.08)	0	0	0	0	0	0	41 (3.51)	35 (2.99)	76 (6.50)	1 (0.08)	3 (0.25)	4 (0.34)
8	35 – 39	0	1 (0.08)	1 (0.08)	0	0	0	0	2 (0.17)	2 (0.17)	26 (2.22)	21 (1.79)	47 (4.02)	4 (0.34)	3 (0.25)	7 (0.59)
9	40 – 44	2 (0.17)	1 (0.08)	3 (0.25)	0	0	0	1 (0.08)	3 (0.25)	4 (0.34)	24 (2.05)	31 (2.65)	55 (4.70)	0	1 (0.08)	1 (0.08)
10	45 – 49	0	2 (0.17)	2 (0.17)	0	0	0	0	0	0	33 (2.82)	24 (2.05)	57 (4.88)	0	0	0
11	50 – 54	2 (0.17)	0	2 (0.17)	0	0	0	2 (0.17)	3 (0.25)	5 (0.42)	21 (1.79)	29 (2.48)	50 (4.28)	0	0	0
12	55 – 59	0	1 (0.08)	1 (0.08)	0	0	0	0	2 (0.17)	2 (0.17)	22 (1.88)	20 (1.71)	42 (3.59)	1 (0.08)	0	1 (0.08)

(Contd...)

Table 4.9 *(Contd...)*

Sl. No.	Age Group (in years)	Illiterate			Literate											
					Pre-primary			Primary			Secondary			H.S.L.C.		
		Male (%)	Female (%)	Total (%)	Male (%)	Female (%)	Total (%)	Male (%)	Female (%)	Total (%)	Male (%)	Female (%)	Total (%)	Male (%)	Female (%)	Total (%)
1	2	3	4	5	6	7	8	9	10	11	12	13	14	15	16	17
13	60 – 64	0	1 (0.08)	1 (0.08)	0	0	0	2 (0.17)	4 (0.34)	6 (0.51)	22 (1.88)	10 (0.85)	32 (2.73)	0	0	0
14	65 – 69	0	0	0	0	0	0	0	1 (0.08)	1 (0.08)	7 (0.59)	7 (0.59)	14 (1.19)	0	0	0
15	70 – 74	0	2 (0.17)	2 (0.17)	0	0	0	2 (0.17)	1 (0.08)	3 (0.25)	15 (1.28)	8 (0.68)	23 (1.96)	0	0	0
16	75 – 79	0	1 (0.08)	1 (0.08)	0	0	0	0	0	0	3 (0.25)	3 (0.25)	6 (0.51)	0	0	0
17	80 – 84	4 (0.34)	2 (0.17)	6 (0.51)	0	0	0	0	1 (0.08)	1 (0.08)	4 (0.34)	0	4 (0.34)	0	0	0
18	85 – 89	1 (0.08)	0	1 (0.08)	0	0	0	1 (0.08)	0	1 (0.08)	0	0	0	0	0	0
Grand Total (%)		51 (4.36)	54 (4.62)	105 (8.98)	12 (1.02)	14 (1.19)	26 (2.22)	66 (5.65)	72 (6.16)	138 (11.81)	430 (36.81)	375 (32.10)	805 (68.92)	14 (1.19)	11 (0.94)	25 (2.14)

Table 4.9 *(Contd...)*

Sl. No.	Age Group (in years)	Literate											
		H.S.			Graduate			Post-Graduate			Total		
		Male (%)	Female (%)	Total (%)	Male (%)	Female (%)	Total (%)	Male (%)	Female (%)	Total (%)	Male (%)	Female (%)	Total (%)
1	2	18	19	20	21	22	23	24	25	26	27	28	29
1	0 – 4	0	0	0	0	0	0	0	0	0	3 (0.25)	5 (0.42)	8 (0.68
2	5 – 9	0	0	0	0	0	0	0	0	0	43 (3.68)	38 (3.25)	81 (6.93)
3	10 – 14	0	0	0	0	0	0	0	0	0	51 (4.36)	53 (4.53)	104 (8.90)
4	15 – 19	2 (0.17)	1 (0.08)	3 (0.25)	0	0	0	0	0 (5.47)	0 (5.82)	64 (11.30)	68	132
5	20 – 24	4 (0.34)	1 (0.08)	5 (0.42)	5 (0.42)	4 (0.34)	9 (0.77)	2 (0.17)	0	2 (0.17)	76 (6.50)	62 (5.30)	138 (11.81)
6	25 – 29	10 (0.85)	2 (0.17)	12 (1.02)	4 (0.34)	3 (0.25)	7 (0.59)	0	2 (0.17)	2 (0.17)	80 (6.84)	47 (4.02)	127 (10.87)
7	30 – 34	3 (0.25)	2 (0.17)	5 (0.42)	6 (0.51)	1 (0.08)	7 (0.59)	0	0	0	51 (4.36)	41 (3.51)	92 (7.87)
8	35 – 39	3 (0.25)	2 (0.17)	5 (0.42)	3 (0.25)	1 (0.08)	4 (0.34)	1 (0.08)	0	1 (0.08)	37 (3.16)	29 (2.48)	66 (5.65)
9	40 – 44	1 (0.08)	0	1 (0.08)	2 (0.17)	0	2 (0.17)	0	0	0	28 (2.39)	35 (2.99)	63 (5.39)
10	45 – 49	0	0	0	0	0	0	0	0	0	33 (2.85)	24 (2.05)	57 (4.88)
11	50 – 54	1 (0.08)	0	1 (0.08)	0	0	0	0	0	0	24 (2.05)	32 (2.73)	56 (4.97)
12	55 – 59	0	1 (0.08)	1 (0.08)	0	0	0	0	0	0	23 (1.96)	23 (1.96)	46 (3.93)

(Contd...)

Table 4.9 *(Contd...)*

Sl. No.	Age Group (in years)	Literate											
		H.S.			Graduate			Post-Graduate			Total		
		Male (%)	Female (%)	Total (%)	Male (%)	Female (%)	Total (%)	Male (%)	Female (%)	Total (%)	Male (%)	Female (%)	Total (%)
1	2	18	19	20	21	22	23	24	25	26	27	28	29
13	60 – 64	0	0	0	1 (0.08)	0	1 (0.08)	0	0	0	25 (2.14)	14 (1.19)	39 (3.33)
14	65 – 69	0	0	0	0	0	0	0	0	0	7 (0.59)	8 (0.68)	15 (1.28)
15	70 – 74	1	0	1	0	0	0	0	0	0	18 (1.54)	9 (0.77)	27 (2.31)
16	75 – 79	0	0	0	0	0	0	0	0	0	3 (0.25)	3 (0.25)	6 (0.51)
17	80 – 84	0	0	0	0	0	0	0	0	0	4 (0.34)	1 (0.08)	5 (().42)
18	85 – 89	0	0	0	0	0	0	0	0	0	1 (0.08)	0	1 (0.08)
Grand total (%)		25 (2.14)	9 (0.77)	34 (2.91)	21 (1.79)	9 (0.77)	30 (2.56)	13 (0.25)	2 (0.17)	5 (0.42)	571 (48.8)	492 (42.12)	1063 (91.01)

Table 4.10 : Distribution of the population of the village Lirmen by age, sex and level of education

Sl. No.	Age Group (in years)	Illiterate			Literate											
					Pre-primary			Primary			Secondary			H.S.L.C.		
		Male (%)	Female (%)	Total (%)	Male (%)	Female (%)	Total (%)	Male (%)	Female (%)	Total (%)	Male (%)	Female (%)	Total (%)	Male (%)	Female (%)	Total (%)
1	2	3	4	5	6	7	8	9	10	11	12	13	14	15	16	17
1	0 – 4	8 (1.28)	12 (1.92)	20 (3.20)	3 (0.48)	5 (0.80)	8 (1.28)	0	0	0	0	0	0	0	0	0
2	5 – 9	0	0	0	3 (0.48)	2 (0.32)	5 (0.80)	16 (2.56)	13 (2.08)	29 (4.64)	0	0	0	0	0	0
3	10 – 14	0	0	0	0	0	0	4 (0.64)	3 (0.48)	7 (1.12)	20 (3.20)	21 (3.36)	41 (6.57)	0	0	0
4	15 – 19	0	0	0	0	0	0	0	0	0	37 (5.92)	38 (6.02)	75 (12.01)	1 (0.16)	1 (0.16)	2 (0.32)
5	20 – 24	0	0	0	0	0	0	1 (0.16)	1 (0.16)	2 (0.32)	32 (5.12)	30 (4.80)	62 (9.93)	6 (0.96)	2 (0.32)	8 (1.28)
6	25 – 29	0	0	0	0	0	0	0	0	0	36 (5.76)	19 (3.04)	55 (8.81)	1 (0.16)	1 (0.16)	2 (0.32)
7	30 – 34	0	0	0	0	0	0	0	0	0	24 (3.84)	22 (3.52)	46 (7.37)	1 (0.16)	3 (0.48)	4 (0.64)
8	35 – 39	0	1 (0.16)	1 (0.16)	0	0	0	0	1 (0.16)	1 (0.16)	13 (2.08)	8 (1.28)	21 (3.36)	4 (0.64)	3 (0.48)	7 (1.12)
9	40 – 44	1 (0.16)	0	1 (0.16)	0	0	0	0	2 (0.32)	2 (0.32)	14 (2.24)	19 (3.04)	33 (5.28)	0	1 (0.16)	1 (0.16)
10	45 – 49	0	0	0	0	0	0	0	0	0	16 (2.56)	10 (1.60)	26 (4.16)	0	0	
11	50 – 54	0	0	0	0	0	0	1 (0.16)	3 (0.48)	4 (0.64)	14 (2.24)	21 (3.36)	35 (5.60)	0	0	0
12	55 – 59	0	0	0	0	0	0	0	0	0	12 (1.92)	14 (2.24)	26 (4.16)	1 (0.16)	0	1 (0.16)

(Contd...)

Table 4.10 *(Contd...)*

Sl. No.	Age Group (in years)	Illiterate			Literate											
					Pre-primary			Primary			Secondary			H.S.L.C.		
		Male (%)	Female (%)	Total (%)	Male (%)	Female (%)	Total (%)	Male (%)	Female (%)	Total (%)	Male (%)	Female (%)	Total (%)	Male (%)	Female (%)	Total (%)
1	2	3	4	5	6	7	8	9	10	11	12	13	14	15	16	17
13	60 – 64	0	0	0	0	0	0	2 (0.32)	4 (0.64)	6 (0.96)	14 (2.24)	7 (1.12)	21 (3.36)	0	0	0
14	65 – 69	0	0	0	0	0	0	0	0	0	3 (0.48)	6 (0.96)	9 (1.44)	0	0	0
15	70 – 74	0	0	0	0	0	0	1 (0.16)	1 (0.16)	2 (0.32)	11 (1.76)	3 (0.48)	14 (2.24)	0	0	0
16	75 – 79	0	0	0	0	0	0	0	0	0	2 (0.32)	2 (0.32)	4 (0.64)	0	0	0
17	80 – 84	0	0	0	0	0	0	0	1 (0.16)	1 (0.16)	2 (0.32)	0	2 (0.32)	0	0	0
18	85 – 89	0	0	0	0	0	0	1 (0.16)	0	1 (0.16)	0	0	0	0	0	0
Grand total (%)		9 (1.44)	13 (2.08)	22 (3.52)	6 (0.96)	7 (1.12)	13 (2.08)	26 (4.16)	29 (4.64)	55 (8.81)	250 (40.06)	220 (35.25)	470 (75.32)	14 (2.24)	11 (1.76)	25 (5.00)

(Contd...)

Table 4.10 (Contd...)

Sl. No.	Age Group (in years)	Literate											
		H.S.			Graduate			Post-Graduate			Total		
		Male (%)	Female (%)	Total (%)	Male (%)	Female (%)	Total (%)	Male (%)	Female (%)	Total (%)	Male (%)	Female (%)	Total (%)
		18	19	20	21	22	23	24	25	26	27	28	29
1	0 – 4	0	0	0	0	0	0	0	0	0	3 (0.48)	5 (0.80)	8 (1.28)
2	5 – 9	0	0	0	0	0	0	0	0	0	19 (3.04)	15 (2.40)	34 (5.24)
3	10 – 14	0	0	0	0	0	0	0	0	0	24 (3.84)	24 (3.84)	48 (7.69)
4	15 – 19	2 (0.32)	1 (0.32)	3 (0.16)	0 (0.48)	0	0	0	0	0	40 (6.41)	40 (6.41)	80 (12.82)
5	20 – 24	3 (1.28)	1 (0.48)	4 (0.16)	3 (0.64)	2 (0.48)	5 (0.32)	0 (0.80)	0	0	45 (7.21)	36 (5.76)	81 (12.98)
6	25 – 29	6 (0.96)	1 (0.16)	7 (1.12)	0	0	0	0	1 (0.16)	1 (0.06)	43 (6.89)	22 (3.52)	65 (10.41)
7	30 – 34	3 (0.48)	2 (0.32)	5 (0.80)	2 (0.32)	1 (0.16)	3 (0.48)	0	0	0	30 (4.80)	28 (4.48)	58 (9.29)
8	35 – 39	2 (0.32)	1 (0.16)	3 (0.48)	1 (0.16)	1 (0.16)	2 (0.32)	1 (0.16)	0	1 (0.16)	21 (3.36)	14 (2.24)	35 (5.60)
9	40 – 44	1 (0.16)	0	1 (0.16)	2 (0.32)	0	2 (0.32)	0	0	0	17 (2.72)	22 (3.52)	39 (6.25)
10	45 – 49	0	0	0	0	0	0	0	0	0	16 (2.56)	10 (1.60)	26 (4.16)
11	50 – 54	1 (0.16)	0	1 (0.16)	0	0	0	0	0	0	16 (2.56)	24 (3.84)	40 (6.41)
12	55 – 59	0	0	0	0	0	0	0	0	0	13 (2.08)	14 (2.24)	27 (4.32)

(Contd...)

Table 4.10 *(Contd...)*

Sl. No.	Age Group (in years)	Literate											
		H.S.			Graduate			Post-Graduate			Total		
		Male (%)	Female (%)	Total (%)	Male (%)	Female (%)	Total (%)	Male (%)	Female (%)	Total (%)	Male (%)	Female (%)	Total (%)
		18	19	20	21	22	23	24	25	26	27	28	29
13	60 – 64	0	0	0	1	0	1	0	0	0	17 (2.72)	11 (1.76)	28 (4.48)
14	65 – 69	0	0	0	0	0	0	0	0	0	3 (0.48)	6 (0.96)	9 (1.44)
15	70 – 74	0	0	0	0	0	0	0	0	0	12 (1.92)	4 (0.64)	16 (2.56)
16	75 – 79	0	0	0	0	0	0	0	0	0	2 (0.32)	2 (0.32)	4 (0.64)
17	80 – 84	0	0	0	0	0	0	0	0	0	2 (0.32)	1 (0.16)	3 (0.48)
18	85 – 89	0	0	0	0	0	0	0	0	0	1 (0.16)	0	1 (0.16)
	Grand total (%)	18 (2.88)	6 (0.96)	24 (3.84)	9 (1.44)	4 (0.64)	13 (2.08)	1 (0.16	1 (0.16)	2 (0.32)	324 (51.92)	278 (44.55)	602 (96.47))

Table 4. 11 : Distribution of the population of the village Yajang-A by age, sex and level of education

Sl. No.	Age Group (in years)	Illiterate			Literate											
					Pre-primary			Primary			Secondary			H.S.L.C.		
		Male (%)	Female (%)	Total (%)	Male (%)	Female (%)	Total (%)	Male (%)	Female (%)	Total (%)	Male (%)	Female (%)	Total (%)	Male (%)	Female (%)	Total (%)
1	2	3	4	5	6	7	8	9	10	11	12	13	14	15	16	17
1	0 – 4	18 (4.34)	18 (4.34)	36 (8.96)	0	0	0	0	0	0	0	0	0	0	0	0
2	5 – 9	0	0	0	5 (1.20)	5 (1.20)	10 (2.40)	14 (3.38)	15 (3.62)	29 (7.00)	0	0	0	0	0	0
3	10 – 14	0	0	0	0	0	0	12 (2.89)	9 (2.17)	21 (5.07)	8 (1.93)	13 (3.14)	21 (5.07)	0	0	0
4	15 – 19	0	0	0	0	0	0	0	1 (0.24)	1 (0.24)	20 (4.83)	19 (4.58)	39 (9.42)	0	0	0
5	20 – 24	0	0	0	0	0	0	3 (0.72)	2 (0.48)	5 (1.20)	20 (4.83)	19 (4.58)	39 (9.42)	0	0	0
6	25 – 29	0	1 (0.24)	1 (0.24)	0	0	0	0	1 (0.24)	1 (0.24)	24 (5.79)	12 (2.89)	36 (8.69)	0	0	0
7	30 – 34	0	0	0	0	0	0	0	0	0	13 (3.14)	11 (2.65)	24 (5.79)	0	0	0
8	35 – 39	0	1 (0.24)	1 (0.24)	0	0	0	0	0	0	9 (2.17)	10 (2.41)	19 (4.58)	0	0	0
9	40 – 44	0	0	0	0	0	0	0	1 (0.24)	1 (0.24)	7 (1.69)	10 (2.41)	17 (4.10)	0	0	0
10	45 – 49	0	0	0	0	0	0	0	0	0	14 (3.38)	13 (3.14)	27 (6.52)	0	0	0
11	50 – 54	1 (0.24))	0	1 (0.24)	0	0	0	0	0	0	7 (1.69)	7 (1.69)	14 (3.38)	0	0	0
12	55 – 59	0	1 (0.24)	1 (0.24)	0	0	0	0	2 (0.48)	2 (0.48)	9 (2.17)	5 (1.20)	14 (3.38)	0	0	0

(Contd...)

Table 4.11 *(Contd...)*

Sl. No.	Age Group (in years)	Illiterate			Literate											
					Pre-primary			Primary			Secondary			H.S.L.C.		
		Male (%)	Female (%)	Total (%)	Male (%)	Female (%)	Total (%)	Male (%)	Female (%)	Total (%)	Male (%)	Female (%)	Total (%)	Male (%)	Female (%)	Total (%)
1	2	3	4	5	6	7	8	9	10	11	12	13	14	15	16	17
13	60 – 64	0	0	0	0	0	0	0	0	0	7 (1.69)	2 (0.48)	9 (2.17)	0	0	0
14	65 – 69	0	0	0	0	0	0	0	0	0	4 (0.96)	1 (0.24)	5 (1.20)	0	0	0
15	70 – 74	0	2 (0.48)	2 (0.48)	0	0	0	0	0	0	3 (0.72)	3 (0.72)	6 (1.44)	0	0	0
16	75 – 79	0	1 (0.24)	1 (0.24)	0	0	0	0	0	0	1 (0.24)	1 (0.24)	2 (0.48)	0	0	0
17	80 – 84	2 (0.48)	0	2 (0.48)	0	0	0	0	0	0	0	0	0	0	0	0
18	85 – 89	0	0	0	0	0	0	0	0	0	0	0	0	0	0	0
Grand Total		21 (5.07)	24 (5.79)	45 (10.86)	5 (1.20)	5 (1.20)	10 (2.41)	29 (7.00)	31 (7.48)	60 (14.49)	146 (35.26)	126 (30.43)	272 (65.70)	0	0	0

(Contd...)

Table 4.11(Contd...)

Sl. No.	Age Group (in years)	Literate											
		H.S.			Graduate			Post-Graduate			Total		
		Male (%)	Female (%)	Total (%)	Male (%)	Female (%)	Total (%)	Male (%)	Female (%)	Total (%)	Male (%)	Female (%)	Total (%)
		18	19	20	21	22	23	24	25	26	27	28	29
1	0 – 4	0	0	0	0	0	0	0	0	0	0	0	0
2	5 – 9	0	0	0	0	0	0	0	0	0	19 (4.58)	20 (4.83)	39 (9.42)
3	10 – 14	0	0	0	0	0	0	0	0	0	20 (4.83)	22 (5.31)	42 (10.14)
4	15 – 19	0	0	0	0	0	0	0	0	0	20 (4.83)	20 (4.83)	40 (9.66)
5	20 – 24	1 (0.24)	0	1 (0.24)	2 (0.48)	2 (0.48)	4 (0.96)	2 (0.48)	0	2 (0.48)	28 (6.76)	23 (5.55)	51 (12.31)
6	25 – 29	4 (0.96)	1 (0.24)	5 (1.20)	3 (0.72)	3 (0.72)	6 (1.44)	0	0	0	31 (7.48)	17 (4.10)	48 (11.59)
7	30 – 34	0	0	0	4 (0.96)	0	4 (0.96)	0	0	0	17 (4.10)	11 (2.65)	28 (6.76)
8	35 – 39	1 (0.24)	1 (0.24)	2 (0.48)	1 (0.24)	0	1 (0.24)	0	0	0	11 (2.65)	11 (2.65)	22 (5.31)
9	40 – 44	0	0	0	0	0	0	0	0	0	7 (1.69)	11 (2.65)	18 (4.34)
10	45 – 49	0	0	0	0	0	0	0	0	0	14 (3.38)	13 (3.14)	27 (6.25)
11	50 – 54	0	0	0	0	0	0	0	0	0	7 (1.69)	7 (1.69)	14 (3.38)
12	55 – 59	1 (0.24)	1 (0.24)	0	0	0	0	0	0	0	9 (2.17)	8 (1.93)	17 (4.10)

(Contd...)

Table 4.11(Contd...)

Sl. No.	Age Group (in years)	Literate											
		H.S.			Graduate			Post-Graduate			Total		
		Male (%)	Female (%)	Total (%)	Male (%)	Female (%)	Total (%)	Male (%)	Female (%)	Total (%)	Male (%)	Female (%)	Total (%)
		18	19	20	21	22	23	24	25	26	27	28	29
13	60 – 64	0	0	0	0	0	0	0	0	0	7 (1.69)	2 (0.48)	9 (2.17)
14	65 – 69	0	0	0	0	0	0	0	0	0	4 (0.96)	1 (0.24)	5 (1.20)
15	70 – 74	1 (0.24)	0	1 (0.24)	0	0	0	0	0	0	4 (0.96)	3 (0.72)	7 (1.69)
16	75 – 79	0	0	0	0	0	0	0	0	0	1 (0.24)	1 (0.24)	2 (0.48)
17	80 – 84	0	0	0	0	0	0	0	0	0	0	0	0
18	85 – 89	0	0	0	0	0	0	0	0	0	0	0	0
	Grand Total (%)	7 (1.69)	3 (0.72)	10 (2.41)	10 (2.41)	5 (1.20)	15 (3.62)	2 (0.48)	0	2 (0.48)	199 (48.06)	170 (41.06)	369 (89.13)

Table 4.12 : Distribution of the population of the village-Yajang-B by age, sex and level of education

Sl. No.	Age Group	Illiterate			Literate											
					Pre-primary			Primary			Secondary			H.S.L.C.		
	(in years)	Male (%)	Female (%)	Total (%)	Male (%)	Female (%)	Total (%)	Male (%)	Female (%)	Total (%)	Male (%)	Female (%)	Total (%)	Male (%)	Female (%)	Total (%)
1	2	3	4	5	6	7	8	9	10	11	12	13	14	15	16	17
1	0 – 4	10 (7.69)	8 (6.15)	18 (13.84)	0	0	0	0	0	0	0	0	0	0	0	0
2	5 – 9	4 (3.07)	3 (2.30)	7 (5.38)	1 (0.76)	2 (1.53)	3 (2.30)	4 (3.07)	1 (0.76)	5 (3.84)	0	0	0	0	0	0
3	10 – 14	1 (0.76)	0	1 (0.76)	0	0	0	3 (2.30)	4 (3.07) (5.38)	7 (5.38) (5.38)	4 (3.07) (10.76)	3 (2.30)	7 (5.38)	0	0	0
4	15 – 19	0	0	0	0	0	0	0	4 (3.07)	4 (3.07)	4 (3.07)	4 (3.07)	8 (6.15)	0	0	0
5	20 – 24	0	0	0	0	0	0	0	1 (0.76)	1 (0.76)	3 (2.30)	2 (1.53)	5 (3.84)	0	0	0
6	25 – 29	0	1 (0.76)	1 (0.76)	0	0	0	1 (0.76)	0	1 (0.76)	4 (3.07)	7 (5.38)	11 (8.46)	0	0	0
7	30 – 34	1 (0.76)	0	1 (0.76)	0	0	0	0	0	0	4 (3.07)	2 (1.53)	6 (4.61)	0	0	0
8	35 – 39	0	0	0	0	0	0	0	1 (0.76)	1 (0.76)	4 (3.07)	3 (2.30)	7 (5.38)	0	0	0
9	40 – 44	1 (0.76)	0	1 (0.76)	0	0	0	1 (0.76)	0	1 (0.76)	3 (2.30)	2 (1.53)	5 (3.84)	0	0	0
10	45 – 49	0	2 (1.53)	2 (1.53)	0	0	0	0	0	0	3 (2.30)	1 (0.76)	4 (3.07)	0	0	0
11	50 – 54	1 (0.76)	0	1 (0.76)	0	0	0	1 (0.76)	0	1 (0.76)	0	1 (0.76)	1 (0.76)	0	0	0
12	55 – 59	0	0	0	0	0	0	0	0	0	1 (0.76)	1 (0.76)	2 (1.53)	0	0	0

(Contd.)

Table 4.12 : *(Contd...)*

Sl. No.	Age Group (in years)	Illiterate			Literate											
					Pre-primary			Primary			Secondary			H.S.L.C.		
		Male (%)	Female (%)	Total (%)	Male (%)	Female (%)	Total (%)	Male (%)	Female (%)	Total (%)	Male (%)	Female (%)	Total (%)	Male (%)	Female (%)	Total (%)
1	2	3	4	5	6	7	8	9	10	11	12	13	14	15	16	17
13	60 – 64	0	1 (0.76)	1 (0.76)	0	0	0	0	0	0	1 (0.76)	1 (0.76)	2 (1.53)	0	0	0
14	65 – 69	0	0	0	0	0	0	0	0	1 (0.76)	1 (0.76)	0	0	0	0	0
15	70 – 74	0	1 (0.76)	1 (0.76)	0	0	0	1 (0.76)	0	1 (0.76)	1 (0.76)	2 (1.53)	3 (2.30)	0	0	0
16	75 – 79	0	0	0	0	0	0	0	0	0	0	0	0	0	0	0
17	80 – 84	2 (1.53)	1 (0.76)	3 (2.30)	0	0	0	0	0	0	2 (1.53)	0	2 (1.53)	0	0	0
18	85 – 89	1	0	1	0	0	0	0	0	0	0	0	0	0	0	0
Grand total (%)		21 (16.15)	17 (13.07)	38 (29.23)	1 (0.76)	2 (1.53)	3 (2.30)	11 (8.46)	12 (9.23)	23 (17.69)	34 (26.15)	29 (22.30)	63 (48.46)	0	0	0

Table 4.12(Contd...)

Sl. No.	Age Group (in years)	Literate											
		H.S.			Graduate			Post-Graduate			Total		
		Male (%)	Female (%)	Total (%)	Male (%)	Female (%)	Total (%)	Male (%)	Female (%)	Total (%)	Male (%)	Female (%)	Total (%)
1	2	18	19	20	21	22	23	24	25	26	27	28	29
1	0 – 4	0	0	0	0	0	0	0	0	0	0	0	0
2	5 – 9	0	0	0	0	0	0	0	0	0	5 (3.84)	3 (2.30)	8 (6.15)
3	10 – 14	0	0	0	0	0	0	0	0	0	7 (5.38)	7 (5.38)	14 (10.76)
4	15 – 19	0	0	0	0	0	0	0	0	0	4 (3.07)	8 (6.15)	12 (9.23)
5	20 – 24	0	0	0	0	0	0	0	0	0	3 (2.30)	3 (2.30)	6 (4.61)
6	25 – 29	0	0	0	1 (0.76)	0	1 (0.76)	0	1 (0.76)	1 (0.76)	6 (4.61)	8 (6.15)	14 (10.76)
7	30 – 34	0	0	0	0	0	0	0	0	0	4 (3.07)	2 (1.53)	6 (4.61)
8	35 – 39	0	0	0	1 (0.76)	0	1 (0.76)	0	0	0	5 (3.84)	4 (3.07)	9 (6.92)
9	40 – 44	0	0	0	0	0	0	0	0	0	4 (3.07)	2 (1.53)	6 (4.61)
10	45 – 49	0	0	0	0	0	0	0	0	0	3 (2.30)	1 (0.76)	4 (3.07)
11	50 – 54	0	0	0	0	0	0	0	0	0	1 (0.76)	1 (0.76)	2 (1.53)
12	55 – 59	0	0	0	0	0	0	0	0	0	1 (0.76)	1 (0.76)	2 (1.53)

(Contd...)

Table 4.12(Contd...)

Sl. No.	Age Group (in years)	Literate											
		H.S.			Graduate			Post-Graduate			Total		
		Male (%)	Female (%)	Total (%)	Male (%)	Female (%)	Total (%)	Male (%)	Female (%)	Total (%)	Male (%)	Female (%)	Total (%)
	2	18	19	20	21	22	23	24	25	26	27	28	29
13	60 – 64	0	0	0	0	0	0	0	0	0	1 (0.76)	1 (0.76)	2 (1.53)
14	65 – 69	0	0	0	0	0	0	0	0	0	0	1 (0.76)	1 (0.76)
15	70 – 74	0	0	0	0	0	0	0		0	2 (1.53)	2 (1.53)	4 (3.07)
16	75 – 79	0	0	0	0	0	0	0	0	0	0	0	0
17	80 – 84	0	0	0	0	0	0	0	0	0	2 (1.53)	0	2 (1.53)
18	85 – 89	0	0	0	0	0	0	0	0	0	0	0	0
	Grand total (%)	0	0	0	2 (1.53)	0	2 (1.53)	0	1 (0.76)	1 (0.76)	48 (36.92)	44 (33.84)	92 (70.76)

through one parent. It is often exogamous. It provides mutual security, government, marriage regulations, religion and ceremonies, property regulations and social control. Some authorities require not only a rule of descent but also a definite place of residence or locality and social integration" (cited in Doshi and Jain, 2001).

Clan can be defined as an exogamous division of a tribe, the members of which are held to be related to one another by some common ties, may be belief in descent from common ancestors, possession of a common totem or habitation of a common territory (Vidyarthi and Rai, 1976).

According to Encyclopaedia of Anthropology (1776), a clan is a kinship group whose members trace their descent from a common ancestor.

Webster defines clan as 'A social group comprising a number of households the heads of which claim descent from a common ancestor......' (cited in Murdock, 1965).

The grouping of clan is well defined in Ao society though they are complicated in nature. Clan system is the fundamental social fabric of the Nagas. Every aspect of their custom and culture is normally based on it. On the other hand, distribution of clan is the centre of their unity and division too.

Clan among the Aos is known as *kidong*. As they follow the patriarchal system, the names and title of their children are drawn from father's line. Even after the marriage, the title of the wife does not change as in case of other society. Clan hold is the basic unit of their social organisation like many other tribal populations. Marriage within the same clan is highly restricted. When it takes place incidentally, they are punished according to their customary laws, which is very severe in nature. Thus, clans among the Aos are exogamous and patrilineal.

As noted earlier, Aos are divided into three linguistic groups, namely Chungli, Mongsen and Chungki group and the distribution of clans and names is not uniform in these three groups. The distribution of clans may differ from chungli and mongsen system and also from the chungki system. It may also differ from village to village or range to range.

Mills (1926), while discussing about the clan system of Ao Nagas categorized as follows :

Chongli Clans

The principal chongli clans are given below grouped under their phratries.

Phongen Phratry

Pongenr, Yimsungr, Aotung, Wozukamr, Lungkungr, Tsitir, Charir, Chongli Aiyir, Yongpur, Hobir.

Longkam Phratry

Lungkamr, Azupongr, Makampongr, Mangkotsungmen, Mozur, Shomisensenzyar, Saiyichang, Ratuchang, Shompuchang, Lamtur, Azukamr.

Chami Phratry

Chamir, Chamitsur or Tsuwar, Chamichang, Mongkamchang, Tamachang, Mutsubu, Sampur, Longrur, Tutangunshi, Amang, Merang, lamtu-ungr, Yatenr, Chichir or Michipar, Chaochir, Chisar.

Mongsen Clans

First Phratry

Aiyir, Tsungsotang Aiyir, Yimchenchar, Alapachar, Achamr, Yungpur, Mongsen Tsitir, Walingr, Longtangr, Lungramr, Atsungchangr.

Second Phratry

Mutir, Mongsentsungr, Mongsen Lamtur, Mongsen Sampur, Longchuchar, Sanglichar or Molungr, Kabzar.

Third Phratry

Ochichar, Longwar, Nungsachar, Kichuchar, Asumpachar, Lungtsuchar, Ningsangchar, Anichar.

Changki Clans

In Chanki group there appears to be no division into phratries at all.

Lungchari, Ungtsiri, Metamsungba, Losanglari, Amri, Changkiri, Alingri, Metsiri.

During the present investigation, the people have been found to be distributed in a total of 10 clans (Table 4.13). It will be seen from Table 4.13 that majority of the people (305; 26.11) belong to the *Longkumer* clan. It is followed by *Aier* (243;20.80), *Longchar* (224;19.17), *Jamir* (176;15.06), *Lamtor* (75;6.42), *Imchen* (69;5.90), *Walling* (51;4.36), *Pongen* (10;0.85), *Ozukum* (10;0.85) and *Tsudir* clan (5;0.42).

Considering the villages under study independently, it has been observed from Tables 4.14, 4.15 and 4.16 that there are 8 clans in the village Lirmen. Majority of the people (224; 35.89) belong to *Longchar* clan. It is followed by *Longkomer* (213; 34.13), *Imchen* (68; 10.89), *Walling* (51; 8.17), *Jamir* (30; 4.80), *Aier* (29; 4.64), *Lamtor* (4; 0.64) clan.

In the village Yajang-A there are 6 clans and majority of the people (180; 43.47) belong to *Aier* clan. It is follwed by *Jamir* (96; 23.18), *Longkomer* (71; 17.14), *Lumtor* (58; 14.00), *Ozukum* (8; 1.93), *Imchen* (1; 0.24) clan. Similarly in the village Yajang-B there are 6 clans and majority of the people (50; 38.46) belong to *Jamir* clan. It is followed by

Aier (34; 26.15), *Longkomer* (21; 16.15), *Lumtor* (13; 10.00), *Pongen* (10; 7.69), *Ozukum* (2; 1.53) clan.

Table 4.13 : Distribution of the population of the villages under study by sex and clan affiliation

Sl. No.	*Name of the clan*	*Number of individuals*		
		Male (%)	*Female (%)*	*Total (%)*
1	*2*	*3*	*4*	*5*
1	Jamir	92 (7.87)	84 (7.19)	176 (15.26)
2	Aier	130 (11.13)	113 (9.67)	243 (20.87)
3	Longkomer	168 (14.38)	137 (11.72)	305 (26.11)
4	Longchar	129 (11.04)	95 (8.13)	224 (19.17)
5	Lemtor	36 (3.08)	39 (3.33)	75 (6.42)
6	Imchen	29 (2.48)	40 (3.42)	69 (5.90)
7	Walling	27 (2.31)	24(2.05)	51 (4.36)
8	Tsudir	3 (0.25)	2 (0.17)	5 (0.42)
9	Pongen	5 (0.42)	5 (0.42)	10 (0.85)
10	Ozukum	3 (0.25)	7 (0.59)	10 (0.85)
Grand total		622 (53.25)	546 (46.74)	1168 (100.00)

Table 4.14 : Distribution of the population of the village Lirmen by sex and clan affiliation

Sl. No.	*Name of the clan*	*Number of individuals*		
		Male (%)	*Female (%)*	*Total (%)*
1	*2*	*3*	*4*	*5*
1	Jamir	16 (2.56)	14 (2.24)	30 (4.80)
2	Aier	11 (1.76)	18 (2.88)	29 (4.64)
3	Longkomer	117 (18.75)	96 (15.38)	213 (34.13)
4	Longchar	129 (20.67)	95 (15.22)	224 (35.89)
5	Lemtor	2 (0.32)	2 (0.32)	4 (0.64)
6	Imchen	28 (4.48)	40 (6.41)	68 (10.89)
7	Walling	27 (4.32)	24 (3.84)	51 (8.17)
8	Tsudir	3 (0.25)	2 (0.17)	5 (0.42)
	Grand total	333 (53.36)	291 (46.63)	624 (100.00)

Table 4.15 : Distribution of the population of the village Yajang-A by sex and clan affiliation

Sl. No.	Name of the clan	Number of individuals		
		Male (%)	Female (%)	Total (%)
1	2	3	4	5
1	Jamir	44 (10.62)	52 (12.56)	96 (23.18)
2	Aier	105 (25.36)	75 (18.11)	180 (43.47)
3	Longkomer	41 (9.90)	30 (7.24)	71 (17.14)
4	Lemtor	26 (6.28)	32 (7.72)	58 (14.00)
5	Imchen	1 (0.24)	0	1 (0.24)
6	Ozukam	3 (0.72)	5 (1.20)	8 (1.93)
Grand total		220 (53.14)	194 (46.85)	414 (100.00)

Table 4.16 : Distribution of the population of the village Yajang-B by sex and clan affiliation

Sl. No.	Name of the clan	Number of individuals		
		Male (%)	Female (%)	Total (%)
1	2	3	4	5
1	Jamir	32 (24.61)	18 (13.84)	50 (38.46)
2	Aier	14 (10.76)	20 (15.38)	34 (26.15)
3	Longkomer	10 (7.69)	11 (8.46)	21 (16.15)
4	Pongen	5 (3.84)	5 (3.84)	10 (7.69)
5	Lemtor	8 (6.15)	15 (3.84)	13 (10.00)
6	Ozukam	0	2 (1.53)	2(1.53)
	Grand total	69 (53.07)	61 (46.92)	130 (100.00)

Marriage (As an institution)

Marriage is generally used as a term for a social institution. The institution of marriage, quite like that of the family, is universal. There cannot be a family without marriage. As such it may be defined as a relation of one or more men to one or more women which is recognised by custom or law and involves certain rights and duties both in case of the parties entering the union and in the case of the children born of it (Westermarck,1926).

According to Encyclopaedia of Social Sciences (1932), marriage denotes those unequivocally sanctioned unions which persist beyond sensual satisfaction and thus come to underlie family life.

According to Wells (1970), "Marriage is an institution: a pattern of rules and customs in respect of some objective or (objectives). It may be defined as the pattern of recognized usages governing establishment and continuance of family group."

Marriage is thus a legally and socially sanctioned union between one or more husbands and one or more wives that accords status to their offspring and is regulated by laws, rules, customs, beliefs and attitudes that prescribe the rights and duties of the partners. As an institution it creates a number of well known roles: husband, wife, father, child, grandfather, mother-in-law, which in most societies have more or less clear patterns of expectations attached to them.

The marriage ceremonies differ from tribe to tribe among the tribal population. In every society, marriage is well defined according to their culture, religion, custom and tradition. There is no written literature on Ao marriage system but they follow a well established practice. Marriage practice is guided by unwritten customary laws. They have been following this from generation to generation. As noted earlier, Aos are divided into three distinct linguistic groups, namely Chungli, Mongsen and Chungki group. However, the dialect though they speak is not the barrier that may prohibit the rules of marriage between them. Marriage among the Aos is known as *kiyimba*, without which a man or woman is considered as an incomplete person. Among the Ao, the system of marriage is more or less a social contract. They consider the tie of marriage as permanent until or unless it is dissolved by divorce or by demise.

The Ao people generally follow some rules of marriage and during the present investigation it has been observed that all the people are familiar with these rules of marriage and they strictly follow these rules as they are under their customary law. These rules of marriage are:

Marriage within the same clan is strictly prohibited. They cannot marry a girl from their own clan. In this regard Jamir and Lanunungsung (2005), while discussing about the Ao Naga marriage system gave the following chart (Fig.4.1) of grouping of clan under which marriage is permissible.

Marriageable (Group A – Group C)

Marriageable (Group A – Group B) | Marriageable (Group B – Group C)

Group(A) (Tongpok)	Group (B) (Longpok)	Group (C) (Longjakrep)
Aier	Azuponger	Anetdong
Imchen	Lemtur	Jamijang/Tamaipong
Imsong	Longchar	Jamitzuti
Lisen	Longkumer	Kichuchar
Ozukum	(Mozur/Motir/Meyur/	Ladongchir
Pongen	Soya/Wozunba)	Longri
Tzuti	Mekumpong	Metsubu
Yimvu etc.	Nokdir	Mongka
	Ratujang	Mongkum
	Sayir	Nungdunger
	Shimpojang	Ongshi
	Tanujang	Salong
	Walling etc.	Sempu
		Tzuwar
		Yaden etc.

Fig.4.1 : Grouping of Marriageable Clans: A Model

Source: Jamir and Lanununsang (2005).

As demonstrated above, marriage within the same clan is highly restricted. It means to say that group (A) can marry only with anyone of from group (B) and (C) list but not from the same clan group and *vice versa* as shown in the chart. However, there may be certain variation in different villages.

According to their customs and traditions, monogamy is the only accepted norm recognized by the society. No person, whether rich or poor can violate this rule. A married person may marry another woman if he so desires, but it can be possible only after divorcing the first wife, because the woman whom he married is his legal wife in the eyes of the society and they are regarded as having one soul until divorce or death separates them.

Joint family system is not found in Ao society as after the marriage, the newly married couple lives separately in a new house constructed by the husband.

Ao society is patrilineal in nature and as a result the names and title of their children are drawn from the father's line. Even after the marriage, the title of the wife does not change as in case of other society. In their society, using of the surname of her husband is restricted.

Tribal endogamy marriage has become a normal practice among them.

The system of dowry is not prevalent among the Aos. However, the presentation of gift on the day of wedding is a common practice either in cash or kind.

In their society, they prescribe the rule of marriage both for widows, widowers as also for divorcees. Generally, a widow may remarry after one year of her husband's death but a divorcee may remarry soon after the divorce is granted.

The people under investigations generally follow the above-mentioned rules as these are under their customary law.

Age of Marriage

In Ao society, there is no hard and fast rule about the exact age of marriage for the boys and girls but pre-puberty marriage and child marriage is not prevalent among them. According to Ao customary law, every male who is of sound mind and who has reached the age of puberty is qualified for marriage. In traditional Ao society, the age of marriage for a boy was between eighteen and twenty five years and for a girl was between sixteen and twenty years. The main considerations of determining the age of marriage are: both the boy and girl must be adults before their marriage. In their practice, a boy must be able to do all sorts of household works. He should show his capacities and ability to independently manage a household and raise food and cash crops in the *jhum* field. The couple must be able to do the work independently and should live in separate house. Besides, in the earlier days, due to head hunting and inter-village fighting, it was a dangerous task to live in a separate house as these frequently disturbed their socio-political life. As a matter of fact, in those days, every householder has to be morally and physically fit to prevent any attack.

But at present with the coming of Christianity, modernization and education, the head hunting practice among them is already abolished and the inter-village fighting are no more practiced. At present the most important condition for a boy is to possess a separate house constructed by him. This is the prerequisite condition for the boy for his marriage. Now-a-days the prime age of marriage for a boy is 27-35 and that of for a girl is 22-25.

Distribution, of the people under investigation by age, sex and marital status has been presented in Table 4.17.

From the analysis of marital status of the people of villages under study (Table 4.17), it is seen that there are a total of 681 (58.30%) unmarried and 450 (38.52%) married persons. Among the unmarried ones, there are 384 (32.87%) males and 297 (25.42%) females. Similarly, among the married persons there are 225 (19.26%) males and females. Further, there are 36 (3.08%) widow and widower (widow—13, 1.11%; widower—23, 1.96%) in the population. There is not a single case of divorcee is found during the present investigation.

A cursory glance of Table 4.17 reveals that none of the boys and girls below 15 years of age in the population is married. In other words child marriage is not in practice.

The highest number of married males (32; 2.73%) and that of married females (32; 2.73%) are found in the age groups (35-39), (45-49) and (40-44) years respectively.

Considering the marital status of the villages under study independently (Tables 4.18, 4.19 and 4.20), it is seen that there are a total of 375 (60.09%) unmarried and 228 (36.53%) married persons in the Lirmen village. Among the unmarried ones, there are 212 (33.97%) males and 163 (26.12%) females. Similarly, among the married persons there are 114 (18.26%) males and 114 (18.26%) females. Further, there are 21 (3.36%) widow and widowers (widow—14, 2.24%; widower-7, 1.12%) in the village.

In the village Yajang-A, there are a total of 235 (56.76%) unmarried and 167 (40.33%) married persons. Among the unmarried ones, there are 133 (32.12%) males and 102 (24.63%) females. Similarly, among the married persons there are 83 (20.04%) males and 84 (20.28%) females. Further, there are 12 (2.89%) widow and widowers (widow—8, 1.93%; widower—4, 0.96%) in the village.

Similarly, in the village Yajang-B, there are a total of 71 (54.61%) unmarried and 56 (43.07%) married persons. Among the unmarried ones, there are 39 (30.00%) males and 32 (24.61%) females. Similarly, among the married persons there are 28 (21.53%) males and 28 (21.53%) females. Further, there are 3 (2.30%) widow and widowers (widow—1, 0.76%; widower—2, 1.53%) in the village.

Engagement of Marriage and the Procedure of Solemnization

In the traditional Ao society marriage took place because of contact and mutual admiration between an adult boy and a grown up girl through free mixing. In such case the female

Table 4.17 : Distribution of the population of the villages under study by age, sex and marital status

Sl. No.	Age group (in years)	Un-married			Married			Widowed			Divorced			Total (M+F) (%)
		Male (%)	Female (%)	Total (%)	Male (%)	Female (%)	Total (%)	Male (%)	Female (%)	Total (%)	Male (%)	Female (%)	Total (%)	
1	2	3	4	5	6	7	8	9	10	11	12	13	14	15
1	0 – 4	39 (3.33)	44 (3.76)	83 (7.10)										83 (7.10)
2	5 – 9	47 (4.02)	40 (3.42)	87 (7.44)										87 (7.44)
3	10 – 14	52 (4.45)	53 (4.53)	105 (8.98)										105 (8.98)
4	15 – 19	64 (5.47)	66 (5.65)	130 (11.13)		2 (0.17)	2 (0.17)	0	0	0	0	0	0	132 (11.30)
5	20 – 24	72 (6.16)	50 (4.28)	122 (10.44)	4 (0.34)	12 (1.02)	16 (1.36)	0	0	0	0	0	0	138 (11.81)
6	25 – 29	68 (5.82)	28 (2.39)	96 (8.21)	12 (1.02)	21 (1.79)	33 (2.82)	0	0	0	0	0	0	129 (11.04)
7	30 – 34	33 (2.82)	11 (0.94)	44 (3.76)	19 (1.62)	29 (2.48)	48 (4.10)	0	1 (0.08)	1 (0.08)	0	0	0	93 (7.96)
8	35 – 39	5 (0.42)	2 (0.17)	7 (0.59)	32 (2.73)	27 (2.31)	59 (5.05)	0	2 (0.17)	2 (0.17)	0	0	0	68 (5.82)
9	40 – 44	2 (0.17)	2 (0.17)	4 (0.34)	27 (2.31)	32 (2.73)	59 (5.05)	1 (0.08)	1 (0.08)	2 (0.17)	0	0	0	65 (5.56)
10	45 – 49	1 (0.08)	0	1 (0.08)	32 (2.73)	23 (1.96)	55 (4.70)	0	3 (0.25)	3 (0.25)	0	0	0	59 (5.05)
11	50 – 54	1 (0.08)	1 (0.08)	2 (0.17)	23 (1.96)	26 (2.22)	49 (4.19)	2 (0.17)	5 (0.42)	7 (0.59)	0	0	0	58 (4.96)
12	55 – 59	0	0	0	20 (1.71)	21 (1.79)	41 (3.51)	3 (0.25)	3 (0.25)	6 (0.51)	0	0	0	47 (4.02)

(Contd...)

Table 4.17 *(Contd...)*

Sl. No.	Age group (in years)	Un-married			Married			Widowed			Divorced			Total
		Male (%)	Female (%)	Total (%)	Male (%)	Female (%)	Total (%)	Male (%)	Female (%)	Total (%)	Male (%)	Female (%)	Total (%)	(M+F) (%)
1	2	3	4	5	6	7	8	9	10	11	12	13	14	15
13	60 – 64	0	0	0	23 (1.96)	10 (0.85)	33 (2.82)	2 (0.17)	5 (0.42)	7 (0.59)	0	0	0	40 (3.42)
14	65 – 69	0	0	0	7 (0.59)	8 (0.68)	15 (1.28)	0	0	0	0	0	0	15 (1.28)
15	70 – 74	0	0	0	15 (1.28)	8 (0.68)	23 (1.96)	3 (0.25)	4 (0.34)	7 (0.59)	0	0	0	30 (2.56)
16	75 – 79	0	0	0	3 (0.25)	4 (0.34)	7 (0.59)	0	0	0	0	0	0	7 (0.59)
17	80 – 84	0	0	0	6 (0.51)	2 (0.17)	8 (0.68)	2 (0.17)	0	2 (0.17)	0	0	0	10 (0.85)
18	85 – 89	0	0	0	2 (0.17)	0	2 (0.17)	0	0	0	0	0	0	2 (0.17)
	Grand Total (%)	384 (32.87)	297 (25.42)	681 (58.30)	225 (19.26)	225 (19.26)	450 (38.52)	13 (1.11)	24 (2.05)	37 (3.16)	0	0	0	1168 (100.00)

Table 4.18 : Distribution of the population of the village Lirmen by age, sex and marital status

Sl. No.	Age group (in years)	Un-married			Married			Widowed			Divorced			Total (M+F) (%)
		Male (%)	Female (%)	Total (%)	Male (%)	Female (%)	Total (%)	Male (%)	Female (%)	Total (%)	Male (%)	Female (%)	Total (%)	
1	2	3	4	5	6	7	8	9	10	11	12	13	14	15
1	0 – 4	11 (1.76)	17 (2.72)	28 (4.48)	–	–	–	–	–	–	–	–	–	28 (4.48)
2	5 – 9	19 (3.04)	15 (2.40)	34 (5.44)	–	–	–	–	–	–	–	–	–	34 (5.44)
3	10 – 14	24 (3.84)	24 (3.84)	48 (7.69)	–	–	–	–	–	–	–	–	–	48 (7.69)
4	15 – 19	40 (6.41)	40 (6.41)	80 (12.82)	–	–	–	–	–	–	–	–	–	80 (12.82)
5	20 – 24	44 (7.05)	35 (5.60)	79 (12.66)	1 (0.16)	1 (0.16)	2 (0.32)	0	0	0	0	0	0	81 (12.98)
6	25 – 29	43 (6.89)	18 (2.88)	61 (9.77)	0	4 (0.64)	4 (0.64)	0	0	0	0	0	0	65 (10.41)
7	30 – 34	25 (4.00)	11 (1.76)	36 (5.76)	5 (0.80)	17 (2.72)	22 (3.52)	0	0	0	0	0	0	58 (9.29)
8	35 – 39	4 (0.64)	1 (0.16)	5 (0.80)	17 (27.24)	13 (2.08)	30 (4.80)	0	1 (0.16)	1 (0.16)	0	0	0	36 (5.76)
9	40 – 44	2 (0.32)	1 (0.16)	3 (0.48)	16 (2.56)	20 (3.20)	36 (5.76)	0	1 (0.16)	1 (0.16)	0	0	0	40 (6.41)
10	45 – 49	0	0	0	16 (2.56)	9 (1.44)	25 (4.00)	0	1 (0.16)	1 (0.16)	0	0	0	26 (4.16)
11	50 – 54	0	1 (0.16)	1 (0.16)	14 (2.24)	18 (2.88)	32 (5.12)	2 (0.32)	5 (0.80)	7 (1.12)	0	0	0	40 (6.41)
12	55 – 59	0	0	0	11 (1.76)	13 (2.08)	24 (3.84)	2 (0.32)	1 (0.16)	3 (0.48)	0	0	0	27 (4.32)

(Contd...)

Table 4.18 : *(Contd...)*

Sl. No.	Age group (in years)	Un-married Male (%)	Un-married Female (%)	Un-married Total (%)	Married Male (%)	Married Female (%)	Married Total (%)	Widowed Male (%)	Widowed Female (%)	Widowed Total (%)	Divorced Male (%)	Divorced Female (%)	Divorced Total (%)	Total (M+F) (%)
1	2	3	4	5	6	7	8	9	10	11	12	13	14	15
13	60 – 64	0	0	0	16 (2.56)	7 (1.12)	23 (3.68)	1 (0.16)	4 (0.64)	5 (0.80)	0	0	0	28 (4.48)
14	65 – 69	0	0	0	3 (0.48)	6 (0.96)	9 (1.44)	0	0	0	0	0	0	9 (1.44)
15	70 – 74	0	0	0	11 (1.76)	3 (0.48)	14 (2.24)	1 (0.16)	1 (0.16)	2 (0.32)	0	0	0	16 (2.56)
16	75 – 79	0	0	0	2 (0.32)	2 (0.32)	4 (0.64)	0	0	0	0	0	0	4 (0.64)
17	80 – 84	0	0	0	1 (0.16)	1 (0.16)	2 (0.32)	1 (0.16)	0	1 (0.16)	0	0	0	3 (0.48)
18	85 – 89	0	0	0	1 (0.16)	0	1 (0.16)	0	0	0	0	0	0	1 (0.16)
	Grand Total (%)	212 (33.97)	163 (26.12)	375 (60.09)	114 (18.26)	114 (18.26)	228 (36.53)	7 (1.12)	14 (2.24)	21 (3.36)	0	0	0	624 (100.00)

Table 4.19 : Distribution of the population of the village-Yajang-A by age, sex and marital status

Sl. No.	Age group (in years)	Un-married Male (%)	Un-married Female (%)	Un-married Total (%)	Married Male (%)	Married Female (%)	Married Total (%)	Widowed Male (%)	Widowed Female (%)	Widowed Total (%)	Divorced Male (%)	Divorced Female (%)	Divorced Total (%)	Total (M+F) (%)
1	2	3	4	5	6	7	8	9	10	11	12	13	14	15
1	0 – 4	18 (4.34)	18 (4.34)	36 (8.69)	–	–	–	–	–	–	–	–	–	36 (8.69)
2	5 – 9	19 (4.58)	20 (4.83)	39 (9.42)	–	–	–	–	–	–	–	–	–	39 (9.42)
3	10 – 14	20 (4.83)	22 (5.31)	42 (10.14)	–	–	–	–	–	–	–	–	–	42 (10.14)
4	15 – 19	20 (4.83)	18 (4.34)	38 (9.17)	0	2 (0.48)	2 (0.48)	0	0	0	0	0	0	40 (9.66)
5	20 – 24	26 (6.28)	14 (3.38)	40 (9.66)	2 (0.48)	9 (2.17)	11 (2.65)	0	0	0	0	0	0	51 (12.31)
6	25 – 29	21 (5.07)	8 (1.93)	29 (7.00)	10 (2.41)	10 (2.41)	20 (4.83)	0	0	0	0	0	0	49 (11.83)
7	30 – 34	7 (1.69)	0	7 (1.69)	10 (2.41)	10 (2.41)	20 (4.83)	0	1 (0.24)	1 (0.24)	0	0	0	28 (6.76)
8	35 – 39	0	1 (0.24)	1 (0.24)	11 (2.65)	10 (2.41)	21 (5.07)	0	1 (0.24)	1 (0.24)	0	0	0	23 (5.55)
9	40 – 44	0	1 (0.24)	1 (0.24)	7 (1.69)	10 (2.41)	17 (4.10)	0	0	0	0	0	0	18 (4.34)
10	45 – 49	1 (0.24)	0	1 (0.24)	13 (3.14)	11 (2.65)	24 (5.79)	0	2 (0.48)	2 (0.48)	0	0	0	27 (6.52)
11	50 – 54	1 (0.24)	0	1 (0.24)	7 (1.69)	7 (1.69)	14 (3.38)	0	0	0	0	0	0	15 (3.62)
12	55 – 59	0	0	0	8 (1.93)	7 (1.69)	15 (3.62)	1 (0.24)	2 (0.48)	3 (0.72)	0	0	0	18 (4.34)

(Contd...)

Table 4.19 : *(Contd...)*

Sl. No.	*Age group (in years)*	*Un-married*			*Married*			*Widowed*			*Divorced*			*Total*
		Male (%)	*Female (%)*	*Total (%)*	*Male (%)*	*Female (%)*	*Total (%)*	*Male (%)*	*Female (%)*	*Total (%)*	*Male (%)*	*Female (%)*	*Total (%)*	*(M+F) (%)*
1	*2*	*3*	*4*	*5*	*6*	*7*	*8*	*9*	*10*	*11*	*12*	*13*	*14*	*15*
13	60 – 64	0	0	0	6 (1.44)	2 (0.48)	8 (1.93)	1 (0.24)	0	1 (0.24)	0	0	0	9 (2.17)
14	65 – 69	0	0	0	4 (0.96)	1 (0.24)	5 (1.20)	0	0	0	0	0	0	5 (1.20)
15	70 – 74	0	0	0	2 (0.48)	2 (0.48)	4 (0.96)	2 (0.48)	3 (0.72)	5 (1.20)	0	0	0	9 (2.17)
16	75 – 79	0	0	0	1 (0.24)	2 (0.48)	3 (0.72)	0	0	0	0	0	0	3 (0.72)
17	80 – 84	0	0	0	2 (0.48)	0	2 (0.48)	0	0	0	0	0	0	2 (0.48)
18	85 – 89	0	0	0	0	0	0	0	0	0	0	0	0	0
Grand Total (%)		133 (32.12)	102 (24.63)	235 (56.76)	83 (20.04)	83 (20.04)	166 (40.09)	4 (0.96)	9 (2.17)	13 (3.14)	0	0	0	414 (100.00)

Table 4.20 : Distribution of the population of the village Yajang-B by age, sex and marital status

Sl. No.	Age group (in years)	Unmarried			Married			Widowed			Divorced			Total
		Male (%)	Female (%)	Total (%)	Male (%)	Female (%)	Total (%)	Male (%)	Female (%)	Total (%)	Male (%)	Female (%)	Total (%)	(M+F) (%)
1	2	3	4	5	6	7	8	9	10	11	12	13	14	15
1	0 – 4	10 (7.69)	9 (6.92)	19 (14.61)	–	–	–	–	–	–	–	–	–	19 (14.61)
2	5 – 9	9 (6.92)	5 (3.84)	14 (10.76)	–	–	–	–	–	–	–	–	–	14 (10.76)
3	10 – 14	8 (6.15)	7 (5.38)	15 (11.53)	–	–	–	–	–	–	–	–	–	15 (11.53)
4	15 – 19	4 (3.07)	8 (6.15)	12 (9.23)	–	–	–	–	–	–	–	–	–	12 (9.23)
5	20 – 24	2 (1.53)	1 (0.76)	3 (2.30)	1 (0.76)	2 (1.53)	3 (2.30)	0	0	0	0	0	0	6 (4.61)
6	25 – 29	4 (3.07)	2 (1.53)	6 (4.61)	2 (1.53)	7 (5.38)	9 (6.92)	0	0	0	0	0	0	15 (11.53)
7	30 – 34	1 (0.76)	0	1 (0.76)	4 (3.07)	2 (1.53)	6 (4.61)	0	0	0	0	0	0	7 (5.38)
8	35 – 39	1 (0.76)	0	1 (0.76)	4 (3.07)	4 (3.07)	8 (6.15)	0	0	0	0	0	0	9 (6.92)
9	40 – 44	0	0	0	4 (3.07)	2 (1.53)	6 (4.61)	1 (0.76)	0	1 (0.76)	0	0	0	7 (5.38)
10	45 – 49	0	0	0	3 (2.30)	3 (2.30)	6 (4.61)	0	0	0	0	0	0	6 (4.61)
11	50 – 54	0	0	0	2 (1.53)	1 (0.76)	3 (2.30)	0	0	0	0	0	0	3 (2.30)
12	55 – 59	0	0	0	1 (0.76)	1 (0.76)	2 (1.53)	0	0	0	0	0	0	2 (1.53)

(Contd...)

Table 4.20 : *(Contd...)*

Sl. No.	Age group (in years)	Unmarried			Married			Widowed			Divorced			Total
		Male (%)	Female (%)	Total (%)	Male (%)	Female (%)	Total (%)	Male (%)	Female (%)	Total (%)	Male (%)	Female (%)	Total (%)	(M+F) (%)
1	2	3	4	5	6	7	8	9	10	11	12	13	14	15
13	60 – 64	0	0	0	1 (0.76)	1 (0.76)	2 (1.53)	0	1 (0.76)	1 (0.76)	0	0	0	3 (2.30)
14	65 – 69	0	0	0	0	1 (0.76)	1 (0.76)	0	0	0	0	0	0	1 (0.76)
15	70 – 74	0	0	0	2 (1.53)	3 (2.30)	5 (3.84)	0	0	0	0	0	0	5 (3.84)
16	75 – 79	0	0	0	0	0	0	0	0	0	0	0	0	0
17	80 – 84	0	0	0	3 (2.30)	1 (0.76)	4 (3.07)	1 (0.76)	0	1 (0.76)	0	0	0	5 (3.84)
18	85 – 89	0	0	0	1 (0.76)	0	1 (0.76)	0	0	0	0	0	0	1 (0.76)
	Grand Total (%)	39 (30.00)	32 (24.61)	71 (54.61)	28 (21.53)	28 (21.53)	56 (43.07)	2 (1.53)	1 (0.76)	3 (2.30)	0	0	0	130 (100.00)

dormitory *tsuki* and male dormitory *ariju* played the most important role in facilitating the marriage between boys and girls.

With the advent of Christianity, a tremendous change has taken place in the system of Ao marriage. The people under investigation are Christians by religion and the most socially accepted marriage among them is the Christian marriage in the Church. Usually, the boy himself or the parents of the boy identify the girl. After selecting the girl, the permission from both the parents is required and confirmation takes place in the family level. As a normal practice, the boy's parents or the boy himself approaches the girl. After that, the Church authority is informed and the official engagement is fixed on an appointed date in the residence of the girl's parents. The parents declare officially that their children are now engaged and the day of marriage is fixed. The Church ascertains the membership of the boy and the girl and their clan affiliation as to whether they can marry or not. If they belong to the same clan, the Church authority does not allow them to marry.

Among the Ao people there is a standing rule for marriage which is followed by the Churches as per the directive of the Ao Baptist Christian Association. According to this rule, from the day of engagement, the Church authority normally gives a time of 90 days restriction before which couple cannot fix wedding day. However, in certain cases there are relaxations of such rules according to situation and local convenience. Then, the main celebration takes place in the Church generally in pursuance of the provisions in Sections 25 and 51 of the Indian Christian Marriage Act, 1872 (Jamir and Lanunungsung, 2005)

The most favourable months of marriage are November, December and January. As in this time, they become free from the Agricultural work and the weather becomes clear at this time.

Christianity not only changes the engagement of marriage

but also change the procedure of solemnization of marriage. The people under investigation solemnized their marriage in the Church. The Pastor conducts the marriage ceremony on the appointed day. As the congregation gathers, the bridegroom waits for the arrival of the bride and her party. The crowd welcomes the bride and her party by standing and the bridal march follows. After then, a song is sung or a word of prayer is offered and as soon as the song ends, the Pastor initiates the main solemnization in a most conventional way. He gives a lesson on Marriage from the Biblical point of view. In his lesson, he expresses the value of marriage, aim of marriage and the role of husband and wife after marriage.

Then, he encourages the bridegroom and bride to join their right hands and first approach the bridegroom to promise that he will be a faithful husband so long they shall live. The groom promises it before God and the witness present in the Church. In the same way, the Pastor again approaches the bride to promise that she will be a faithful wife so long as they shall live. The bride also promises it before God and the witness present in the Church.

After promising individually, the Pastor approaches both the bride and groom simultaneously that they will co-operate each other in any case until death. Both the husband and wife accept this and give a reply as "Yes we do".

After completing this, the exchange of ring follows. Having all these formalities the Pastor on behalf of the Church authority and ABAM (Ao Baptist Church Association) and looking to heaven for divine sanction, he, pronounces them husband and wife in the presence of God and the assembled witnesses. Then he gives a Marriage certificate which is received by the bride with a speech "What thereafter God had joined together let not man put as under". After a word of thanks giving prayer, the marriage solemnization ends in the Church.

As soon as the marriage solemnization ends, all people come with the newly married couple, in the bridegroom's residence where the reception and wedding feast follows. Depending on the economic condition, the number of items in the feast is also vary. But the meat of pig and cow is common for all of them.

Divorce and Adoption

Though divorce is very rare in Ao society but their custom recognizes divorce after the marriage. There are certain causes of divorce. These causes are common to both husband and wife and either of them. But as long as such a divorce is not obtained, the marriage subsists and therefore an Ao cannot perform a second marriage until divorce. Divorce among them is very simple as it does not require going to court. A divorce can take place through mutual agreement in the presence of other members of the family. A divorce is allowed even during pregnancy if the question of divorce arises due to the pregnant women's fault. First, the clan members decide the divorce case in presence of both the parties and finally, a petition is given to the village council (*putu menden*) which is the final authority in the matter.

Unlike divorce, adoption is also recognised by their society. The adopted son is considered as being born in the new family and he looses his tie with the old family. Generally, the purpose of adoption is for the parents who adopt any child to get help and support in all domestic affairs and especially when they become aged. A widow or unmarried woman also can adopt a child so that the adopted child might look after her during her old age.

During the present investigation, not a single case of divorce or adoption has been observed.

Thus it is apparent that, after the inception of Christianity, the Ao Nagas do not practice the traditional way of engagement of marriage and ceremony. Today, the most socially accepted marriage is the Christian marriage in the Church. This kind of marriage is mostly honoured and recognised by their society now. Marriage without getting a certificate from the Church is not well recognised in their society and exclude from the Church member. Though the people now follow the Christian procedural practice of marriage but the traditional rules of marriage still exists among them.

Inheritance of Property

From very early times, the rights to own and inherit property by an individual or clan or community are largely decided by the tradition and customs of the society. Like patrilineal non-tribal societies, succession and inheritance of property take place through the male line in patrilineal tribal societies also. In such societies, traditionally a woman is kept out of the decision making process in matters relating to ownership or transfer of property (Devi, 2002). The Aos too follow patriarchal and patrilineal family system where major shares of the property go to the sons rather than the daughters.

Concept of Property

In most legal, social and scientific usages, the term property refers to rights of ownership of possession of something (Encyclopaedia of Anthropology, 1976).

The customary laws of Aos define rights and obligations about ownership of various things at the levels of community, clan and private and by gender. The major properties both movable and immovable in the context of their culture according to the members of villages under study are: land, both ancestral and self-acquired and the products of land; residential houses that may be in the village or town; granary; ornaments and clothing; utensils; livestock; weapons; machineries etc.

The Ao society being patrilineal the father is the head of the family. The ancestral property is jointly owned by male clan members and nobody can sell any part of the ancestral property. If anybody violates this law, he will be completely debarred from owning the ancestral land. Father being the sole owner over the self-acquired properties, uses the property in accordance with his desires and wishes of the members of his family. All the children born to him and his wife are entitled to enjoy and share jointly both the ancestral and self-acquired property. As soon as his sons marry and form a separate family of their own, they are entitled to own the ancestral property and also the father's acquired property jointly but no longer remain depended on the father's family.

Modes of the Devolution and Succession

In Ao society, the people distribute their wealth either on divorce or on death of parents.

In case of divorce, one-third of the property go to the person who wants to divorce and the rest two-thirds left to the person who do not accept the divorce. This may take place both in case of husband and wife. If a husband wants to divorce against the wishes of his wife, then he is allowed to take only dao, spear, war shield, gun and his own clothing. Similarly, if the wife does not want to stay with her husband, then she is allowed to carry only her personal clothing and some other minor items. Generally, it is the duty of the husband to look after the children after divorce.

In case of death of the father, the remaining undistributed property goes to the next male heir, in order of seniority. Under the Ao customary rules of inheritance, property develops upon the heirs by succession and inheritance is always in male line. As the daughter after their marriage come under the care of a different clan and family, they are not entitled to own the properties of her father. However, the father can give the daughter a share of property except the ancestral landed properties as a gift if he desires. Such gift may be treated as her private property. If the father gives the land permanently to his daughter then later on it will be inherited by her son. She can also sell it or give it to others if she so desires and generally in such case the first preference is given to her brothers. But there is another practice which is called *sungko* gift and in this practice the daughter can enjoy the land of her father only during her lifetime and after her death, the land returns to father's clan.

Regarding succession of property among the sons, all the sons may jointly hold ownership of the ancestral and self-acquired property of their deceased father besides division of the property. As a general rule, sons whether from the same mother or not get the parental property equally. However, the eldest son is given the first privilege to select his preferred portion. In the absence of sons, the brothers, brother's son, cousins, nearest kinsmen and so on in that order inherits the property of the brother.

With regard to succession of property among the daughters, they inherit the personal property belonging to a female, namely her ornaments, clothes, utensils, furniture, tools and so on and so forth. However, a portion of ornaments may be divided with her brothers. In absence of a daughter, the property passes to women and men of the clan of the deceased. The components of women's property are: gifts at the time of marriage by parents and relatives, ornaments, dress and property acquired by inheritance. For such matter a woman possesses absolute right of disposal, as these are her individual property.

The widow of the deceased has no right of inheritance but receives a portion of paddy, furniture, clothes and utensils mainly for the purpose of her maintenance. She is entitled to live in the same house and also to cultivate the land and enjoy the resources from the land of her husband throughout her lifetime unless she remarries. On her death the same will be inherited by the heirs of her husband.

Thus it has been observed that under the Ao customary

rules of inheritance, property devolves upon the heirs by succession and inheritance is always in the male line. Daughters are not entitled to own the properties of their fathers as they come under the care of a different clan and family after their marriage. A woman gets only her personal property such as ornaments, clothes etc. so on. But she can get land as a gift by her father's money and during her lifetime, the sons can receive it if they make a will; otherwise it goes to her father's clan.

Village Council and Village Administration

The Nagas are more democratic in nature and practice than the other tribal communities. Naga villages are more homogeneous, self-sustaining and independent and distinct in terms of village administration.

Before the introduction of British administration in Ao area, they had their own way of administration which was village centred and had its own way of maintaining law and order and dispensing justice. In earlier days, during the establishment of a village, an organisation called *putu menden* is also established. Its members are selected by consensus of the respective clans and the members hold office for one generation. Generally among the chongli group this system of government is known as *putu menden* and among the mongsen group it is known as *samen menjen*. The word *putu* refers to 'generation' and *menden* means 'seat'. This *putu menden/shamen menjen* is the highest authority of a Ao village and all the members exercise their supreme power collectively in their village administration.

There is a great difference between chongli and mongsen system of *putu menden/shamen menjen*. However, the general principle is almost same even though the structure and composition are a little bit different. The ruling term of a *putu* is thirty years in the case of chongli system while in the case of mongsen system it is more flexible with a tenureship of six years. The size of *putu menden* varies from village to village depending on the size of population and the number of clans.

After the introduction of the Nagaland Village and Area Council Act of 1978 and the Village Development Boards Model Rules, 1980, it is the responsibility of the village council to look after the overall developmental aspects of the villages in Nagaland. The Village Development Board is a development branch under the village council. The Act encourages uniform pattern of village administrative system throughout the state of Nagaland. However, the existence of traditional system of village administration like 'Putu Menden' is recognised by the said Act (Jamir and Lanunungsung, 2005).

Thus, in every Ao village there are two village level political organisations, viz., traditional village council and statutory village authority. The existence of these two political organisations should not be understood as a two tier political organisation. In fact, the former represents the continuation of the traditional political organisation and the latter, the introduction of local self-government by the state. The village authority type of local self-government among the tribals of Nagaland is in lieu of the Panchayati Raj introduced in the plains. Election of the village authorities in Nagaland was held in 1978. The year 1978, therefore, represents a point of transition in the village level political organization of the Aos. Though the statutory village authority is becoming more important in village administration these days, the traditional council still exists.

The statutory village authority, i.e. the present village council is made up of a chairman, a secretary and members. In the traditional system, the office bearers in the village council are selected from among men only, women are debarred from taking up such positions and this system is still followed by them in the present village council. In the time of election the villagers first choose members in accordance with the prevailing customary practices and usages. Generally, in the selection of members each clan available in the village represents one member and the members should not be Government service holder. Depending on the population of the village, the number of members also varies. From the selected members, the members choose one as a chairman of the village council. The village council selects and appoints a secretary who may or may not be the member of the council. If the secretary is not a member of the village council, he shall have no voting rights. These village council members are approved by the State Government. The headmen are also selected by the villagers and the headmen are the members of the village council. The numbers of headmen in a village also vary depending on the population of the village. The secretary of the village authorities or councils are generally educated than the other members. This is necessary due to the fact that a secretary is required to maintain proper records of the proceedings and resolutions of the village authority.

During the present investigation, it has been recorded that the village Lirmen has ten village council members and one secretary. Out of these ten members, one is chairman who also acts as headman. There are also three more headmen from these members. Thus, in Lirmen village, there are all total four headmen. The village Yajang-A has forty eight members. Out of these one is chairman, two are headmen and one is secretary. The village Yajang-B has eleven members out of these one is chairman, one is headman and one is secretary.

The Aos have not outright given up the traditional village council following the introduction of village authority system. They have remained something of old organisation while accepting the new model of local self-government. According to the village council members in the traditional council, *unger* was the highest rank which is followed by *shimen* and *sosang*. These traditional office bearers are still exists in the modern village council but their position is now somewhat different. Thus, one way of striking an adjustment between the old and the new has been through the introduction of certain officials of traditional village council into the statutory village authority. In Table 4.21 the model of the village council of Lirmen village has been given.

Table 4.21 : Members of Lirmen village council

Sl. No.	*Name*	*Educational level*	*Officė hold*
1.	B. Shila Walling	Matriculate	Chairman, Headman
2.	L. Bendang Longchar	Under Matric	Headman, Vice-chairman
3.	Tongpang Longchar	Under Matric	Headman
4.	Imkong Longkumar	Under Matric	Headman
5.	Supong Lonkumar	Under Matric	Member (*Sosang*)
6.	Tekatong Imchen	Under Matric	Member (*Sosang*)
7.	Jempongjang Longur	Under Matric	Member (*Samen*)
8.	Rongsenchiba Longsa	Under Matric	Member (*Samen*)
9.	Tekachiba Imchen	Under Matric	Member (*Unger*)
10.	Sungpong Longchar	Under Matric	Member (*Unger*)
11.	Bangerkumba Imchen	Matruculate	Secretary

Both the traditional and modern village council is based on democratic principles of choosing leaders by consensus. To fulfil the required membership, sometimes two members are chosen from one clan. During the present investigation it has been observed that the people of Lirmen follow five years ruling term and the people of Yajang-A and Yajang-B follow 30 years ruling term. When a seat becomes vacant, the chairman shall call upon the village concerned to choose a member. Vacancy of a member in village council is filled up by the same clan representative and generally the lower rank member takes the position of the upper rank.

Christianity has become a major influence in the life of the Aos. Church based organizations are present in every village. But the spheres of the Church and the village council or village authority have formally remained separate. The Church is concerned mainly with religious activities. However, there are certain areas where Church also assumes some administrative and reform-oriented roles. The Church plays an important role in the regulation of marriage. For example, marriage by elopement is still common among the Aos. This type of marriage is against the Christian code. The Church encourages negotiations and agreement of opinion between the parents of prospective groom and bride. Church membership of those who elope without the approval of the parents and the Church are cancelled. Though the Church is primarily concerned with religion, it works together with village authority in matter of social control and maintenance of moral standard of the people.

Ariju and Village Administration

The *ariju*, popularly known as 'dormitory' or 'bachelor's house' (*morang*) is one of the most significant social institutions found among the Aos in the past. It is one of the oldest and strongest means of social control. As a unique institution, it serves as the agent of social security with trained and disciplined personnel. Before the coming of modern schools and colleges, there was no formal learning institution in Naga society. Hence, it occupied a unique place of learning centre in Naga society. This bachelor's house is not only a sleeping place for bachelors but it serves the needs of society such as social security, promotion of culture and training centre of master craftsmanship.

Literally, *ariju* refers to 'fortress' from where the looming of enemies is carefully watched. *arr* means, the enemies and *ju* means to guard or watch. Thus, *ariju* means, 'watch place of enemy' in the real sense of the term.

With the coming of Christianity and modern education the *ariju* has lost its importance and usefulness, as its principal objectives were to guard the village against the attack of head hunters of the earlier days. However, during the present investigation it has been noted that though the traditional form of *ariju* is not found among the people but the age group system in *ariju* is still exists among the people under study. Generally, all the male members of the villages are divided into age group system. This age group system is also varying from one linguistic group to another. However, the most common to all the groups is that each age group (*zunga*) has to remain in the same status for three/four years before they are upgraded to a higher status.

The *ariju* of Lirmen village consists of the following seven age groups (*zunga*) namely:

Join
Peri
Jangdak
Lanu Jankdak
Yimpoug Yakba
Ariju Shingo
Ayim Shingo

The membership of *ariju* is extended to all the male members irrespective of their status since they are entitled into its system at the age of 13-15 years. The members first enter into the *ayim shingo* stage and stay there four years then in the same order upgraded to the last stage, i.e. *join*. As the members go out from the *join* they observe a feast with the meat of pig/cow. All the *ariju* members arrange this feast and they only invite the village headmen in this feast.

There is also one secretary and treasurer in the *ariju*. The secretary may be from anyone of the age group but the treasurer must be from the *join*. The *join* age group acts as a leader and they are assisted by *peri*. In case of weakness of the *join* and *peri*, *jangdak* help in running the *ariju*. But in such case, the *jangdak* have to complete four years period without which they cannot go to the upper level.

After completion of four years in the *join* the members go out from *ariju* and after that they take the stage of *mong ana*. Again after four years, completion in *mong ana* they get the stage *olangoin*. From the *olangoin* stage a few members are selected as village council member and those who are not selected, remain in the *olangoin* stage. This *olangoin* is just like advisers who give advice both to the village council members and *ariju*. When there is any dispute between village council members and *ariju*, the *olangoin* solve the problem. After *olangoin*, the last stage is *batier* stage and all the aged persons come under this stage.

On the other hand, the village Yajang-A and Yajang-B has the following *five* age groups in the *ariju*:

Lanumapang
Pongsen
Litsilam
Tenapang
Songpo

The system is somewhat different from the Lirmen village as they are linguistically different. In this system the membership of *ariju* starts from 15 years. The members first enter into the *songpo* stage and remain there 3 years. After completing 3 years they enter into *tenapang* stage and in the same order they enter into the remaining stages, i.e. *litsilam*, *pongsen* and *lanumapang* with an interval of 3 years in each stage. The *lanumapang* is the last stage of *ariju* and after crossing this stage the members become the members of village council. Those who are not included in village council, remain in the *lanumapang* stage. All the aged persons come under the *pujir* category which is the last stage and after entering in this stage everyone get free from socio-religious and economic duties.

Thus, in case of village administration, the *ariju* also plays an important role. Both village council member and *ariju* member simultaneously run the village administrative works. The *ariju* member performs all the village level works and sometimes they also serve as a wage earner during the time of clearing of forest for *jhum* cultivation. Besides in everyday, there are two male members in each village, who look after the village and send message here and there. They also inform about any accident, death and any village level problem and dispute to the village council. These working persons are known as *nokimonger*. Except village council member, Pastor and *batier/pujir* category, all the village male members have to perform this duty. Generally, from each household one member go in a day. They follow a rotation and always two members from different household go for this duty. If someone violates this rule, he will be fined in cash or kind by the village council. Those who are reading outside the village and those who are Government service holder are also excluded from this duty.

During the present investigation, it has also been observed that there is a yearly meeting *sungmangpong* in mongsen and *imcharo* in chongli which is held in the month of October after completion of harvesting. The meeting is held in the residence of *unger* which is conducted by the village council and *lanumapang/olangoin* category members. The meeting is like an audit function of one financial year. The period is from October to October. In this meeting the village council members examine the expenditures report of the secretary and allow to pay the additional expenditures occurred in the time of occasional visit of V.D.P. persons. Again, in this meeting, on the basis of whole year expenditures from October to October, the village council members prepare their estimated price list of the production commodities for next year budget. The selection of new land for *jhum* cultivation and date of community fishing are also decided by the village council members in this meeting:

Thus, it is apparent that the village council (*putu menden*) is the highest authority in a Ao village and all the members exercise their supreme power collectively in their village administration. They settle the village level disputes in accordance with the customary laws which are not in written form and differ from village to village.

5

RELIGIOUS LIFE

Religion is a term generally used to describe man's relation to the supernatural powers and various organized systems of belief and worship in which these relations have been expressed. There are no people, however primitive, who are without religion. Religion interacts significantly with other cultural institutions to such an extent that no social phenomenon presents a larger range of expression and implication (Troisi, 1979).

Religion plays an important role in the life of a man in a society. It involves some sort of emotional bond that binds the individuals together. Generally, the people abide by the religious prescriptions without raising much questions (Sharma, 2002).

Religion is the expression of manner and mode of adjustment affected by people with their conceptions of the supernatural (Devi, 2004). There is no single society in the universe which does not have a religion. In view of social cohesion and control, religion is of great importance apart from law. Hence, religion is accepted by all as divine course.

The Ao Nagas have their own religion. Though Aos are Christian by religion at present but traditionally they were animist. In these days of pervasive spread of Christianity among the Ao Nagas, it is very difficult to acquire from the villagers a detailed and consistent picture of the pre-Christian religious life. At this stage even the elderly villagers (informants) cannot provide a clear account of the supernatural world: the concept of soul, the other world and beliefs and rituals associated with propitiation and appeasement of deities and spirits. The very lack of information, even for satisfying historical interest, is an indication of the deep penetration of Christian faith among the people. In the present study, though it is not necessary to provide a detailed account of the traditional religion, which no longer prevails, certain aspects are summarized here to assess the nature of change.

Traditional Religion

The traditional religion of the Ao Nagas was animism. Their religion based on oral doctrine propitiating deities and spirits, but worship for images or idols were not practiced. As far as it is possible to gather information from the villagers, the Ao Nagas had several Gods having different duties and functions both in earth and heaven. These Gods were, namely *Kotaksungba, Anungtsungba, Longkitsungba, Meyutsungba, Teroktsungba, Lijaba* and sacrifices were offered to appease them.

In their dialect heaven means *Kotakli* and *Kotaktsungba* is the God of heaven. His dwelling place is heaven. He is the controller and giver of sunshine and rain on earth and sometimes he is addressed as the maker of the earth as well.

Anungtsungba is the God of sky and his name is used interchangeably with God of heaven *Kotaktsungba*. He is also the controller of sunshine and rain.

Longkitsungba is the God of cavern and sometimes his name is used interchangeably with *Meyutsungba,* who is the God of heaven. *Longkitsungba* is also the judge in heaven.

Meyutsungba is also the God of heaven where to the souls of the death go after they cross this earthly home. He is also the entertainer and the supreme judge in heaven. He awards every soul favour or punishment according to his work on earth, be it good or bad. Those who lead a life of righteousness on earth are awarded with a heavenly home to live eternally after his death. But for un-righteous men who lead a life of dishonesty are sent to a place of eternal torment.

Lijaba is also one of the most important Gods. He is the creator, sustainer and controller of this earth and it is he who also supplies the material blessings to mankind. It is mostly to him that the people offered sacrifices and worship and particular days are observed in his honour. For his honour Ao people also observe *Moatsu* for six days and *Tsungrem Mong* for three days.

Teroktsungba is God of Gods, the creator of the Universe-the sun, the moon, the stars and the planets. He is the controller of the Universe. His dwelling place is above the skies. It was to him that their forefathers offered worships, prayers, praises, honours and different sacrifices like mithun, cock, hen, etc. and sometimes even human beings were sacrificed to him for the longevity of lives on earth, getting riches and for recovery from illness and for bearing children and avoiding bad luck.

From time immemorial the Ao Nagas have had a clear concept of life after death. They had the faith that unlike all other living creatures human beings had an imperishable soul which continued to survive even after our physical body is perished. They believed the existence of a heavenly home where the souls of men eternally lived together in the presence of God.

In the past there was no fixed worshipping place and there was no professional priesthood in the Ao villages. The oldest man in the village performed the religious ceremonies. *Gennas* (means something prohibited or taboo) and different ceremonies were observed by them. However, these systems are not observed after the advent of Christianity to their land. Today, the traditional religion is of academic interest only. Christianity has made tremendous advances.

With regard to the religion of the Ao Nagas, Aier (1990)

opined, "We the Ao Nagas have got a religion of our own which is in many ways, similar to the Jewish old religion in our way of worship, sacrifice and concept of God, priesthood and the use of animals for sacrifice and the observance of genna (*anembong*) and taboo (*ashibang*). However, there lies a great difference in between these two, because of the fact that from time immemorial they had their own script, a language in which they have preserved their religion in black and white; whereas we were not having their own script and as such we could not have a written religion. Of course, there is a long tale which tells us that we, the Ao Nagas have had a written script of our own and our forefathers had kept it written on dry leather, but the same had been eaten by a dog and thus our script was lost once for all. We believe there is much truth in it. Nevertheless, our unwritten religious practices remained very firm and effective, binding on us throughout all ages, even up to the dawn of Christianity and in some ranges of our Ao country it was very popularly used even up to the middle of present century. Of course, even today there are few people in our area who faithfully adhere to their old religious rites and practices. But in all the villages of the lower ranges of Ao country Christianity rapidly swallowed the old religion in a very short time and slowly but steadily the rest of the villages in the upper ranges were also captured. Thus the time old religion is being disappeared from the villages before it is properly preserved and written down by educated people among the Aos."

Christianity among the Ao Nagas

Christianization of the Aos cannot be properly understood without some reference to the advent of Christianity in Nagaland. As opined by different authors such as Sangma (1987), Singh (1972), Rev. Miles Bronson was the first Missionary to the Nagas. According to the views of the same authors, after the coming of Christianity many changes have taken place in the indigenous Naga practices and religion which was regarded as animism and it had been replaced by the religion which American missionaries brought during the middle of the nineteenth century.

When the Christianity came, the Nagas gradually accepted it and it might be because of the absence of other religion. There was no other religion, except, the traditional Naga religion before the Christianity was brought to Ao area by the American Baptist missionaries. The American Baptist missionaries were the first among the missionaries to enter the Naga Hills in 1888 and they worked among the Namsangias. Rev. Miles Bronson taught them Christianity and the art of cultivating tea. He was followed by Dr. Clark among the Ao Nagas at Molungyimjen village in 1876. These two missionaries visited these Naga tribes before the areas inhabited by them were annexed by the British. But in the Angami areas, the missionary work was not possible until complete annexation as the Angamis offered the strongest opposition to the British ever since the two came into contact and a virtual war situation persisted till the end. Due to disturbed situation, the British Government also did not allow the missionaries to visit the Angamis.

It was Major Jenkins, agent to the Governor General, North East Frontier who invited the American Baptist Foreign Society in Burma to undertake a 'Mission of Civilization' among the warlike tribes on the Assam frontier in 1836. He also promised the society all possible official and personal help. Accordingly, they sent Rev. Nathan Brown and Rev. O.T. Cutler to Sadiya to start mission works among the tribes of Assam in 1836. Later, they shifted their mission centre to Jaipur and subsequently to Sibsagar. Rev. Miles Bronson was deputed to work among Singphos at Jaipur. While he was at Jaipur, he took interest in Nagas of the vicinity who were known as Namsangias, named after village Namsang. He visited Namsang village in 1838 and there he established a school and a Church with the help of the chief and their villagers. The mission school was attended by the sons of the chiefs. But hardly Brownson's family had settled at Namsang, his whole family fell ill and he left the village in October 1841. After that he did not return to the Nagas. Therefore, the works among the Nagas ceased for many years. Brownson might not be successful from missionary point of view but the credit goes to him as the pioneer of western education and Christianity among the Nagas. He paved the way for future missionaries to work in the Naga field.

Another Baptist missionary, Rev. E.W. Clark, came to Sibsagar in 1869 for missionary work. During his stay there, he met some of the Ao Nagas who came down to plain area for trade, and he took great interest to teach Christianity among the Ao Nagas who were living near Sibsagar district. He was able to win some converts and bring the surrounding villages under his influence. In 1851 the first Ao Naga, a villager from Merenkong, was baptized, though he was later killed during a visit to his village in a hostile attack.

To carry out the mission, Clark induced an Assamese evangelist and a school teacher named Godhula Babu. Thus, the actual missionary work among the Ao Nagas began only in 1871 with the arrival of Godhula (an Assamese Christian) at Dekhahaimung (Molungyimchen), an Ao village. The Nagas, in the initial stages, suspected Godhula to be an agent of the British Tea Company at Amguri which was encroaching upon their territory, and so they adopted an unfriendly attitude. Godhula, however, persevered and was able to win their confidence by his devotion to the missionary cause. It was his singing of Christian hymns in Assamese that attracted the villagers most. In April 1872, Godhula brought nine Ao Nagas who wished to become Christian and they were baptized in Sibsagar Church by Rev. Clark on 18th December, 1872. The Rev. E.W. Clark himself went to Dekhahaimung (Molungyimjen) in 1876 and baptized 15 more Ao Nagas. On 2nd March, 1876, Clark settled at Molungyimjen and established a school and taught the Nagas with his preaching activities. But the Christians in that village faced many difficulties from non-Christian in their village. The Nagas were suspicious of Clark and his motives because they found that his teachings challenged their age-old customs. The new religion forbade drinking of rice beer, sleeping in the *morung*, work on Sundays and participation in sacrifices. These prohibitions were the very antithesis of Naga way of life.

The villagers' hostile attitude forced Clark to move away from Dekhahaimung along with his new converts. They went to a place nine miles north-east and established a new village as Christian village at Molung on 24th October, 1876, which was distinguished from the animist village. Molung became the mission centre for many years and in due course, the number of converts increased and a school was also started. The Rev. Clark wrote the Ao Naga dictionary, a catechism, a hymn book and translated the Gospels of Matthew and John. As Sword said, "The hostility of the natives had turned into friendship for they had in this time learned to love and reserve him—village after village surrendered to Christ." In 1885 the Clarks were reinforced by the arrival of Dr. S. W. Rivenburg a medical missionary and his wife. But the Rivenburgs left for Kohima in 1887 to replace the Rev. C D King there. In 1889 the Ao area was annexed. The mission centre was then shifted to a more central location at Impur, near Mkokchung on 4th October, 1894 and Impur became a renowned mission centre not only for the Ao Nagas but also for other tribes of Naga Hills. This marked the beginning of organised Christian missionary work in the Naga Hills. The Church started growing after passing through many difficulties and continuing labour. The first Association of the Ao Naga Church was held at Molung on 12th and 13th March, 1897.

Impur was to become, in the year to come, the nerve centre of Christian activities among the Naga tribes. The missionaries made their impact through (a) evangelistic work, (b) educational work and (c) medical relief work.

The evangelists, with Impur as their base, went from village to village preching the gospel of Christ. The people were exhorted to embrace Christianity lest they had to burn in the 'hell fire'. It was impressed upon them that all the heathens, as the non-Christians were called, would have to pass through hellfire an written in the Bible. This teaching fell on credulous ears because the Nagas found in it a confirmation of their traditional belief in a great fire which would end the world. A large number of Nagas accepted the new faith to avoid the terrible ordeal. Christian endeavour or societies were organised and an attempt was made to harness the youth. Regular Bible classes were organized at Impur and these were attended by representatives from the local Churches. It was emphasized that every soul was directly responsible to God and it was for the people to accept Jesus Christ as the Saviour and Lord.

Education was an important instrument of conversion and it formed a preparation evangelica. As mentioned earlier, about the starting of a school at Molung by the Clarks which could be said to have been the beginning of educational work among the Nagas by the Christian missionaries. The Bible was the text-book in the school, which was supplemented with other books containing Christian teachings. The idea behind that was, every school boy or girl, on leaving the institution, should become a messenger of the Gospel. The medium of instruction in the school was English. In 1898 the Rev. S.A. Perrine started a training school at Impur to train Pastors and lay workers. In the initial stage of the school there was only nine pupils but gradually the number increased. The Perrines were later reinforced with the arrival of Haggards. Haggard taught the art of preaching and Mrs. Haggard taught the craft of sewing. In 1901 the Rev. and Mrs. Dowd also joined at Impur.

Clark had foreseen the great utility of medical work in developing the missionary cause and accordingly he had made a special request for a qualified medical missionary. In response, Dr. S.W. Rivenburg came to Molung in 1885, but he had to leave for Kohima. Among the Aos the first full-time medical missionary was Dr. Bailey. Helping the villagers by giving medicines was greatly appreciated and it went to a long way towards winning their confidence. People from far-off places came to Impur for treatment and they were given a dose of Christianity also. After Dr. Bailey left Impur, the medical work was supervised by the missionary doctors at Jorhat with a trained Ao compounder in charge of the dispensary at Impur.

In this way, having established their base in the Ao area, the Baptist missionaries gradually spread to the other tribal areas of Nagaland.

With regard to the people under study, it has been recorded that the Christianity came to the Lirmen and Yajang-A villages first and then in Yajang-B Village.

In the village Lirmen the influence of Christianity took place in the year 1885 and in the year 1898, seven members of this village were baptized. These seven members were the founder of this village and they came to this village from Waramong, Tibuya and Yimgemkimong. These seven members who were baptized first, namely: Imnayongdang, Inobangba, Nukshilemla, Tekatiba, Mayangtemba, Tongpangluba, Intinangpong.

As noted earlier, the village Yajang-A was established in the year 1882 and the village was formed by the people who were coming from three different places, namely: Waramong, Molong and Lirmen. At the time of establishment of the village, except Molong, the people from Waramong and Lirmen were not Christian. The people from Molong popularised the Christianity and after that all of them embraced Christianity. In 1885 after 3 years of the establishment of the village, the Church was established there.

The village Yajang-B was established in the year 1970 and from the time of establishment, all the people were Christian as all the people came to this place from Yajang-A village. In other words, the people of Yajang-B are the clan members of the village Yajang-A and they had to come to this place due to growth of population in the Yajang-A.

THE CHURCH ORGANIZATION AT THE VILLAGE LEVEL

Each Ao village has a village level Church organization. All the three Ao villages under investigation have their own Churches. A Church is basically a religious institution, yet it has some juridical functions in certain selected spheres like regulation of marriage and its confirmation and religious sacraments. In Mokokchung district, Baptist Churches are predominantly found among the Aos, however in some places, Roman Catholic Churches are found but the number is very less. Thus, most of the people are members of the Baptist Church.

The Baptist Church

The Baptist Church covers 99 per cent of the total Ao population. Under the Japokong range, all Ao villages have the Baptist Church. As the villages under study are under the Japokong range, all these three villages have only the Baptist Church. The Ao people have a Bible written in their language, i.e. in Chongli language, as it is the common official language for all and everyone understand it. They get it from Impur which is mission centre for Ao Baptist Church. The Holly Bible is written in their language entitled as *'Temeshi Lai'* is used by them in Church services. However, the English language version of the Bible is occasionally used by the educated Aos during Church services now-a-days.

In Baptist Church a Pastor is a functionary who assumes the role of a priest at the village level. A Pastor conducts Church services every Sunday and in other religious festivals. He is approached by the villagers to offer prayers for the sick to ensure quick recovery and to facilitate the educational or professional achievements of the villagers. He conducts religious sacraments at house warming ceremony, birth of a child and naming and also at a wedding and death. In the latter, he administers the oath to be taken by the bride and groom. Thus, Pastor plays a role at the village level and exercises considerable religious authority over the villagers. A Pastor's work among the Aos is remunerative. Generally, the village people decide the amount. For instance, the Pastor of Lirmen village gets a salary of Rs. 4000 p.m. The expenditure on the salary is met by the villagers from out of cash contributions made by them at every Sunday prayer service.

A Pastor is assisted by deacons. There are 7 deacons in a Church and each deacon has certain specific duties to perform. The deacons render their services on honorary basis. On every Sunday prayer, the deacons perform their duties rotation- wise. Thus, on Sunday 3/4 deacons are in charge of money collection, one is in charge of congregation and one is dedicated by the Pastor to pray on Sunday on behalf of all.

A village Church is functioned under the supervision of a local Church Board which consists of the Pastor, seven deacons, two active Church members; one is secretary and the other is treasurer and all male, chairperson of the village women's society and an official from the statutory village authority.

Every village Church has a subsidiary women's organisation. It is called 'Women's Society' and its main work is to organise special Church services for women every Thursday morning. The Christian Youth Endeavour (CYE) is another Church based organisation which carries on duties such as holding discussions among the youths on Christianity and teach them good lessons about Jesus Christ. There is a youth director who conducts this fellowship service, i.e. gathering youth of the village in Church on every Sunday afternoon. The youth director gets a salary of Rs. 3000 per month from the Church. The youth also contribute cash separately and this is used for office maintenance of CYD.

There is a nominating committee, the members of which select the Church member. The village people first select the members of the nominating committee and these members of nominating committee are chosen from different disciplines such as one from village council member, one from acting deacon member, one from Christian Youth Endeavour, one from *arogolar,* i.e. from women Church society, one from teaching staff and two either male or female from the villagers.

These nominating committee members with consulting the Pastor choose 7 deacons (male) from the village people. The deacons may be married or unmarried and there is no age limit. However, they should have able mind and have experience about the deacons' duty. These 7 deacons are allotted 7 specific duties. These are:

(a) One is as Assistant Pastor. In absence of the Pastor, he takes the charge. In case of death of a person, the funeral procession is his responsible duty.
(b) All Church properties are come under the responsibility of one deacon.
(c) Christian Youth Department (CYD) is looked after by one deacon.
(d) The women department is also looked after by one deacon.
(e) One is incharge of paddy collection.
(f) One is incharge of Sunday school department for the children.
(g) One incharge of arrangement of meat (pig/cow) in the time of different occasions.

All these positions of deacons must be agreed by the Pastor and without his agreement; no one can be suitable for each specific position.

After selecting the deacons, the nominating committee members again select one secretary and one treasurer from the village people and in this case also both are male persons. If the committee members fail to select these two members, it is the duty of the newly selected deacons to select secretary and treasurers from the villagers.

The committee members then again select two more group members, namely *aien mapongchaer* and *ajak mapongchaer*. Both these groups have specific duties relating to Church and in each group there are three members (male). The *aien mapongchaer* are servants of deacons. When the deacons go for Church meeting outside the village, they carry the luggage. The word *aien* means outside from the village, *mapong* means time and *char* means do. On the other hand, the duty of *ajak mapongchar* is to collect the paddy from house to house of the village people as the word *ajak* means paddy.

After selecting all these, the committee members finally select the women department in Church by consulting with the Associate Pastor Woman. They select 7 women which are known as *denlaklar* in mongsen and *tenzukla* in chongli. Besides, they also select one secretary and one treasurer for women department in Church. To assist the *denlaklar/ tenzukla*, two assistants are also selected namely *ajak mapanglar* and *aien mapanglar*. They are like *aien mapongchar* and *ajak mapongchar* and each consists of 5/3 members.

All the selected members whether deacons or the women department's member, should be agreed by the Pastor and the associated Pastor woman.

Arogo mongdang is the Church general meeting which is held in every year at the end of November. In this meeting one corresponding committee is organised and both male and female can be member of it. Generally, the committee is formed with 5-7 members. In this meeting they discuss about all the Church related problems.

The Aos loyalty to the Church is very strong. The average villager, young or old, man or woman, adheres to the Church rules and seldom fails to make his/her Church contributions. All the three Church leaders, i.e. Pastor, Associate Woman Pastor and Youth director visit to the sick people's house and pray for them. They also visit to the week religious minded people's house and share the words of God and pray for them to strengthen their spiritual life. They also counsel the people who take narcotic and other alcoholic substance. In the death of a person, they go to that particular deceased person's house and comfort them by sharing the words of God.

Every household makes contribution to the Church funds in the form of cash at the time of regular services and also pays out one-tenth of the annual agricultural produce as tithe. Every housewife also contributes a measure of rice annually towards the Church-based women's society.

The village level Church is affiliated to a regional organization called Ao Baptist Church Association which was established in 1897 by a few number of local Churches. It is popularly known as the *Ao Baptist Arogo Mungdang* (ABAM) in Ao which has its headquarters at Impur under Asetkong range in Mokokchung district. This Baptist association is run by an Ao who is designated as secretary. This is in fact, one of the largest Associations in terms of the number of local Churches, baptized members and the area of coverage under the Nagaland Baptist Church Council, Kohima (NBCC). As quoted by Jamir and Lanunungsang (2005), there are over 133 affiliated local Baptist Churches and 44 fellowship Churches with 70,000 baptized member under Ao Baptist Arogo Mungdang (ABAM). The main objective of this organization is to promote/manage the Church growth and development and to endeavour the missions of the Church. It has several working departments such as the Department of Church and Mission, Christian Education, Literature and Research and Finance and Property. Its activities and other business are carried out under the directive of a strong Executive Committee. The Ao Christian Youth Endeavour (ACYE) and *Ao Baptist Tetsur Mungdang* (Women Wing ABTM) are the two main components of ABAM, besides many other standing committee working under it thus this organisation is considered as one of the most powerful and effective agents of change.

The *Watsu Mungdang* is purely a women socio-cultural

organisation established on April 23, 1982 under the banner of Unity and Progress. This organisation came into existence because of the initiative taken up by the Ao Women Baptist Association, Impur that functions under the ABAM. This is the apex body of Ao women organisation dealing with socio-cultural promotion, development and advancement related to the women issue.

IMPACT OF CHRISTIANITY ON THE LIFE OF THE AOs

The impact of Christianity on the Ao Naga culture is tremendous on individual, social and religious levels. The people accepted the new religion as a basis of their progress. Conversion to Christianity changed their lives completely and their lives were transformed into a newer and richer life. Evidently, with this the family life and the village life had become different. Christianity has brought about far-reaching changes in the field of traditional beliefs and practices as well as in customs, habits and social relations. In many ways, their advancement in education and economy are the outcome of conversion. In the following pages, a few visible areas of change are outlined below:

Concept of religion

Among the people, religion means 'worshipping God'. God gives salvation, retention and save the human life. God is the greatest of all and Jesus Christ is the son and spirit is after Jesus. All these three are acting as same and not separated from each other. They believe that after Jesus Christ only the Holy Spirit take care of them and it is now situated in heaven. However, spirit is everywhere and in every person. After Christianity, they do not believe much on malevolent spirit and instead of it, they believe Holy Spirit. According to them, '*tanela temeshi*' is Holy Spirit and it is omni spirit. However, they believe that there is something malevolent and *temenen tanela* is the bad spirit for them. This spirit causes sickness and even death if it is sighted by them. Under Christianity, those who do well, go to heaven after death and those who do not, go to hell. Before the advent of Christianity the Ao Nagas assigned every illness to be the wrath of the devil or evil spirit. When someone fell ill, Divine (Sacred) man had to be consulted and according to the divine man's prescription pigs, dogs, cows, fowls were sacrificed and offered to God with drinks to propitiate the evil spirit. Now-a-days the Christian Nagas do not perform such sacrifice, as their conception about health and disease have undergone much change.

Appearance

Regular bath, wearing clean and pressed clothes and keeping one's appearance tidy were emphasized as part and parcel of being a good Christian. Thus, the people (both men and women) are seen to attend Church services in western dresses. Now all the people are seen to wear all modern dresses. They wear their traditional dresses only at the time of festival and occasional cultural show.

Food and Drink

The conversion of Christianity did not lead to abandonment of traditional food except rice beer (*yi*). At the initial stage of conversion, many elderly persons who grew up in the pre-Christian days did not find it so easy to give up their age-old habit. Some of them complained that *yi* was a part of their traditional food. But Christianity has put a ban on it. Now, in every village there is a strict prohibition from the Church to drink rice beer or other modern alcohol. Violation of this rule by any family or individual, make them liable to a fine in cash or kind, and the Church and village council levy charges against such persons. Now-a-days, instead of rice beer people have switched over to tea drinking. A detail note on food habit of the Aos is given in Chapter VI.

Naming

During the pre-conversion days ritual *kinimong* was observed for six days in case of male child birth and in case of female child it was observed for five days. Now-a-days, the new born whether male or female is blessed and given a name by the elder clan member in presence of the Pastor, who also offers prayers on the day in the house of the new born. This ceremony is observed on the third day from the birth of the new born. If the new born is a girl child then, the ritual *tengrong-atuba* is also observed on that day in which the ear hole of the child is done by an elderly man of the clan.

Marriage

The traditional marriage in Ao society took place because of contact and mutual administration between an adult boy and a grown up girl through free mixing and in this process the female dormitory *tsuki* and male dormitory *ariju* played the most important role. But after Christianity, these dormitory systems no more prevail and Baptist Church does not accept the traditional way of engagement of marriage system of Aos.

Today, the most socially accepted marriage among the Aos is the Christian marriage in the Church. The engagement of marriage and procedure of solemnization has already been noted in earlier chapter (Chapter 4). Marriage by elopement is in defiance of the Church rules and as such the membership of the involved person stand cancelled till the Church confirms such a union. Though their names are removed from the Church register, the couple is expected to attend Church services regularly. If they are found diligent and regular in attendance, the marriage is subsequently confirmed by the Church.

Death

With regard to the disposal of dead, the common feature between the traditional and Christian system is that both the systems provide for disposal by burial. In every village there is a common burial ground.

Under the traditional system after the death and before burial, generally a feast with rice and beef are given by the family members of the deceased. A *genna* was observed for few days after death and within this *genna* period the family members do not work in their agricultural field. They erect stone-structures for their respectable person and old and rich deceased in the burial ground. They were buried in such a way so that they may remember the dead member, generation after generation.

Now, after Christianity, as soon as a death occurs in the village, the village Church bell is rung signifying that a death has occurred in the village. On hearing the sound of the bell, the village elders and youths assemble at the house of the deceased. Some village youths go to the village cemetery to dig a new grave while the other villagers and relatives of the deceased are engaged in clearing the dead body and cover it with new dress. In the meantime some others are engaged in making a wooden coffin. The dead body is kept in the state in the bed and the village Pastor leads the assembled villagers in prayer and hymn singing. The dead body is then taken outside and placed in the wooden coffin as it is ready. The coffin is then taken with a funeral procession to the grave.

After the funeral procession reaches the burial ground, the coffin is placed beside the grave. The lid of the coffin is removed to enable the assembled relatives and villagers to have a last glimpse of the deceased. The Pastor recites portions out of the Bible and hymns are sung by the villagers before the coffin is finally placed in the grave. The Pastor first put a handful of earth in the grave and he is followed by the relatives of the deceased and other villagers.

Household Life

With regard to household life it has been observed that the Church exerts considerable pressure on every person to conform to prescribe social and religious codes of conduct. The fear of incurring God's displeasure for misdeeds; call for confession of one's sin. Such beliefs and practices mould the behaviour of the people these days. The blessing of food before taking a meal is regularly observed by the people.

Though there have been many visible changes in day-to-day behaviour pattern, certain structural principles of social relations have remained same as existed earlier among the people. Thus, the rules of marriage, inheritance of property, land holding pattern etc. continues following their traditional rule.

Festival

The Ao Nagas had several festivals in year and these festivals and religious ceremonies are usually performed throughout the year according to agricultural calendar. Thus, most of the Ao's festivals are centred round to their agricultural activities and celebrated with feasting. During these festivals, dances and music took the main part. These festivals are an essential part of the socio-cultural life of the Aos, which represents a colourful heritage and as an ethnic community. But after Christianity, the Ao Nagas have abandoned most of their traditional festivals; however, they still continue to perform the traditional *moatsu* festival with certain change and modification. In the following pages a detail note on traditional way of celebrating the *moatsu* festival and its changing pattern is given.

Moatsu is the biggest and popular festival of the Ao Nagas and it is held just after completing the seed sowing in the *jhum* field. The word itself is a way of praying to God for the well-being of the whole community of cultivators. So, it takes place just after sowing is over. In this festival they worship *Lijaba* God and according to them he is the creator, sustainer and controller of earth and supplies the material blessings to mankind. Before arrival of J.P. Mills in Mokokchung there was no any distinct date to perform this festival. But after arrival of J.P. Mills in that area, people used to perform this festival uniformly in one time, i.e. from 1-6th of May because all of them complete their seed sowing within the month of April. Merangkong was the origin place of *moatsu* festival.

Moatsu festival is normally observed in the open field or street. It is characterized by dance with colourful traditional dresses, singing, drinking, tug of war and other activities where both men and women including children participate. The dancers with their best ceremonial dresses go round and round in the open street, singing songs of joy and blessings. That is why this is known as the most popular and common festival of Aos.

The starting day of this festival is known as *sungben*. On that day people used to carry firewood for cooking on the days of feasting. Rich families of the village kill fatted pig or cow for consumption. They get interested to distribute meat pieces to their relatives and neighbours. During this period they invite their son, daughter and grandchild to join with them in feasting. On this night each and every person of the family used to remain chaste. The young men of *morung* remain indoors without mixing with girls who sleep at night in group in a widow's house (*tsukitem*). The second day of the festival is '*yati*'. On that day the main feasting is performed for the different groups of people of the village for both the sexes. From the day they wear their traditional dresses and gather each age group people in a particular house where feast is arranged for their own age group (*zungar*). In the feast they take meat of pig or cow with rice beer. The friends and lovers exchange presents to each other on that day.

The *morung* feasting is also performed in the same day.

The whole young groups of the village gather in their respective *morungs*. They enjoy in drinking and feasting for two days. The meat of pig or cow takes important place for the inmates of that particular *morung*. From the evening of the third day both the sexes take part in singing, dancing and the tug of the war. Songs of all types such as love songs, head hunting songs, songs connected with feast of merits, etc. are sung on this occasion. During that period there is a special item of dancing and tug-of-war. For tug-of-war a long and big vine is used as a rope which is made from sword bean creeper collected from the jungle. One end of the rope stands the menfolk and on the other end of the rope stands the womenfolk. Both the groups touch and hold the rope. There they sing a special song of tug-of-war often connected with love songs. It is only for amusement and not a real tug-of-war. Each side allowing intentionally to be pulled over a reasonable distance and then pulling back to other side, chanting responsively and slowly and steadily the menfolk allow the womenfolk to pull downhill shouting a cry of victory to the womenfolk. This is only to show a gesture of respect and consideration to the women-folk. Such game of singing, dancing and tug-of-war continue interchangeably all through the days.

Erection of *moatsu* pillar is another significant activity that is associated with *moatsu* festival and it is a part of this festival. It is not an ordinary pillar but one of the most significant pillars and is associated with deep philosophical meanings. The youngest group of the *arijumen* (*sungpur*) arranges this pillar well before hand in front of the *ariju*. A healthy well grown bamboo turning the eastern side is felled and brought to the village carefully. It is then planted facing the sunrise. It is thirty to forty feet high with branches turning towards the ground like an arch with green leaves. It is well planted in order to carry several persons who participate in the climbing competition. Fifteen to thirty feet of its stem is well polished with pig's fat to make it slippery for the climbers. This pillar signifies the tree of victory, *mangko tong*, the tree where human heads are kept hanging. This post remained in the spot till the final celebration of *moatsu*. The *arijumen* of all age groups take part in the climbing competition one after another and climb up as fast as possible to reach the portion where the leaves or flowers are hung in the air and pluck them. As the competition continues, the female age group, watch with great appreciation. All the competitors try to pluck the leaves and before the leaf reaches the ground, the girls catch the falling leaves singing the song of victory cheering the title of winners.

The last day of *moatsu,* i.e. the sixth day is called *mertsungpangdok*, meaning the formal end of the use of a small metal hoe called *mertsung* used in cultivating the ground to loosen the soil and to cover the grains after sowing. In other words this day of the ceremony marks the end of using hoes as implements in the cultivations for the season. Another kind of tool or implement called *alolem*, a semi-circular instrument for lightly shaving the earth in weeding, is put into service in place of *mertsung*. At last at night all the villages take a piece of cloth like a tail and by taking it in one end they run outside home from one side to another side in the road. They believe that if they do that way the evil spirit and ghost go away from their village. The village council member and the village headman are the leader of this work. Thus the *moatsu* came to end.

But at present the Ao Nagas are totally converted to Christianity and its impact is revealed not only in social life but also in rites and rituals. As such, they observe this traditional festival with certain change and modification. At present, the *moatsu* festival is performed for one day only instead of traditional six days. It may be observed in any one day between 1st May to 3rd May. The day is selected by the village council member which is considered as suitable by the people of a particular area or village. A change is also observed in the procedure of performing the festival. As usual all the families contribute for the festival either in cash/kind. Members of *ariju* are responsible for arrangement of the feast. Some of the villagers offer pig or cow or rice for that occasion. It depends on the economic condition of the family. On the appointed day, they assemble together in the field. It is a must to wear all their traditional dresses and ornaments. They also bill one *ariju* and the *moatsu* pillar in front of the *ariju* as a model for that day. Then an elderly person narrates the tradition of this festival. The idea is to make the younger generations aware about its significance. Then the people with own age group start to perform the traditional *moatsu* associated songs and dances. Some young boys take part in the climbing competition on the *moatsu* pillar. The traditional rule of tug-of-war is also followed by the village youth boys and girls. After completing all these programmes, they together make the big feast with the meat of pig and cow. They also use all their traditional utensils for drinking and eating purposes on that day. However, the traditional rice beer is avoided due to Christianity. In the evening the adult male persons use to proceed in different directions with their own age group to door to door of that particular area to enjoy themselves by singing and dancing. Every household offers them something to eat and drink according to availability of the items at that time. They also express their views through songs on that day which is a traditional rule that they are practising now. The entire idea behind this community gathering/feast is to renew social relation and interacting among the members and offering a tribute to their ancestors.

Under Christian religion, people are seen to celebrate many special days every year such as Christmas, New Year, Father's Day, Mother's Day, Good Friday, Easter Sunday, Fasting Day etc.

Dance and Music

Christianity has brought about considerable changes also in the field of dance and music. The traditional dance and music are unimportant now-a-days. Only few elderly persons can sing the traditional songs. During my fieldwork, it has been observed that the people sing hymns set to western tune. The devotional music has also affected the general style of music among the people. There is also a strong impact of Western popular music among them. Generally, the educated boys and girls are seen to listen such types of Western songs. However, there is now a clearly discernible trend of reviving the old dance and music for presenting 'tribal culture' to the outside world on formal occasions.

In all the three villages, the youths have taken up effective measures to revive and preserve traditional dance and music at least for presentation on formal occasions and to participate in dance competition organised by Government Departments.

The traditional musical instruments are not available among them. They use only the drum as traditional musical instrument at dance performances. For the young people the guitar is the ubiquitous musical instrument.

The foregoing discussions thus indicate that during the last few decades or so Christianity has penetrated deep into the life and culture of the Ao Nagas. Modern formal education which came along with Christianity has been consistently working as a major force, often as a catalyst, in bringing about socio-economic changes.

6

ECONOMIC LIFE

The economic and social aspects of a community are always interdependent. Both depend upon the nature and potential of human resources. Economic well-being generates factors favourable to education, health and many other skills, etc. In order to achieve a higher quality of life, there should always be a proper socio-economic well-being.

Economic life includes the activities associated with the fulfilment of material needs of the people. Every community has its own way to meet the basic needs for the existence of its members. On the other hand, the economy of a group is constituted by the various economic activities, which in fact are multifaceted, varied and complex.

Production is the basic economic activity of human being and the mode of production plays an important role in shaping the social structure, the psychology and ideology of a community. The quality and content of economic pursuits determine the economic status of the group in relation to the wider society.

The economic condition of a group of people determines their overall standard of living, which in turn is reflected in their health condition. The health status of a community highly depends upon the economic condition of the people. People from higher economic condition generally possess a better health status as they are expected to get better accessibilities and facilities regarding maintenance of health as well as health care services. Thus, economic condition and health are interdependent.

With regard to the population under investigation, it may be noted here that the people have predominantly agricultural economy. They are traditionally shifting cultivators. However, since after their settlement in the foot hills regions in the recent past, they have acquired plots of land suitable for wet cultivation. Thus they have two types of cultivation—*jhum* or dry in the hills and wet or permanent in the plains. Much of the Ao traditional social, cultural and economic behaviour is centred round the dry cultivation called *tongonglo*. However, the cultural and religious practices associated with dry cultivation have mostly been given up in the wake of Christianity. The adoption of wet cultivation in the adjoining plain tracts has made dry cultivation in the hills increasingly unimportant.

In the following pages, an attempt has been made to outline the contemporary character of Ao economy in which dry cultivation has come to be supplemented by various new types of economic activities and their overall economic condition including food habit and living condition.

Occupation

Occupation determines, to a great extent one's mode of living, thinking and behaviour etc. Therefore, it is necessary to have an idea about the different occupational pursuits of the people under investigation.

The main occupation of the people is cultivation. Nearly all adult members in a household are engaged in agricultural activities in one way or another. Very young children and aged persons are however exempted from tasks in the field. The men and women have specific areas of specialization in economic activities including agriculture. The women are primarily the house-keepers in Ao society. However, like other tribes of Nagaland, among the Ao, the women play a very important role in shifting cultivation. Their principal task in the field includes preparation of the soil, sowing, weeding and harvesting. Felling of trees, clearing of jungle and firing are masculine tasks.

Agriculture being the primary occupation of the people, under investigation, all the people concentrates all their endeavours upon this main economic activity. Now-a-days, however, with the inroad of education as well as because of increase in the population, some of the people have gradually been taking up some other non-traditional occupations. As for instance, for some people service and business are the primary occupations. However, agricultural pursuits are also maintained alongside by some of them. Other categories of occupation are housewife (domestic preoccupation) and students. Individuals who are too young and too old are being conveniently grouped under the category 'dependents'.

An idea about the distribution of the population under investigation by sex and occupation has been presented in the Table 6.1.

It will be seen from Table 6.1 that there are a total of 667 (57.10%) individuals whose primary occupation is agriculture. Out of these 343 (29.36%) males and 324 (27.73%) females.

The table further shows that there are 10 (0.85%) males whose primary occupation is agriculture and secondary occupation is business. There are all total 39 (3.33%) people who have service (Government) as their primary occupation. Out of these 33 (2.82%) males and 6 (0.51%) females. Again there are only 3 (0.25%) males whose primary occupation is service and secondary occupation is agriculture. Only 8 (0.68%) males have business as their primary occupation and 18 (1.54%) males have business as primary and agriculture as secondary occupation. Besides, there are 220 (18.83%) individuals (114; 9.76% males and 106; 9.07% females) who are categorized as student and 38 (3.25%) individuals (22; 1.88% males and 16; 1.36% females) who are primarily student and subsidiarily involve in agriculture. There are only 23 (1.96%) females which remain only as housewife. There are 142 (12.15%) individuals (71; 6.07% males and 71; 6.07% females) which are in the dependent category.

Village-wise distribution of the population by sex and

occupation has been presented in Tables 6.2, 6.3 and 6.4. The tables show a similar trend and there does not seem to exist any observable difference in the three villages. However, the fact that in the village Yajang-A, no individuals are found in the category of primary service and secondary agriculture and in the category of only business. In the same way in the village Yajang-B no individuals are found in the primary business and secondary agriculture.

Table 6.1: Distribution of the population of the village under study by sex and occupation

Sl. No.	*Occupation*		*Male (%)*	*Female (%)*	*Total (%)*
	Primary	*Subsidiary*			
1	*2*	*3*	*4*	*5*	*6*
1	Agriculture	–	343 (29.36)	324 (27.73)	667 (57.10)
2	Agriculture	Business	10 (0.85)	–	10 (0.85)
3	Service	–	33 (2.82)	6 (0.51)	39 (3.33)
4	Service	Agriculture	3 (0.25)	–	3 (0.25)
5	Business	–	8 (0.68)	–	8 (0.68)
6	Business	Agriculture	18 (1.54)	–	18 (1.54)
7	Student	–	114 (9.76)	106 (9.07)	220 (18.83)
8	Student	Agriculture	22 (1.88)	16 (1.36)	38 (3.25)
9	Housewife	–	–	23 (1.96)	23 (1.96)
10	Dependent	–	71 (6.07)	71 (6.07)	142 (12.15)
	Grand Total (%)		622 (53.25)	546 (46.74)	1168 (100.00)

Table 6.2 : Distribution of the population of the Lirmen village by sex and occupation

Sl.No.	*Occupation*		*Male (%)*	*Female (%)*	*Total (%)*
	Primary	*Subsidiary*			
1	*2*	*3*	*4*	*5*	*6*
1	Agriculture	–	186 (29.80)	184 (29.48)	370 (59.29)
2	Agriculture	Business	6 (0.96)	–	6 (0.96)
3	Service	–	26 (4,16)	4 (0.64)	30 (4.80)
4	Service	Agriculture	2 (0.32)	–	2 (0.32)
5	Business	–	7 (1.12)	–	7 (1.12)
6	Business	Agriculture	15 (2.40)	–	15 (2.40)
7	Student	–	63 (10.09)	54 (8.65)	117 (18.75)
8	Student	Agriculture	8 (1.28)	9 (1.44)	17 (2.72)
9	Housewife	–	–	19 (3.04)	19 (3.04)
10	Dependent	–	20 (3.20)	21 (3.36)	41 (6.57)
	Grand Total (%)		333 (53.36)	291 (46.63)	624 (100.00)

Table 6.3 : Distribution of the population of the Yajang-A village by sex and occupation

Sl. No.	Occupation		Male (%)	Female (%)	Total (%)
	Primary	Subsidiary			
1	2	3	4	5	6
1	Agriculture	–	131 (31.64)	115 (27.77)	246 (59.42)
2	Agriculture	Business	2 (0.48)	–	2 (0.48)
3	Service	–	5 (1.20)	2 (0.48)	7 (1.69)
4	Service	Agriculture	–	–	–
5	Business	–	–	–	–
6	Business	Agriculture	3 (0.72)	–	3 (0.72)
7	Student	–	38 (9.17)	42 (10.14)	80 (19.32)
8	Student	Agriculture	12 (2.89)	5 (1.20)	17 (4.10)
9	Housewife	–	–	2 (0.48)	2 (0.48)
10	Dependent	–	29 (7.00)	28 (6.76)	57 (13.76)
	Grand Total (%)		220 (53.14)	194 (46.85)	414 (100.00)

Table 6.4 : Distribution of the population of the Yajang-B village by sex and occupation

Sl. No.	Occupation		Male (%)	Female (%)	Total (%)
	Primary	Subsidiary			
1	2	3	4	5	6
1	Agriculture	–	26 (20.00)	25 (19.23)	51 (39.23)
2	Agriculture	Business	2 (1.53)	–	2 (1.53)
3	Service	–	2 (1.53)	–	2 (1.53)
4	Service	Agriculture	1 (0.76)	–	1 (0.76)
5	Business	–	1 (0.76)	–	1 (0.76)
6	Business	Agriculture	–	–	4 (3.07)
7	Student	–	13 (10.00)	10 (7.69)	23 (17.69)
8	Student	Agriculture	2 (1.53)	2 (1.53)	4(3.07)
9	Housewife	–	–	2 (1.53)	2 (1.53)
10	Dependent	–	22 (16.92)	22 (16.92)	44 (33.84)
	Grand Total (%)		69 (53.07)	61 (46.92)	130 (100.00)

Agriculture

Agriculture is the source of livelihood for more than half of the world's population (Encyclopaedia of Britannica, 1768). The shifting cultivation is particularly acute in the North-Eastern states of India like Mikir and North Cachar Hills of Assam, Arunachal Pradesh, Nagaland, Mizoram, Manipur, Meghalaya and Tripura, where, about six lakhs of Tribals are dependent on Jhum for their livelihood. It is a widely prevalent traditional form of cultivation of land on hill slopes in the hill areas of Nort-East India. Soil conservation survey reveals that except the Angami and Checkasang, all the Naga tribes indulge in the practice of shifting cultivation to sustain themselves (Singh and Joshi, 1990). Thus, traditional system of agriculture is the main occupation of the every Naga tribe. Having found no other suitable alternative farming, they mostly practice shifting cultivation in large scale.

In order to understand the cultural ethos of Naga tribes and jhuming as their material base, it is essential to examine these operations in detail. In the following pages a detail description of method of cultivation among people under investigation has been given.

Pattern of Landholding

Land is the most important natural resource from which the Ao derived their subsistence. The land among the Ao is mostly hilly although there are small portions of valley in certain blocks. Generally, at the time of establishing a new village, the founding leaders used to reserve certain portion of land for residential sites as well as jhum lands in the village. Shifting cultivable land is kept secured by the village community and the residential sites are aligned in rows and also at different places. Each clan possesses the land both for residential and for the purpose of cultivation. Again, in the vicinity of the village, there are protected pockets of lands for forest, bamboo groves and pastures owned by different clans. All the distant lands which individuals or clan cannot claim belong to the village. Each village has certain areas of common land such as sites for worship, cemetery, water tanks, ground etc.

In Nagaland, no non-Naga can own the land as per the Act of Indian Article 371 (A). It means that land can neither be sold out to the outsider nor can they buy it (Jamir & Lanunungsang, 2005). Among the Aos the boundaries of the land are well demarcated as inter-tribal boundary, inter-village boundary and boundary line with individuals, groups, clan and families within their own villages. Generally, they use stone pillars, natural sources, streams, rivers, big trees, mountains and hillocks etc. as identity marks of the land boundary. They do not have land survey record because the land in Nagaland is yet to be surveyed. However, boundaries are well established and they are known by the villagers.

All the land disputes arising in the village are referred to the village council (*putu menden*) who gives the verdicts in presence of both the parties according to their customary law. Generally, they try to settle their land disputes cases in their clan level first and if fail, the matter is referred to the *putu menden* for final judgment.

As the people under investigation, usually practice shifting cultivation, they require vast tracts of land, which is cultivated by the members of each clan within the jurisdiction of their own land. This is the most traditional system of cultivation where a group of farmers occupy a particular portion of land every year.

In the villages under study the jhum cycle is ideally of ten years duration. Under the prevailing system, a field is put under cultivation for two years continuously and then abandoned for ten years in favour of another new tract. However, in Lirmen village, the cycle comes to 7 years sometimes, if they get suitable tract near about and no mind to go to a far place.

A few households now possess wet fields in the plains and dry jhum in the hills. Though the Aos have adopted wet cultivation during the last few decades, they still continue their traditional shifting cultivation. Table 6.5 shows the land holding pattern among the Aos in the three villages.

Table 6.5 : Pattern of landholding according to villages under study

Sl. No.	Name of village	No. of households	Dry field	Wet field	Both dry and wet field	Landless
1	2	3	4	5	6	7
1	Lirmen	130	100	18	7	5
2	Yajang-A	101	60	2	37	2
3	Yajang-B	28	19	1	7	1
	Total (%)	259 (100.00)	179 (69.11)	21 (8.10)	51 (19.69)	8 (3.08)

It will be seen from Table 6.5 that out of 259 households, 179 (69.11%) households cultivate jhum cultivation, 21 (8.10%) households cultivate wet cultivation and 51 (19.69%) households practise both jhum and wet cultivation. There are only 8 (3.08%) households as landless.

Considering the villages independently, it has been seen that in the village Lirmen, out of 130 households, 100 households practise jhum cultivation, 18 households practise wet cultivation and 7 households practise both jhum cultivation and wet cultivation. There are 5 households as landless.

Similarly, in the village Yajang-A, out of 101 households, 60 households have jhum cultivation, 2 households practise wet cultivation and 37 households practise both jhum and wet cultivation. There are only 2 households as landless.

In the village Yajang-B, there are 28 households, out of which 19 households practise jhum cultivation, 1 household practises wet cultivation and 7 households practise both jhum and wet cultivation. There are only one household as landless.

Methods of Cultivation

Agriculture is a household level enterprise. Those persons who share food from the family hearth also contribute their labour to various agricultural activities. Agricultural activities start in the month of December or January and harvesting is completed in the month of October-November. The methods of two types of cultivation—dry or *tongonglo* and wet or *tzulu* are described below.

Dry Cultivation

The usual process of shifting cultivation demands the selection of a patch of land on hill slope. The selection of land is normally done in the October month. The auspicious task of selection of field and delineation of its boundary is the function of village council. The seniormost person on the advice of his junior members distributes the land for cultivation. According to Ao customary practice, no individual farmer is allowed to operate even in his own land for cultivation unless the village council gives consent for that purpose. The idea behind this practice is not only for safety of the entire surrounding environment from fire while burning the field but also to maintain the forest and ecological balance in the locality. Those who do not have suitable land for cultivation also get on rent for one year as tenant. The slope selected for jhuming, being a community land is allotted to each household. At the time of allotment of land, the size of the family and work force available are the standard norms taken into consideration.

Preparation of jhum fields start in January, after the celebration of Christmas and New Year's Day. As the people are Christian, commencement of season's agricultural activities is not associated with the observance of any traditional ritual or ceremonial activities.

However, on starting day, the member of a particular household is to follow certain restriction, i.e. the household who first go to the field must remain chaste the night before, as they have a traditional belief that any violation of this, may bring hardship to the village in the shape of crop failure and epidemics. Generally the village council members select from themselves, who will take the initiative and on that day no other household of the village go to the field.

Clearing of jungle and felling of trees are done by both male and female. The clearing of vegetation is done with the help of dao, bush knives and axes with great manual energy. Slashing and lopping of trees commences in the early hours of the day and continues till sun-set with a rest period in the mid-day in the field. This operation takes one month to complete as it is the task of individual families. Bushes, scrubs and small trees with thin stems are cut but the trees which are at suitable places for use as climbing poles for beans, gourds, pumpkins are often left standing.

After slashing, the felled trees and scrubs are spread over the field and allowed to dry under the scorching heat. The drying period may last for one month until the slashed material is reasonably dry.

After completion of drying of the slashed material, the burning stage of jhum land comes. Burning is done in the month of March and complete in one day. After burning, each household selects a site for his field house, locally known as *athi/aluchen*. After that, in the first week of April seed sowing is started on an auspicious day which is selected by the Pastor. The particular family, who took the initial stage of cutting jungle, performs the seed sowing first and in this matter they also remain chaste at night before. In case of paddy, seeds are sown broadcast over the jhum field. In all other cases seeds are sown in holes made by *murtchung* (iron blade small hole).

As the sowing is over they leave the seeds for one month to become mature. Then in the first week of May on a suitable date they observe the *moatsu* festival which is associated with the jhum cultivation.

Once the crop is sown, the jhumias pay cursory attention to the crop. While paddy matures the Ao undertake weeding two times. Usually, the first weeding is done after one month from the date of sowing and the second weeding is done after one month of the first weeding, while hoeing of vegetables is a must for after every ten to fifteen days. Weeding of crops is done with the help of hoe, locally known as *alulem*. The hoe is usually a small hoop iron with two pieces of bamboo attached to either end crossing to form a handle.

Harvesting is a continuous process which starts from July and lasts up to October. During this period vegetables are ready for harvesting and from thence onwards there is adequate availability of fresh vegetables. The surplus vegetables are given as gifts to the neighbours or bartered with them. When the vegetables are in abundance they are supplied to the markets of neighbouring towns to fetch some amount, out of which kerosene, oils, spices, salt and utensils are purchased. Harvesting of paddy in the jhum field is undertaken jointly by the able-bodied members of the household, often with additional assistance obtained from among the co-villagers on reciprocal basis. Sickle and sharp indigenous knives are the tools used in reaping the crops. The reapers cut the ears with a very short stalk, gathering a bunch in the left hand and cutting with a sickle (*ninok*) thrown over the shoulder into the reaping basket on the back. Women, girls and elderly man reap, while sturdy young men go round with big baskets into which they empty the contents of each reaper's basket, taking what they have collected to the threshing floor. The harvested paddy is threshed in the field itself before the separate grains are brought home in baskets. Threshing and other remaining work, including transportation are performed by the members of the concerned household. The grains thus obtained are measured in measuring baskets and carried up to the granary.

As noted earlier, under the prevailing system, a field is put under cultivation for two years continuously and then abandoned for ten years in favour of another new tract. As a result there are two types of field, one is new field and the other is old field. In this regard, seeds sown in new and old field are also different. As normal practice, crops yield from the new field are used as seeds in the newly prepared field and on the other hand, crops yield from the old field are used as seeds in the old field. The paddy cultivated in the new field is known as '*chakchi*' and that of in the old field is known as '*mosorong*'. '*Mapok*', another variety of paddy is also cultivated, in the new field. Regarding the amount of seeds preservation for the next year cultivation, they follow a common faith. Thus, they preserve that amount of paddy which is harvested in the first round and bring to the threshing floor. The Ao people become busy in the entire year for shifting cultivation as they have activities to perform in both old and new fields in different times. The annual agricultural activities of shifting cultivation of Aos both in old and new field and the crops cultivated in the jhum field are outlined in Tables 6.6 and 6.7.

Table 6.6 : Agricultural calendar (for Jhuming)

Months	*Major activities*
January	Commencement of tree-felling and scrub-cutting in new jhum plots.
February	Cut trees left for drying, and preparation of the old field.
March	Firing of felled trees and vegetation and construction of field house and sowing of seeds in the old field.
April	Sowing of seeds for paddy and vegetables in new plot and first weeding for paddy in the old field.
May	Celebration of *Moatsu* festival and first weeding for paddy and care for standing crops in the new plot.
June	Second weeding for paddy in the new plot and harvesting of vegetables in the old plot.
July August	Harvesting of paddy in the old plot and vegetables in new plot.
September	Harvesting of paddy in the new plot.
October	Plantation of winter crops continues
November December	End of agricultural season and preparation of next year's field, festive seasons.

Table 6.7 : Crop cultivated in jhum field

Name of the crop	
English name	*Local name*
Paddy	Chak
Pumpkin	Korimosa
Tomato	Bengena
Kidney bean	Luli
Gourd	Angseemavio
Arum	Manu
Sweet-potato	Simarshi
Lady's finger	Vendi
Brinjal	Sungarlikok
Onion	Alulasong
Naga onion	Ropsi
Ginger	Sungpok
Chilli	Mircha
Corn	Mandi
Simolualu	Alishi
Tengamora	Tasensa
Bitter gourd	Kura
Cucumber	Jange
Sugarcane	Napa
Majenga	Mongmo

Wet Cultivation

Cultivation of rice in permanent fields in the plains has become an important activity these days among the people under investigation. However, they possess their land for wet cultivation (*tzulu*) in the foothills regions. The people are now aware that wet cultivation is more productive and sedentary. This is due to the close contact with the nearby Assamese people and also modernization. So, whenever they are able to locate plots of flat arable land, they are eager to convert it to wet rice fields.

Though the people now-a-days trying to increase the wet rice cultivation but still the traditional method of cultivation, i.e. shifting cultivation is predominant among them. However, cultivation of paddy in permanent field has been a definite boon to their economy. It has ensured a steady supply of the staple food, rice and has even made possible generation of surplus for sale at times of need for cash. Wet cultivation also has enabled the owners of such plots free themselves from the decision of the village community regarding the date of commencement of agricultural operation on particular plots to be cultivated as are obligatory under shifting cultivation. Use of draught animals, both buffalo and bullock, has also meant a saving on human labour in Agriculture. They use plough with iron share for digging furrows of moderate depth. Generally, the soil in the foothills regions is rich and water logging is never a problem in their fields.

Terrace cultivation is unknown among them and there is not enough water in their area for terracing jhum fields. Thus the only alternative to jhuming is the wet cultivation in the foothills regions.

OTHER ECONOMIC ACTIVITIES

Although agriculture is the main occupation of majority of Aos, it does not confine them throughout the year. They are also engaged in other economic activities like raising vegetable gardens, cattle farming, poultry and livestock keeping, basket making, collection of wood both for the purpose of house construction and fuel, hunting and fishing. In the following pages, these economic activities are given in details.

Trade in Forest Products

Besides the annual agricultural produce in the form of paddy and some other vegetables, the economy of the people is also enriched by certain products collected from the neighbouring forests. The chief among these are firewood, thatch and *tokopat* for roofing, broom stick and some amount of timber used in house construction. Some people sell forest products in the market. Generally the thatch and *tokopat* are sold in village level by the villagers. The open reserve forest areas of a village cater to the firewood requirements of the villagers. The women collect dried twigs, branches and barks of trees to be used as firewood. The sale of firewood collected from the forest has become an important source of earning for many villagers. As they follow the jhum cycle of 10 years duration, greater re-growth of forest is possible and therefore extraction of firewood from their respective jhum fields is not difficult. Firewood selling is a male occupation.

It may however also be mentioned here that sale of timber is not only an individual understanding. To meet certain requirements of the village, timber is extracted from the village reserve forest which is under the control of the village authority. The money obtained from the sale is used for the construction of community building such as Church and school and for village development. Any timber extracted from jhum fields may be individually sold to earn some cash by individual villager.

Other forest products such as thatch and *tokopat* (leaf of a kind of palm tree) are used by the villagers for their own house roofing and in need, they sell these to each other among them. However a few families earn some cash from the sale of broom stick in the nearby market. Whenever they are in need of cash they sell some jhum products such as sweet potato, pumpkin and cucumber etc. They sale their products in the nearby markets and thus, these market places play an important part in the economic life of the people under study.

The cane and bamboo works practised throughout the tract by every household. As Nagaland is rich in bamboo and cane, this abundance has made them common objective to be used for the construction of dwellings, furniture, utensils and other necessaries of daily life. In fact, the people with limited use of metal and almost absence of pottery dependent heavily on bamboo and cane as the only raw materials to make their implements, weapons and articles of everyday life.

Animal Husbandry

The people are fond of rearing animals like pig, fowls, cow etc. to supplement their household income and also to meet the domestic requirements of meat. Water buffalo are kept by few villagers for use as draught animals. Buffalo meat is also consumed by them.

Poultry keeping is universal though number of fowls in a household is not high. There is hardly any buying and selling of poultry within the village. Poultry is reared mainly for occasional domestic consumption and to enrich meals on festive occasions.

The Aos greatly relish pork and so, pigs are kept in most of the households. Pork is taken on the occasions of Christmas, New Year's Day, Wedding celebration, House-warming, etc. Pigs are kept properly barricaded so that these cannot damage the kitchen garden of any villager.

Kitchen Gardening and Horticulture

There are little kitchen gardening activities among the Aos. Vegetables mostly come from the jhum fields. Generally in their residential area they also cultivate orange, pear and pineapple. Some of them also possess these in far area from the residence. Besides, they also cultivate betel-nut and betel leaf in these areas. These are the only commercial horticultures among them.

Hunting and Fishing

The people sustain their economy by hunting and fishing also. The forests of Aos are a fine hunting ground for certain animals such as monkey, bears, deer, jackal, wild bears, elephant etc. As hunting is very important for the livelihood of the Aos, they start practising it from childhood. The youngsters accompany the hunting parties whenever they get an opportunity. They hunt wild birds and animals both individually and in groups. When an animal is killed, the man who makes the fatal attack gets the major share. The rest of the meat is shared equally by all the other members of the hunting team. Generally they use their own indigenous methods for hunting. However as a weapon, gun, spear, etc are used.

The Aos are also expert in fishing and they adopt various methods in the operation. All the people of the three villages under study, go for fishing in their near about river side. Annually they go for community fishing in the month of October. The date and time of commencement is fixed in the annual meeting by the village council. All the ariju members, village council members and other oldest person who have retired from the village administration work, together go for fishing and they start early in the morning and stay there in the night. Community fishing is a masculine task and according to their custom, no female person can participate and observe in this community fishing. Fishing expeditions are carried out in groups of persons by making small dykes in the streams with bamboo and mud and leafy branches. The water thus accumulated is poisoned with the mixture of particular kind of seeds of a tree or by bleaching powder. The catching of fish is done in the morning 3.00 O'clock. Then all the people together have a feast there and come back to their residence. After reaching their residential area, they gather in the ground of the village with their fishes. Then the *ariju* members divide the fishes by age-wise among the people who went for fishing. The highest portion goes to the oldest person among the people. Though the people annually go for community fishing but in general, they go any time for fishing for household consumption.

Consumption Pattern

As a matter of tradition the crops produced in a season by the

Aos are not consumed instantly. The whole production of paddy in a year is primarily meant to last the whole year. Therefore, everybody feels the necessity of storing it in a secured place, away from fire and various agents of mass destruction. In some of the traditional dwelling houses paddy is stored inside containers made of bamboo which are placed at a corner of the house. Now-a-days, the granaries for storing paddy are built little away from the main dwelling house. They stand on wooden platform and mostly iron sheet roofed. Apart from paddy other seasonal crops like gourd, pumpkin etc. are also stored inside the granary. For feeding the domesticated animals they grow some roots and tubers such as simolualu, arum etc. The crops harvested in a year are therefore stored for future use.

Even the meat of animals killed in a hunting expedition or from market is not immediately consumed; a portion is smoked over the family hearth and preserved on a platform above the hearth for future consumption. By continuous exposure to the heat of fire the meat cannot be infected by pests or household flies. Similarly fish and other food items are also preserved in the same fashion. Apart from paddy, pulses and vegetables, juice of fruits are normally preserved for use throughout the year. In preservation of this item no chemical is used.

Every village has devices to face any dire eventualities like famine and fire. For such occasions the village Church and Church based women's society maintain reserve of paddy. Such reserves are built by way of tithe to be contributed by every household at the rate of one-tenth of its agricultural produce. Similarly, the village women's society also builds up a store of paddy through collection from its members.

Normally, the people take three meals a day, one in the early morning, one in the mid-day and another in the evening. A meal consists of cooked rice and a curry, either vegetable or meat or fish and sauce of dry fish and chilli. Use of mustard oil is rare and they prefer generally the boil items. The vegetables and to some extent, the meat are stewed and a small quantity of salt and spices are added to improve the taste. For the working persons in the field, a meal is very necessary in the mid day. For this purpose, when they go to the field they carry these food items in a packet. Though the consumption of rice beer was common in the past, only a few persons have the habit of drinking. Majority of the people do not consume rice beer since after embracing Christianity. The alternative beverage is tea. Fruit juice, is also taken by them. The traditional food items of Aos are fermented fish and fermented pulse. They are also fond of meats like chicken, beef, pork, and meat of dog. Cooking is performed by women mostly however it may also be performed by the male individuals according to their convenience.

Nature of Spending

The daily expenses in a household are generally met from the cash earned through the sale of forest and jhum products. In a few households nearly all day-to-day expenditure is met with salary of the working members. During November and December, many villagers sell some paddy from their stores to sustain the expenses of Christmas which include buying of new clothes for both young and old.

The daily household expenditure cover purchase of various items such as cigarette, bidi, soap, salt, mustard oil, pulses, potato, sugar, kerosene oil, tea leaves, beef and pork etc. They buy these items from the village shop or nearby market. Other contingent expenses of a household include purchase of shirts, trousers, shoes, wrist watches, books and stationery for school and college going children, a few cosmetic items and medicine.

Some of the expenditures are also done by travelling by bus and hired taxi They go by bus and taxi to Mokokchung, Dimapur, Jorhat and so on and they visit these places for shopping, for attending to official matters or for mere recreational purposes. A little expenditure is also done by house tax and by electric bill.

Most of the parents spend some amount of money on children's education. The educational facilities in the villages under study are up to primary and middle level. Therefore, education for the children as long as they stay in the village is not very expensive. However, if one studies outside the village, expenditure on education becomes comparatively high. A few householders have sent their children to Mokokchung, Tuli, Dimapur, Hyderabad for undertaking higher studies. Thus, they have to remit a fair sum of money for every boy and girl studying outside.

Marriage and death also includes some amount of expenditure. The minimum expenditure in negotiated marriage involves the cost of the meat of pig/cow and tea to be offered to the invitees and villagers. Funeral rites do not involve much expenditure. The deceased person's family has to arrange for the burial and a simple post-funeral prayer meeting.

In general, the nature and extent of expenditure varies from one household to another depending on the level of income. The majority of the people live at the bare subsistence level economy. Only a handful of the people enjoy a life better than those of the others because of the regular cash income earned in the form of salary.

Material Life

Material life and economic life are interrelated as well as interdependent. As such, before taking up the concluding item of discussion for the chapter, it will be prudent to have a brief idea about the material life of the people.

In almost every household the usual items for furnishing are wooden chair, bench, table and almirah etc. Some families possess cane and plastic furniture. With regard to utensils, bell-metal pots are used for cooking rice. Various types of basketry made from bamboo and cane are used in kitchen as well as in agriculture and also in carrying firewood and bamboo cylinders filled up with water from down. Stainless steels are also used.

The people possess a variety of consumer goods like wrist watch, wall clocks, bicycles, scooter, bike, radio and in some families even T.V. These are purchased from the neighbouring towns.

Among the food items, rice is the staple food. Their traditional food include mainly steamed rice, fermented fish, sauce of dry fish and chilli and meat of pig, cow, dog etc. Betel nut and leaf chewing is a universal habit among the people.

With regard to dress habits, it may be noted that the male traditional dress consists of a piece of black cloth round their waist which comes up to the knee. Upon this, a number of long narrow lines of beautiful white coloured linear stripe cloth made of cotton thread is used by them to decorate their front part, from lower part of their abdomen to the knee. Sometimes, a jacket type of cotton made small cloth they wear to cover their upper parts. Upon this, a small red coloured decorated scarf they put on their chest from their right shoulder. They wear short necklace *shipu* made of wild boar tusk and a long sized necklace *shiretzuk*, made of cowrie shells and small glass beads. They put *temko*, a headgear, which is black round based made of bear's hair, on which, feathers of hornbill are also fixed. They wear ivory armlets, *kampang* and wristlet of white cowrie shells. A cleaver or axe (*dao*) is fastened by them in a wooden sheath which they keep behind their body with the help of a cotton string round their waist. Regarding the women dress they usually wore short piece of red coloured decorated cloth, which was also vary according to clan and used to come down up to the knee. There was nothing for the upper part except the many stringed beads necklace to partly cover the breasts.

Now as a traditional dress, the women wear a red coloured

decorated cloth from their waist to the knee which is also vary according to their clan. A white blouse with sleeves they wear to cover the upper part. A blue coloured type of cloth is taken by the women in one side of their arm. The necklaces are with numerous strings of red and blue coloured cornelian beads and with most beautiful traditional conical objects look very nice. They decorate the upper part of their ear with brass made large sized rings. A feather of hornbill bird is also used by them to decorate the head. They use a brass made bracelet. The Ao *chaddar* with a decorated stripe in the middle depicting various animals and designs is commonly used by men.

At present, due to advent of modern civilization people are seen to wear all kinds of modern garments. Now the men folks wear all sorts of new fashion dresses such as trousers, shirt, coats, knitted woollen jackets and often a tie and shoe. Even the cultivators now wear short shirts and canvas shoes etc. which are available in the market. The educated girls are not behind the menfolk. They also come forward and use all kinds of modern dresses of skirts, mini, midi, maxi, kurta-pyjama etc. and with high hill shoe. The village girls too wear all sorts of such dresses. The village women use to wear piece of untainted cloth tied round their waist and they use blouse with brassiere. In all cases, blouse of either Western or Indian type or shirts of modern variety are used. This trend has led to the increased demand for modern dresses and has helped the traders to flourish.

Ornaments for personal adornment are very few. Except the elderly women, the women folk and the girls now-a-days wear all available earrings bracelets, necklace, glass bangles and chain etc. in the market. A few economically sound family, use to wear gold and silver jewelleries such as earring, ring, chain etc.

FOOD HABIT

The food habit of a community or a group of people is

determined by the culture as well as the prevailing ecological conditions. Prescription, preference and prohibition of the different food items are guided by the cultural practices and values. The ecology on the other hand is responsible for availability or deficiency of different food items in different environmental settings.

Health has a direct relation with the intake of food and drinks that help one in carrying out the physiological processes for living.

In order to have an understanding of the food habit of the people under investigation, the discussion has conveniently been confined, mainly to a qualitative enumeration of the diet and dietary composition. The discussion, by and large, incorporates data on food items, preparation process, timing, food under special circumstances, food taboos etc.

Food Items

Every human group has some uniqueness with regard to its food habit. The people under study are also not an exception in this sphere. The staple food of the people is rice. They take different varieties of locally available vegetables with rice. The wild roots and shoots as well as the flesh food (viz. pork, chicken, deer, beef, elephant, fish, egg etc.) are their usual delicacies. As a result of the influence of Christianity they have given up the individually prepared rice beer and have switched over to tea drinking. They usually take both black and milk tea. Though rice beer is totally avoided, but they prefer to drink the modern alcohol as available.

Generally, they take rice with meat, fish, vegetables and sauce. All kinds of meat are taken and most of the meat comes from domestic animals such as cow, pig, fowl etc. which are mainly imported from outside the state. Dried fish is a favourite constituent item for chilly curry as well as for sauce. Egg is either purchased from the market or generated at home from the domesticated birds (chicken).

They get vegetables from agricultural products and a good number of families also possess kitchen garden. They use the yields of kitchen garden for domestic consumption. The vegetables both agricultural and kitchen garden include papaya, pumpkin, yam, different types of beans, pea, potatoes, tomatoes, lady's finger, cucumber, reddish, chilli, bitter gourd and different varieties of leafy vegetables etc. Besides in most of the houses there are fruit trees and bamboo grooves. They also collect edible wild leaves and shoots from their surroundings. But, sometimes, when there is acute need, they purchase vegetables from the nearest market. Purchase of vegetables from the market is, however, very rare, mainly because of economic ground. During the present investigation, it has been observed that the common vegetables of their daily menu are papaya, brinjal, bean and different leafy vegetables etc. The use of chilli has been found to be very extensive. They are very fond of food like bamboo shoot, tree bean and fermented fish that they considered very special items. They are also fond of spicy food. Most of the cooking includes meat and fish is done simply by boiling.

A fairly detailed list of their food and drink items has been presented in Table 6.8.

Table 6.8 : List of the common food and drink items of the Aos of the study area

Sl. No.	*Broad categories of items*	*Name of the Items*		
		Local name c = chongli, m = mongseng	*English equivalent*	*Biotanical name*
1	*2*	*3*	*4*	*5*
1	Cereals	Chang (c), Achang (m)	Rice	*
2	Pulses	Mosur	Lentil	Lens escuents
		Naga dal	Mah	
3	Leafy vegetables	Chipi (c), Aan (m)	*	*
		Auwang (c), Achang (m)	Edible fern	Pteridium aguilinum
		Pudina	Mint	Mentha viridis
		Chuni	Coriander	Coriandrum sativum
		Napu	Coriander	Coriandrum sativum
		Manu	Colocasia	Colocasia esculenta

(Contd...)

Table 6.8 : *(Contd...)*

1	*2*	*3*	*4*	*5*
4	Vegetables	Alu	Potato	Solanum tuberosum
		Chimachi (c),	Sweet potato	Batata edulis
		Chimacha (m)	*	*
		Alichi (c), Alicha (m)	Pumpkin	Cucurbita maschata
		Kormocha	Gourd	*
		Aanganchima	Papaya	Curica papaya
		Mamaza	Bean	Glyime soja
		Ajangkon	Bitter gourd	Mormordica charantia
		Kora (c), Khare (m)	Lady's finger	Hibiscus escufentus
		Bhendi	Turnip	Drasica rapa
		Chalgum	Couliflower	Brasicaderaceae
		Naro chibi	Sweetgourd	*
		Changlikok	Long bean	Phaseolus vulgaris
		Loli	Cucumber	Cucumus sativus
		Jangge	Elephant fruit	Dillenia indica
		Rongkongchung		Raphanus-sativus
		Mula		
		Mircha	Chilli	Caosicum
		Bengena	Tomato	Lycopersicum esculentum
		Chunglikok	Brinjal	Solanum melongena
5	Spices	Haldhi	Turmeric	Cucurma-domestica
		Mitche	Salt	*
		Ropsi	Garlic	Allium sativum
		Chongmok	Ginger	Zingiber officinale
		Lachun	Onion	Allium copa
		Gulmorish	Blackpaper	Piper nigrum
		Mong mong (mejenga)	*	*
		Tutsur	Mustard Oil	Brasica compestris
6	Fish	Anju	All locally available fish and dry fish	Pisces
7	Meat	Aak	Pork	*
		Nachi	Beef	*
		Aann	Chicken	*
		Gang	Buffalo	*
		Aaj	Dog	*
		Masu (c), Matchi (m)	Deer	*
		Ber	Bird	*
		Afu	Snake	Reptila species
8	Fruits	Mango	Banana	Musa puradsiaca
		Tate	Mango	Mengifera indica
		Polong	Jack-fruit	Artocarpus integrefolia
		Naring	Orange	Citrus reticulate
		Tenga	Lemon	Citrus aurantifolia
		Mosomi	*	*
		Chupa chubon	*	*
		Letchi	Lichi	Emblica oficinalis
9	Drink	Tzu (c), Atche (m)	Water	*
		Sungo (c), Sunga (m)	Tea	Camellia sinensis
		Yi (c), Ayo (m)	Wine	*
		Mama che (c)	Miilk	*

* English equivalent and scientific names could not be made available

Daily Food Habit

The people generally take three major meals a day, which may be termed as breakfast, lunch and dinner. As the people are mostly agriculturists, they have to go to their jhum field early in the morning. Therefore, the working people both male and female take their meals; one in the morning before going to the agricultural field, one at the lunch time which they carry with them and the other in the evening. During the working hours in the agricultural field they are provided black tea by the adults children of the people. They make it in the field and drink in bamboo pipes. However, the non-working members take their first meal with the working members at the same time. They take the second meal in between 12 a.m. to 1.00 p.m. They also take black/milk tea, sometimes with snacks (if available) two or three times during the day.

Usually, the people take either black tea or milk tea with sugar and biscuits (if available) in the morning after they get up from the bed. They generally, get up at 4/5 a.m. in the morning. Then the women-folk get busy in preparing their meal. After that, all the people (both working and not working) take their meal. The working people also bring with them the required amount of tiffin from the prepared meal to take in the lunch time. The school going children also take their meal with them.

In their morning meal, people generally take rice with vegetables. They take dry fish regularly and also sauce with a mixture of dry fish, tomato, chilli and salt. Sometimes, they also take meat and egg with rice.

However, on Sunday, there is a little bit change in their daily menu. On that day they get up lately, as they do not go to the jhum field and make more items to eat with rice. All the people go to the Church on Sunday for praying and they complete their morning meal before going to the Church. At 11.30 a.m. the Church time is over and they return back to their home. Some people also use to visit to their neighbours on that day as they are free of daily work. At 12 Noon to 1 p.m. they take their lunch with meat/fish. Meat is very common item among them on Sunday.

As noted earlier the working people take some amount of tiffin with them to the jhum field. Sometimes they take both rice and vegetables but sometimes they take only the cooked rice and prepare the other items in the jhum field in the lunch time with the available vegetables and leafy vegetables of the jhum field. They also take black tea there and use bamboo pipes to drink. After returning from their duty, some of them take black tea for refreshment. The non-working persons also take tea with them with snacks (if available). Sometimes they take tea with home made snacks of banana and sweet potato.

The people take their dinner early and finish it by around 8 p.m. and retire to the bed as early as possible. The menu for the dinner is not much differ from the morning meal and lunch.

Consumption of vegetable oil, mustard oil, milk and coffee are very rare among them. In their vegetable curry or other delicacies, they use the locally available onion, ginger and garlic. Chilli as noted earlier is used extensively.

In this context, while discussing about the food habit of the Nagas, Jamir and Lanununsang (2005) wrote "A place of no breakfast, nor lunch or dinner system unlike other places especially in rural society. They take three meals a day, i.e. early in the morning, noon and in the evening without much restriction of food items. This is a place of early rising and early sleeping."

However, a resume of distribution of the food items of the people under investigation may be as follows:

Morning: Black/milk tea with sugar, rice with vegetables, sauce, dry fish, chilli.

Afternoon: Rice with vegetables, dry fish, black tea with or without sugar.

Evening: Rice, sauce, curry (meat, fish or egg or vegetable curry) with the water of bamboo shoot as flavour.

With regard to their food habits, an overall idea (qualitative) may be obtained about the distribution of the proximate principles, vitamins and mineral salts etc. in their food items.

Rice is the only cereal used by the people which is the main source of carbohydrate that provides energy. Potato and different edible wild roots also supply them carbohydrate to some extent. The vegetables, wild edible shoots and leaves also provide them some amount of energy.

The food items of the people that contain protein (i.e. the body building nutrient) include fish, pork, chicken, egg, mutton, beef, bean and some other vegetables. However, these items are taken by the people only as delicacies. Normally, these are not included in their usual daily menu. Besides, meat of duck, pigeon and wild birds and animals also sometimes constitute their occasional delicacy. In most of the families fish is taken frequently in all seasons. They also preserve fish in a unique manner for the days of scarcity of fish in their surroundings and also for the unavailability of nearest market. They also preserve the fleshes of different animals in a unique way. They take the flesh of all wild animals and birds. They also consume some insects (viz. grass-hopper, mantis etc.) and the eggs and larvae of some other insects found in the forest. All these substances also fulfil the need of protein and fat in their body.

As most of the food items are boiled without or with minimum oil, whatever fat they get is also derived from fish, meat, egg etc. Vitamins and other nutrients are obtained from green and leafy vegetables, and locally available fruits.

It may be relevantly emphasized here that ignorance of the need of additional nutrients during pregnancy, post-natal period and after prostrated illness etc., seem to be common feature among the people.

In general, the people do not have any idea of the need of a balanced diet. People are fond of the flesh food (viz. meat and fish) and they believe that these foods contain all the required nutrients for the body. These items are not in regular menu and these are taken less frequently than vegetables. However, dry fish are taken very frequently. These seem to fulfil their need of proximate principles, vitamins and minerals in usual state in their health. But, the prevalent practice of not using the fats and oils in their regular diet seems to create deficiency of the same in their body.

Poverty and ignorance seem to be playing an important role to deprive the people of having balanced diet in terms of nutrients required for their good health.

Process of Food Preparation

The process of food preparation and cooking of different items also been found, by and large, to be culture bound and these vary from society to society. At the same time it is also a fact that the varying preparation techniques have different impact on the nutrition contents of the food items. With regard to the use of fuel for cooking, Rongmei and Kapoor (2005) reported, "In hilly region less households use Liquefied Petroleum Gas (LPG) for their cooking as compared to valley where no burning woods are available free. In case of hilly areas lots of firewoods are obtained from the forest without any cost. So far in valley irrespective of their economic condition ninety per cent use LPG whereas in hilly areas in spite of abundance of firewood available, around fifteen per cent of households with good economic condition use LPG as their cooking fuel." In this context, the people under study mostly use wood as a fuel for cooking. There are only few families, use LPG for cooking.

In the following pages an attempt has been made to have some idea about the process of food preparation that prevails among the Aos under investigation.

Rice (*Chi*)

Boiling of rice in water is prevalent in all the cultural groups. The people under investigation have been found to cook rice in aluminium vessels having narrow mouth with a cover or lid on it. Some of them also use saucepan and pressure cooker. But during the preparation of food for a feast, the big saucepans are used to cook rice. For preparation of rice, at first the water is boiled and then the measured amount of rice (washed and cleaned beforehand) is put there. The boiling continues till the rice is so softened and during the period, occasional stirring with the help of a ladle is necessary to have the entire rice uniformly boiled and softened. However, it has been observed that the amount of water put in the container is measured in such a way that when the rice is properly boiled there does not remain any extra water to be strained. Thus, the Aos do not have the practice of separating the excess water from the prepared rice. In this process they can preserve the total starch contents of the rice as is done the urban areas by using pressure cookers.

Vegetables (*Aunsutsu*)

They generally prefer to take boil vegetables than the fried. At first, the raw vegetables, shoots, roots, leaves etc., are cut into pieces of the required size and then washed properly before cooking. Then in a sauce, required amount of water is added and the cut pieces are added there and cover it with a cover and keep it on hearth having fire. After boiling these vegetables they mix salt and chillies during the time of eating. Sometimes, they also mix dry fish and the water of bamboo shoot for better test.

Pulse (*Naga mah*)

They take pulses (*mah*) very rarely. At first measured amount of lentil is washed and cleaned. It is then boiled in measured amount of water in an aluminium container. After boiling, the container is taken out from above the hearth.

A frying pan/saucepan is then placed on the fire and when it becomes hot, the required amount of mustard oil is poured in it. When the oil is properly hot, the required amount of chopped onion and chilli are poured there to get it fried. Then salt and turmeric powder is added there as required. The boiled lentil is then poured in the pan and allowed to boil again. Sometimes, vegetables like papaya, yam, potato etc. are also added in the preparation of *mah*.

Fish Item (*Anju/Ango*)

Two types of fish items are prepared by the people. At first fresh fish is cut into pieces and then wash only one time. In a aluminium pot they pour water as required and add the cut piece of fish with chilli, salt and the water of bamboo shoot. Then the pot is placed on the hearth of the fire to boil till everything becomes soft to the desired extent. Sometimes, they also add vegetables and the edible leaves there to have a unique taste in the curry.

They have another one method of preparation of fish item which is known as *bangtangsen*. In a bamboo pipe the cut pieces of fish are kept with a mixture of chilli, salt, bamboo shoot. Then the open mouth of bamboo pipe is tied by a leaf (like banana leaf) and keeps the pipe in the hearth of the fire till it becomes ready to be served.

Meat Item (*Shi*)

The flesh of different types of animals and birds is taken by frying or by making curry. At first the chopped flesh is cleaned and washed. Then the pieces are boiled in a saucepan with required amount of water. Before complete boiling, they add the mixture of chilli, onion, garlic, ginger (locally available) in the pan and it is mixed thoroughly with the meat with the help of a ladle. Then, required amount of salt and turmeric powder are added and the pan is covered with a lid. At a regular interval stirring is done with the help of a ladle for three to four times, till it is cooked well. Sometimes they mix locally available leaves as spices. As a flavour they also mix the bamboo shoot water in the meat.

Sauce (*Lun*)

They also prepare a sauce with a mixture of chilli, coriander (local variety) and dry fish and tomato and with salt. This item is usually taken with rice very frequently and in every meal.

Tea (*Sungo/Shinga*)

They buy tea from the neighbouring soaps and town. For the preparation of tea, at first water is boiled in a aluminium kettle or pot. Then the required amount of tea is placed on a filter and the hot water is poured on the cups. In the cup they add sugar and milk (either packed/cow). After few minutes tea is prepared for drink. They drink this liquor throughout the day. Mostly they take tea without milk.

Besides these food items, there are also some food items which are very much fond of by these people. Some of these are *chonglong, mongotakong, alichitakong, anichitakong, akuni* etc.

Chonglong

It is made from an insect which is found in naga badam (almond) tree and other dry/putrefied tree or logs. At first the collected insects are washed in hot water and then it is boiled with bastenga (bamboo shoot) till the water is soaked. After that these are kept in air tight container. At the time of requirement, they slightly warm it and take with rice. It is also used as sauce by mixing it with chilli and salt. They also use it as mouth freshener at the time of fever.

Mongotakong

It is made from any type of banana. First bananas are cut into pieces longitudinally and are kept dry in sunlight and in absence of sunlight it is also dried in fire place. It is taken as snacks with tea.

Alichitakong

It is a kind of potato. It is boiled in water with salt and then sliced and dried in the sunlight for 2-3 days. After properly dried these are kept in the air tight bottle. At the time of eating, they just fry it in oil and with sugar and are taken with tea.

Anichitakong

Takong means keep dry. The matured leaves of arum cultivated in jhum field are collected and these are then wrapped with banana leaves. The packet is then kept under heavy pressure for 3-4 days. Then these are grinded with wooden grinder (*hongki*) and keep it again in the same process for 1-2 days until liquid juice comes out. Then it is made soft by steam or by placing it near the hearth fire for 1-2 hours. After completing this whole process, the soften paste is mixed with chilli, *majenga* (a kind of spice), salt properly and make some small cakes and keep these cakes to dry for 2-3 days in the hearth fire. Sometimes, they make these cakes without mixing with chilli, *majenga* and salt. These cakes are finally kept in *makong* (a basket made of bamboo and cane) over the hearth for future consumption.

Akuni

It is made from a local variety of pulse which is available in their jhum field. At first the measured lentil is boiled in a aluminium saucepan with salt till the water is soaked and then it is kept above the hearth by wrapping it with a leaf (like banana leaf) locally available. They keep it in this way for 5-6 days until a fermented smell comes out from the prepared item. The people very much fond of this item and they take it with rice.

Utensils Used in the Kitchen

The people use different aluminium pots with large mouth such as *ketli, subu* etc. They also use steel utensils for the cooking and serving. Wooden as well as steel/aluminium ladle (*chikok*) are used. They use all steel and fibre dishes, bowls, cups etc. Drinking water is stored in the bucket (*bulti*).

Food under Special Circumstances

As noted earlier, in each cultural group, certain items are prescribed and some others are prohibited on certain specific occasions. The following pages have been devoted to have an understanding of the people's prescription and prohibition of various food items during different phases of life like disease, pre-natal and post-natal period, babyhood, marriage, festival, death etc.

Food during Disease

During the present investigation, it has been observed that the people by and large not very conscious regarding the need of some specific food items during any type of disease. This is due to their ignorance with regard to the correlation between disease and food. That is why there does not exist any restriction, even in case of serious diseases.

However, now-a-days, the educated people seem to have been relatively more conscious regarding the bad effects of certain food items during particular diseases.

In gastric they do not take any sour items. In wound, they do not take meat or fish item and take boil foods. They do not eat arum and brinjal during scabies. In cold and cough they avoid eating the leaves of arum. However, there are some medicinal plants (Chapter 7) which they use at the time of different ailments.

Food during Pregnancy and after Delivery

Among the people, no special food has been found to be provided to the pregnant woman. They take usual day-to-day meal. The people, by and large, are not aware of the fact that an expectant mother needs some extra care in respect of diet, as she takes diet for both herself and the fetus. That is why pregnant woman takes normal meal. Thus, it is quite likely that an expectant mother does not get the required amount of nutrient.

After delivery also, no special food has been found to be provided to the pregnant woman. Only for breast feeding they supply papaya.

Food during Babyhood

For the first year of their life, the infants are totally dependents on breast milk. Sometimes breast feeding is usually continued up to two-three years. After completion of 3/4 months semi-solid food is introduced. These are rice powder mixed with milk. After 6 months they give the baby rice with milk and other items.

Food during Birth Ritual, Marriage Ceremony, Death Ritual and in Festival

In all these rituals and occasions the food items are same. They take meat of pig and cow with rice in these occasions. They are very much fond of meat of pig and cow and in every occasion or ritual they take it as main item. However, depending on the economic condition, the number of food items and quantity may vary. The usual items include rice, vegetables, fish, pork/beef, sauce of chilli and dry fish.

The Mouth Refreshers and Narcotic Substances

The people, irrespective of age and sex have the habit of using betel-nut as an important mouth refreshing item. Most of the people any time chew a piece of betel-nut. It is also invariably offered to the guests and visitors as a mark of affectionate hospitality. The people feel that intake of betel-nut refreshes both the mouth and the mind.

Habitat of smoking *bidi* (tobacco rolled in leaf) among the males is also very common in the villages under study. From younger to older people, all use to smoke heavily and during study it has been observed that everyone smoke a *bidi* while interviewing them. But, the smoking habit is absent among the females.

Though Christianity abandoned them from intake of local alcoholic drinks (rice beer) but they are, both male and female, fond of to take the modern alcoholic drinks. Occasionally, they take it as available.

Food Storing and Preservation

People store the annual jhum product in the granary. Besides, paddy, some other crops, such as pumpkin, gourd etc. are also stored in the granary. The seeds (paddy) to be used in the

Plate No. 1

Views of Lirmen Village

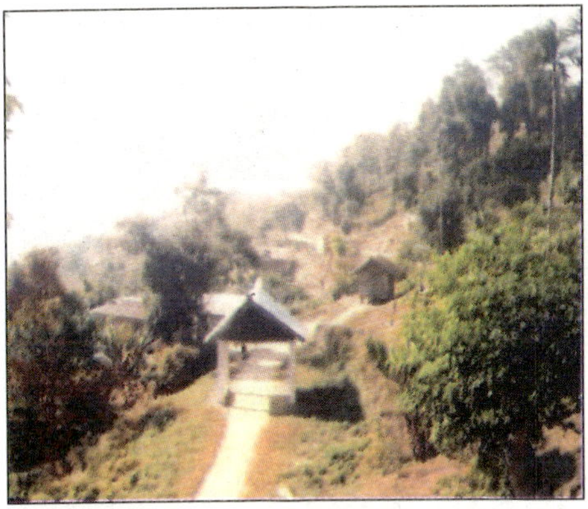

Lirmen Village

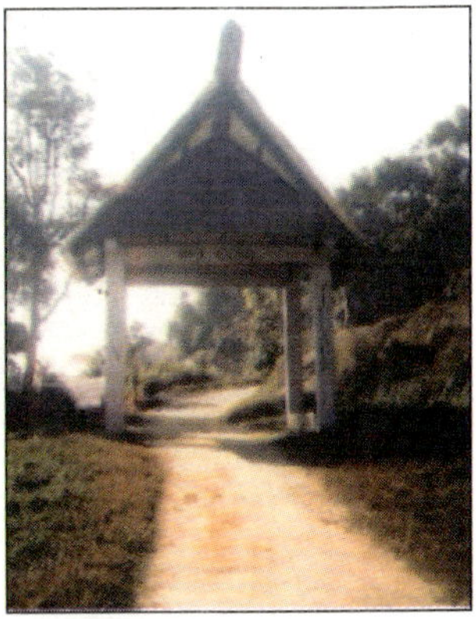

Entrance gate at Lirmen Village

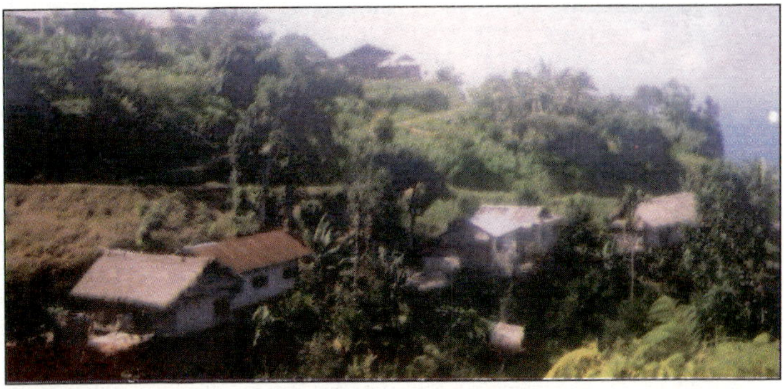

Yajang-A Village

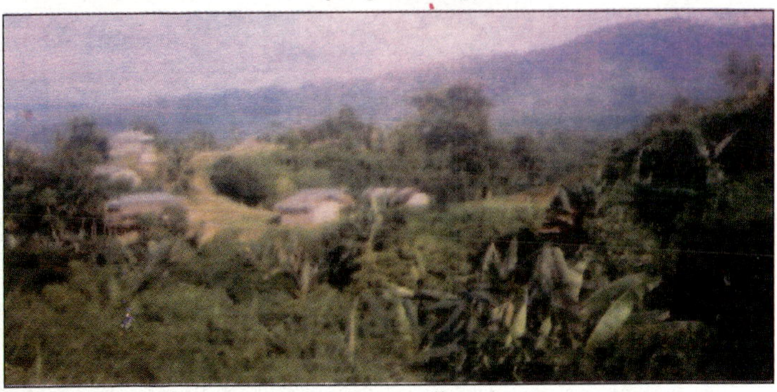

Yajang-B Village

Plate No. 2

Views of Lirmen Village (Contd.)

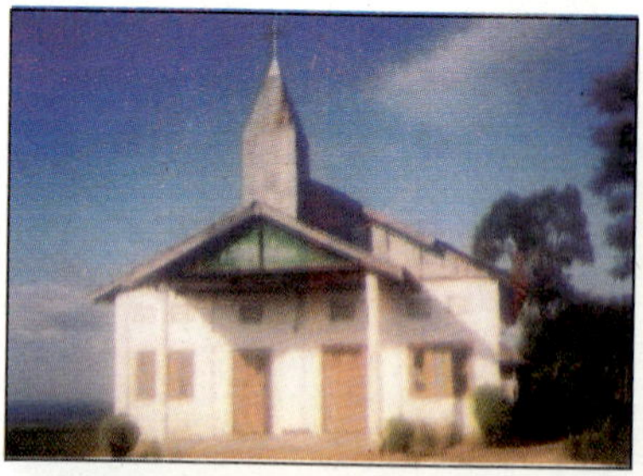

Baptist Church at Yajang-B Village

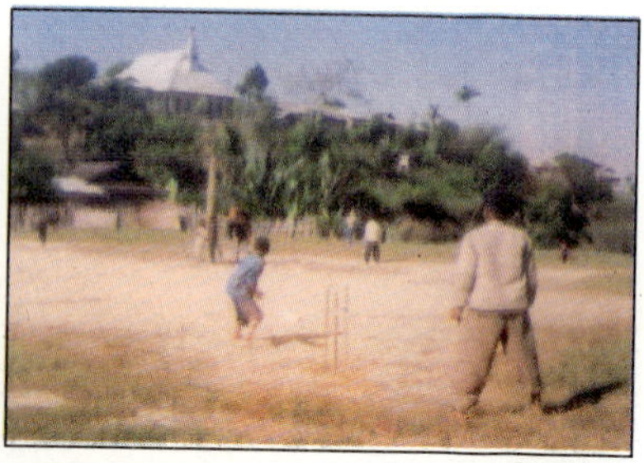

A playground at Yajang-A Village

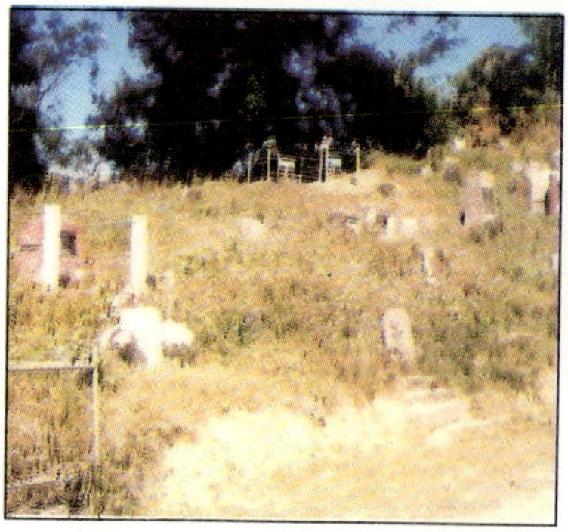

A burial ground at Lirmen Village

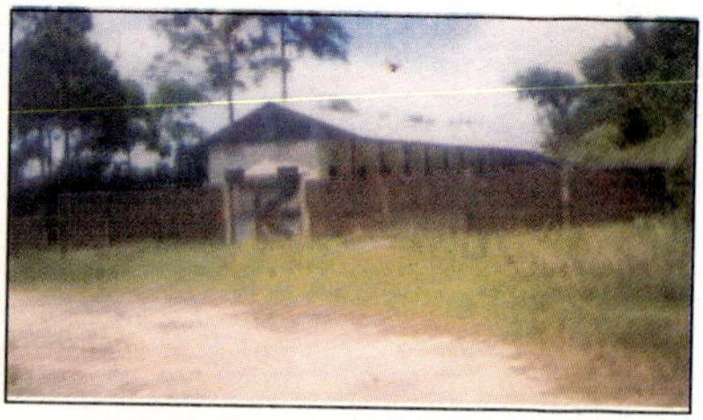

M.E. School at Lirmen Village

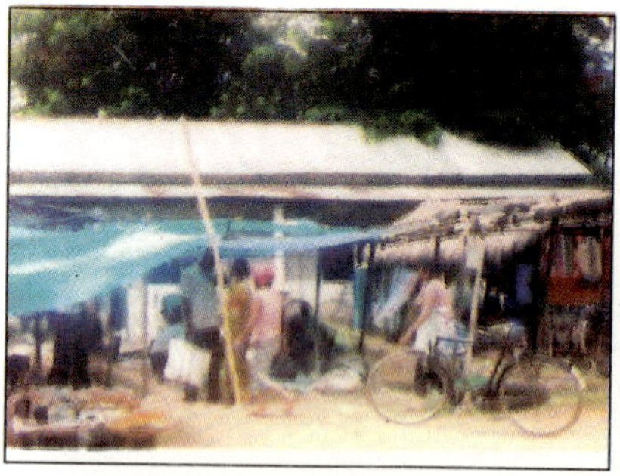

Weekly market at Assam-Nagaland Border

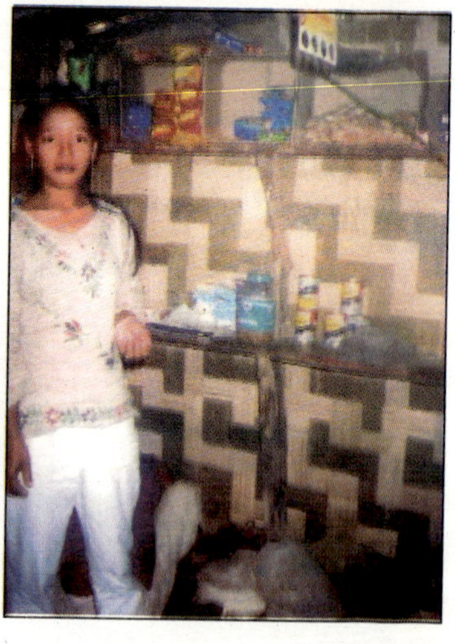

A village shop at Yajang-B Village

Plate No. 3

An Ao Naga Marriage Being Solemnized in the Church

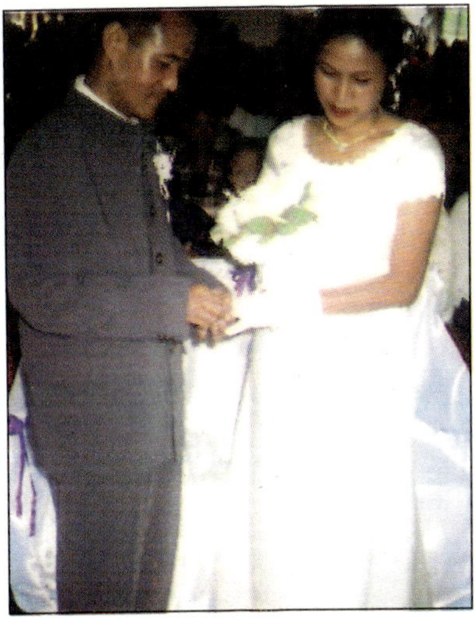

The groom and the birde exchange the wedding ring

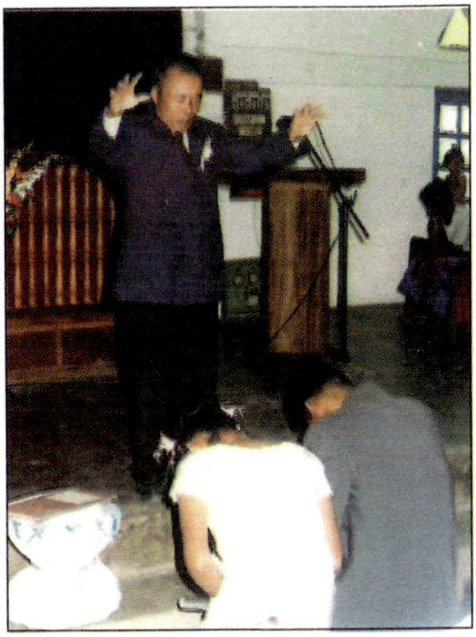

The Pastor blesses the couple and declares them husband and wife

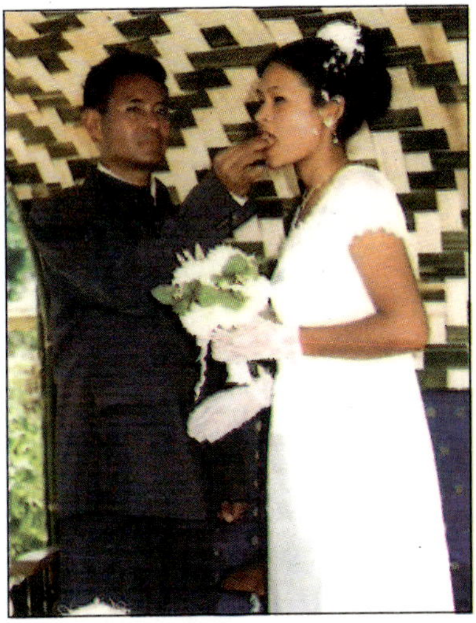

The bride and the groom shares the wedding cake

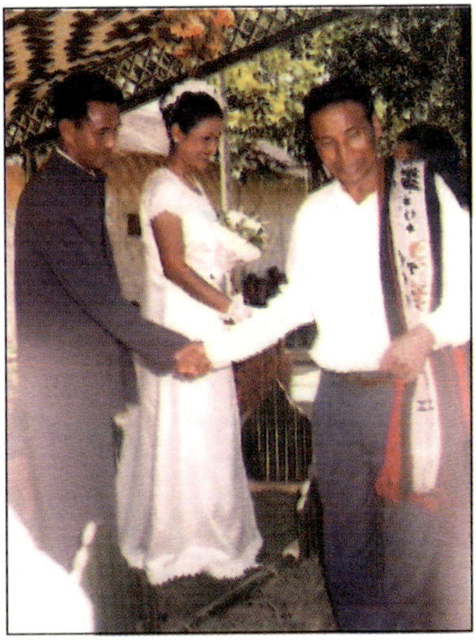

The wedding reception

Plate No. 4

Some Aspects of Religious Life

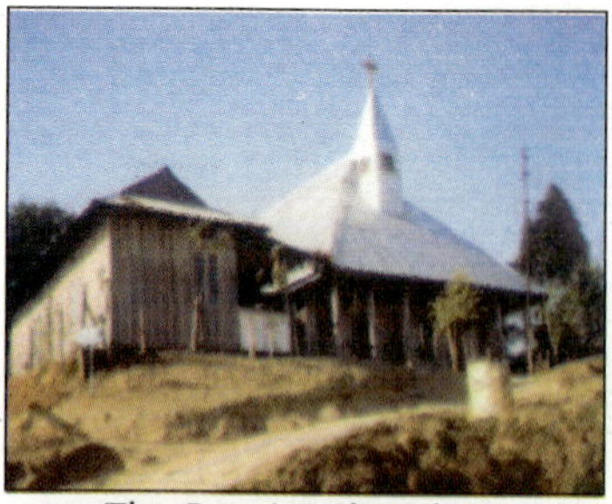

The Baptist Church at Yajang-A Village

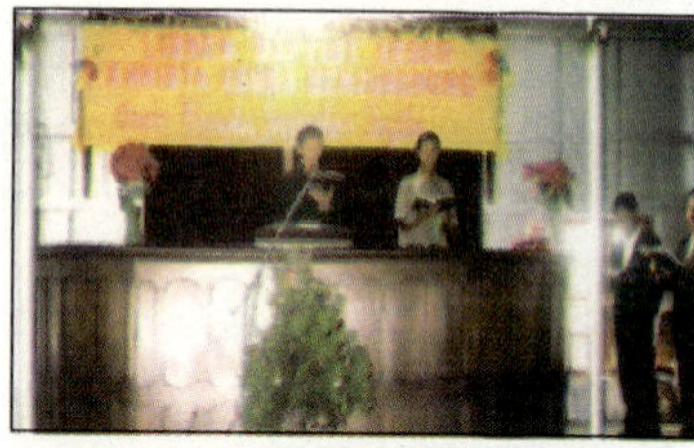

A Christmas prayer in Lirmen Baptist Church

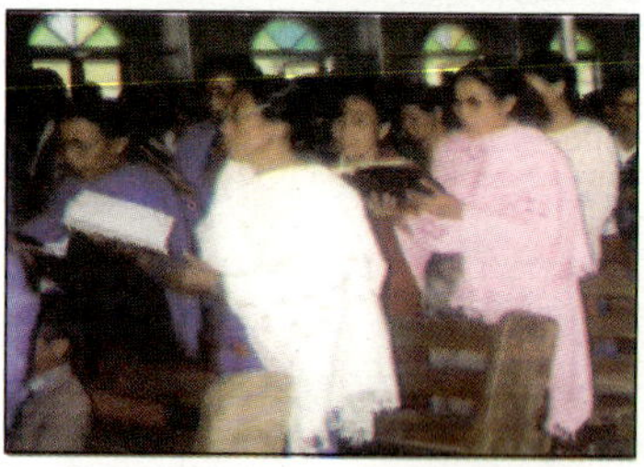

Chrismas service in progress in Lirmen Baptist Church

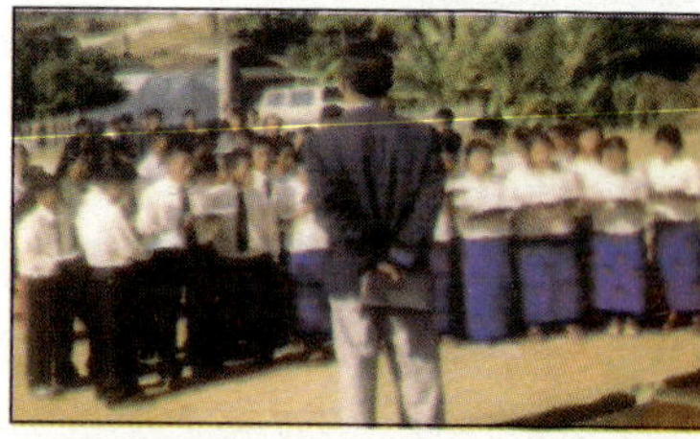

A Christmas carol in progress at Yajang-A Village

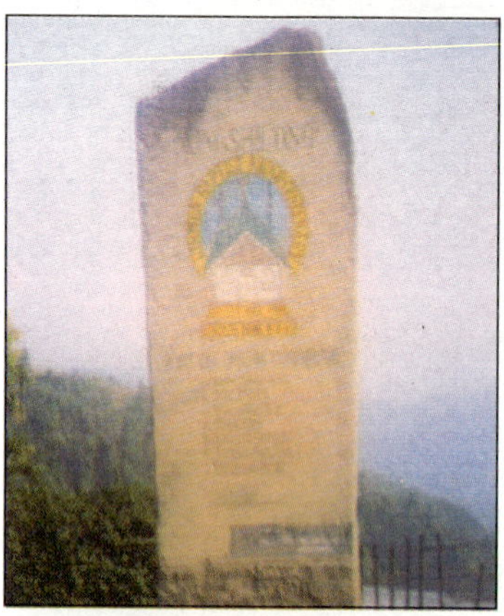

An epitaph depicting the first seven Ao Nagas who were Christianed in Lirmen Village in the year 1898

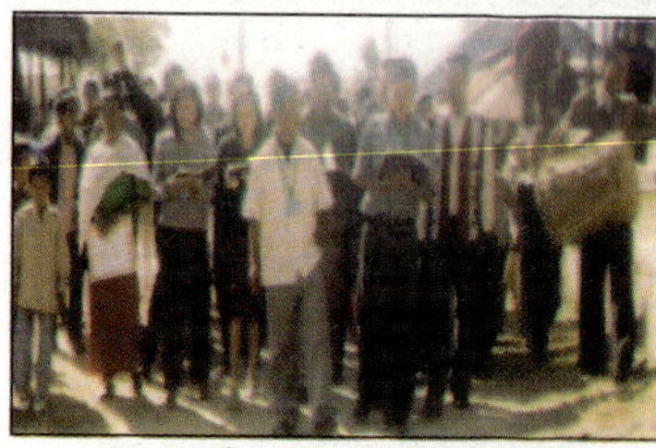

A carol singing group at Lirmen Village

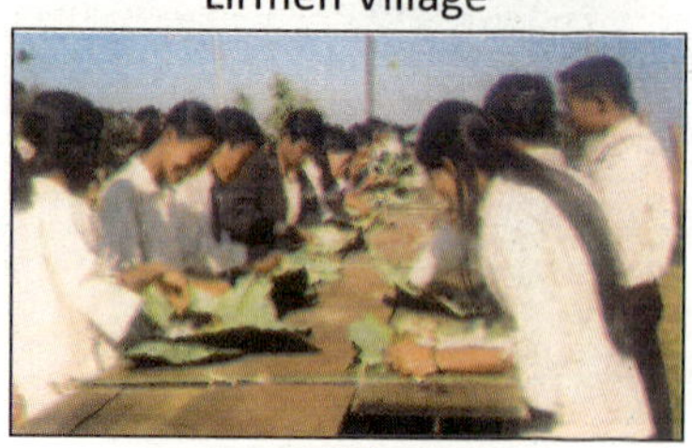

A Christmas feast at Yajang-A Village

Plate No. 5

Views of Moatsu Festival

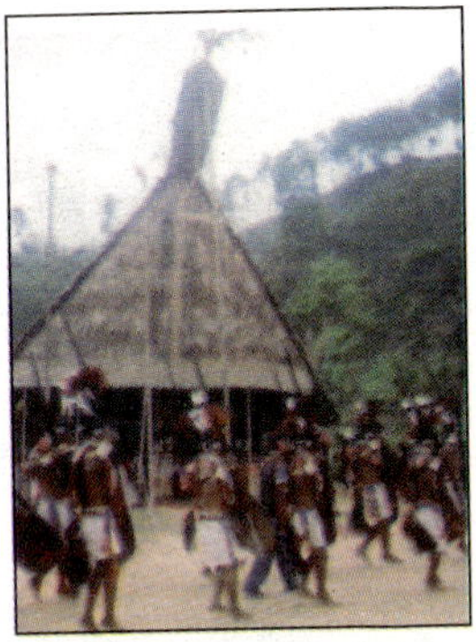

A moatsu dance in front of morung

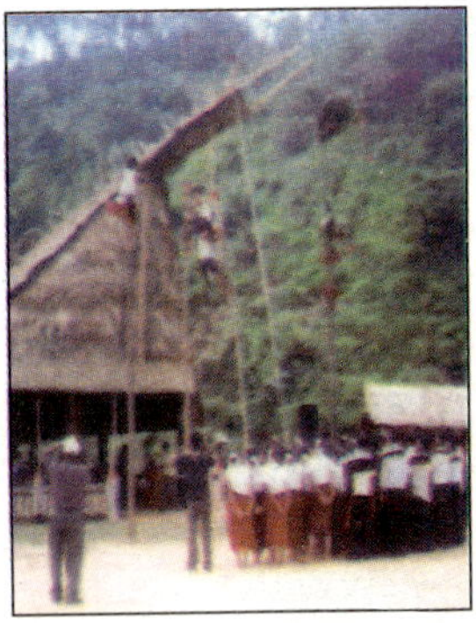

A moatsu pole climbing competition among the youths

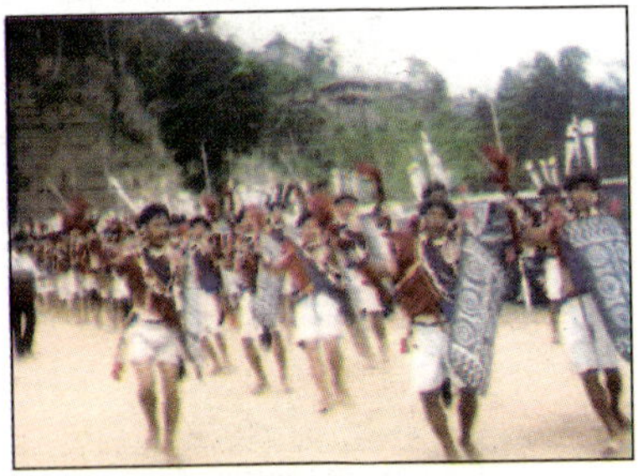

The dancers in their forms

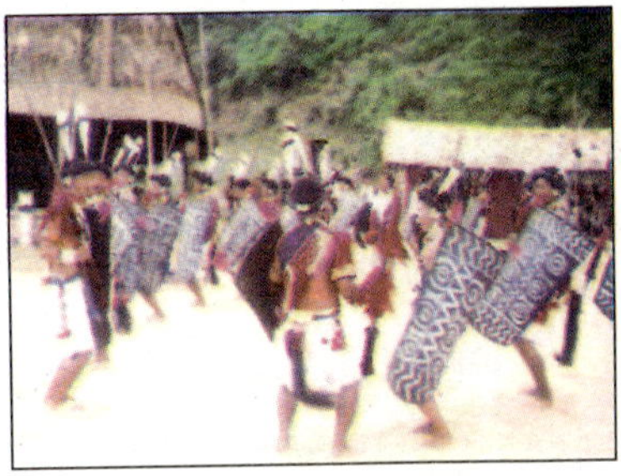

Moatsu dance in progress

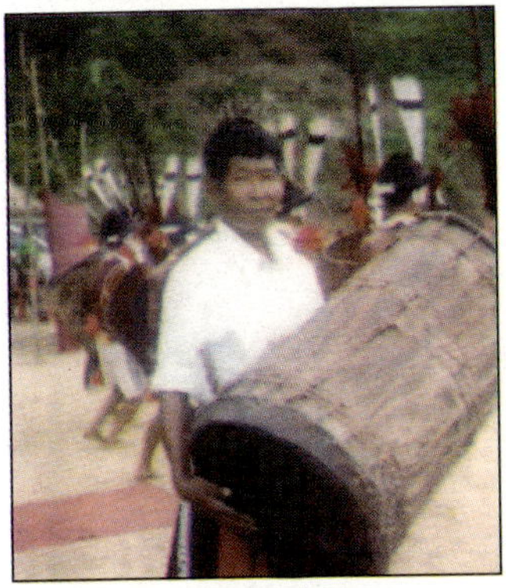

An Ao Naga drummer

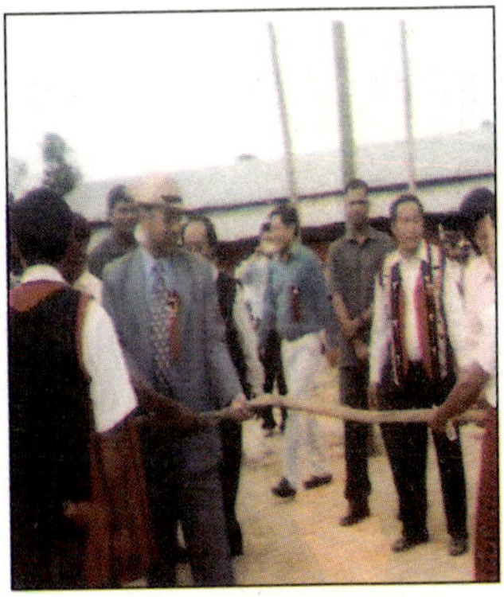

A tug of war competition

Plate No. 6

Reflecting Jhum Cultivation

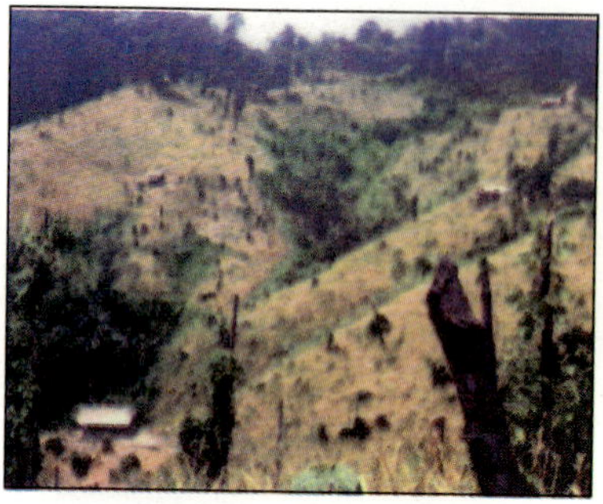

A view of the jhum field at Yajang-A Village

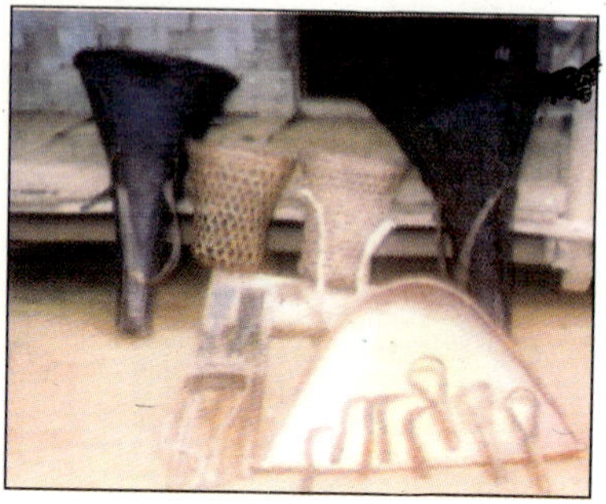

Traditional agricultural implements

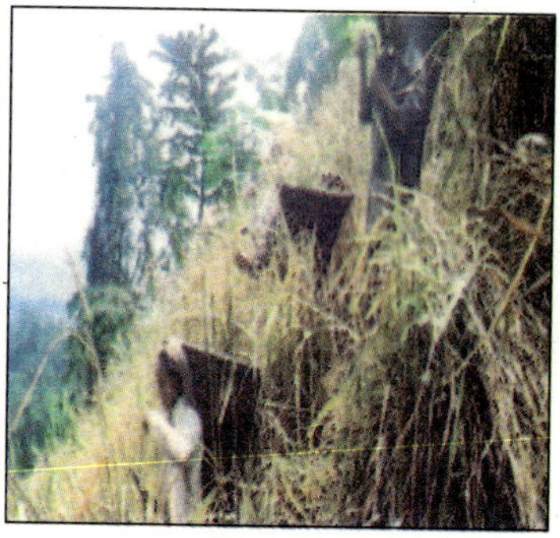

Harvesting the jhum

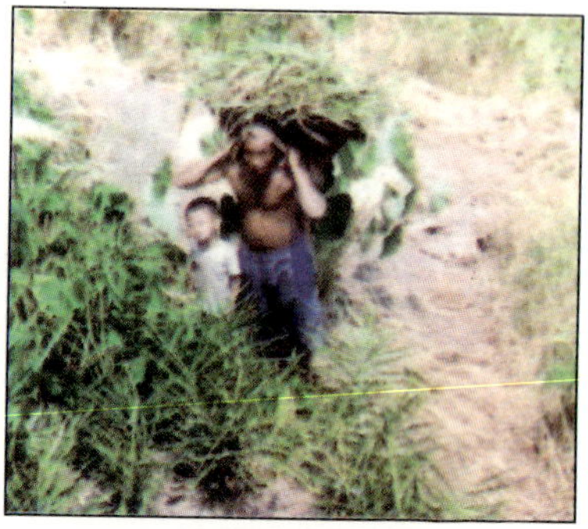

A man transporting the harvested paddy stalk

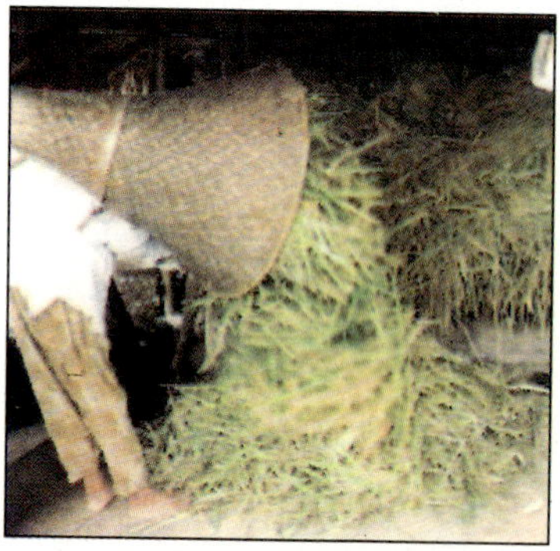

A view of the threshing floor

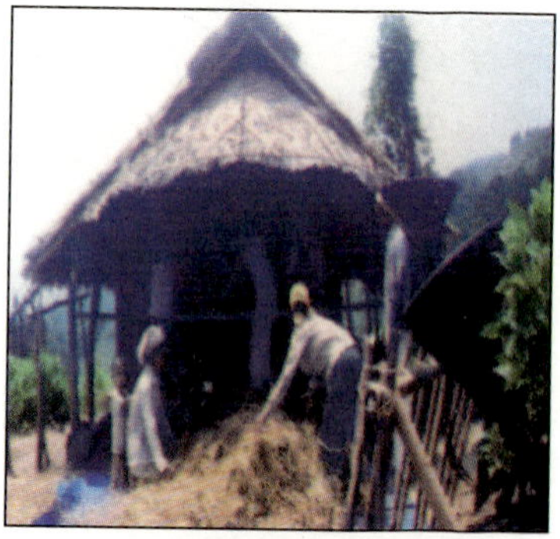

Threshing is in progress

Plate No. 7

Reflecting Traditional Dress and Ornaments

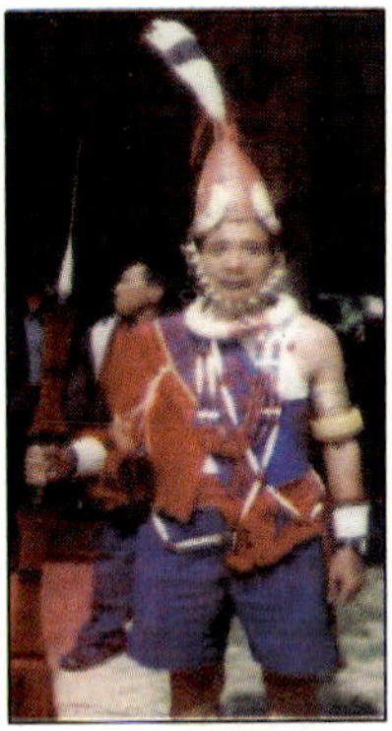

An old man in traditional dress

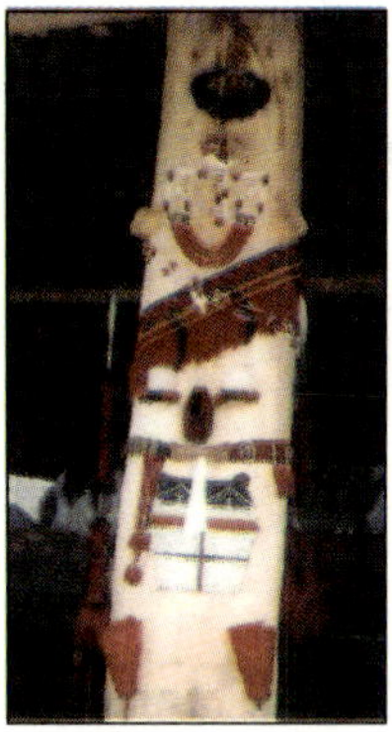

Traditional ornaments

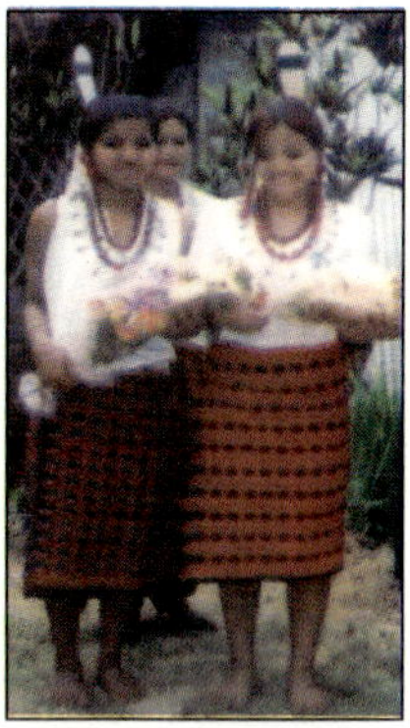

Girls in traditional dress

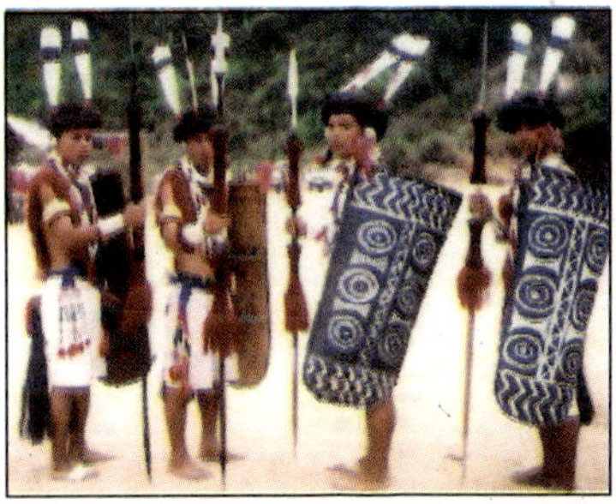

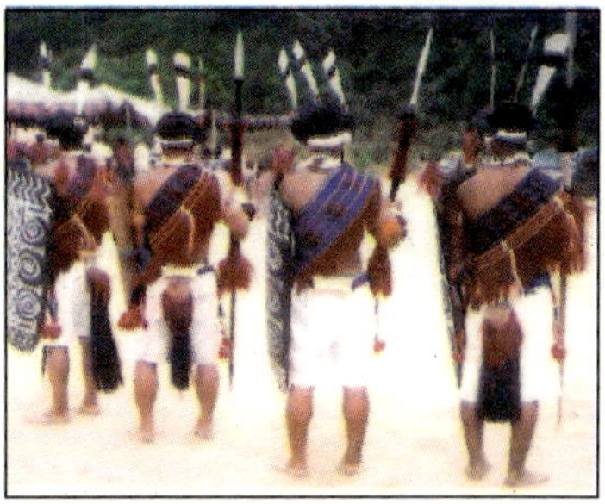

Boys in traditional dress

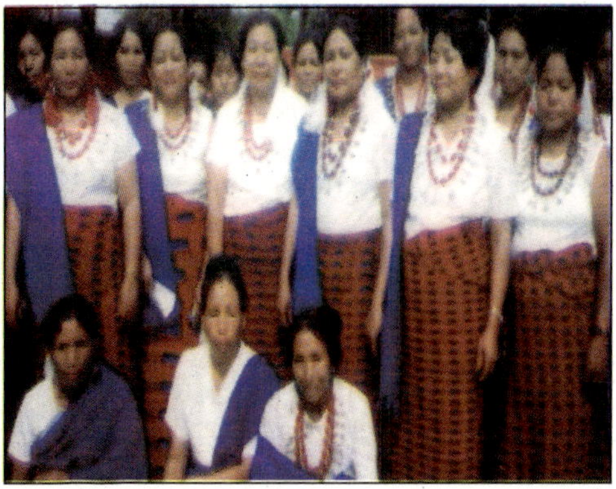

Women in traditional dress

Plate No. 8

Reflecting Food Habit

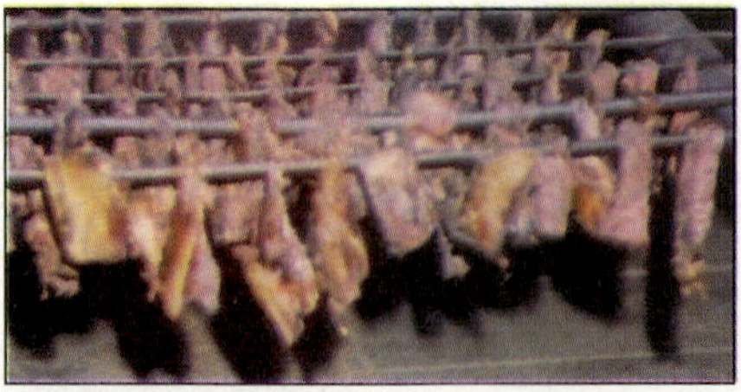

Meat

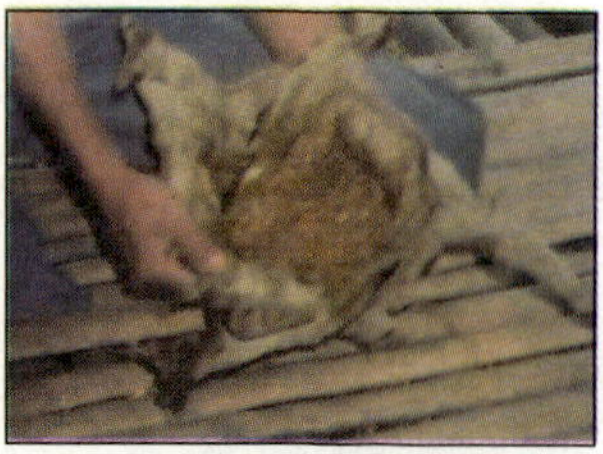

Fermented pulse (Akuni)

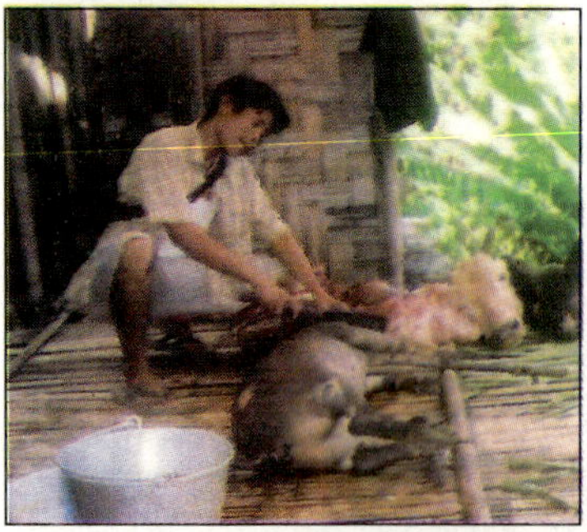

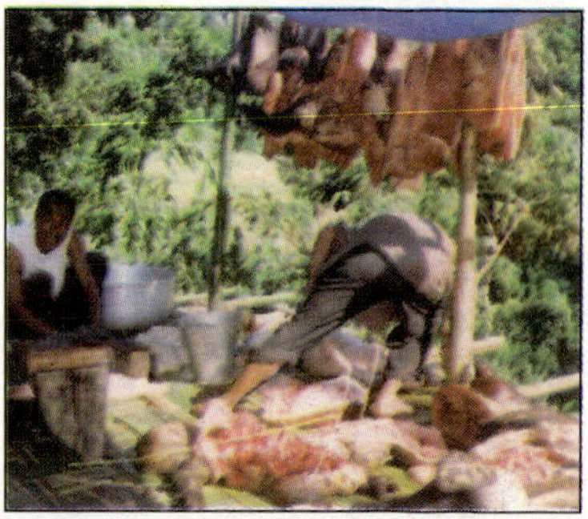

Pork and beef are chopped for a marriage feast

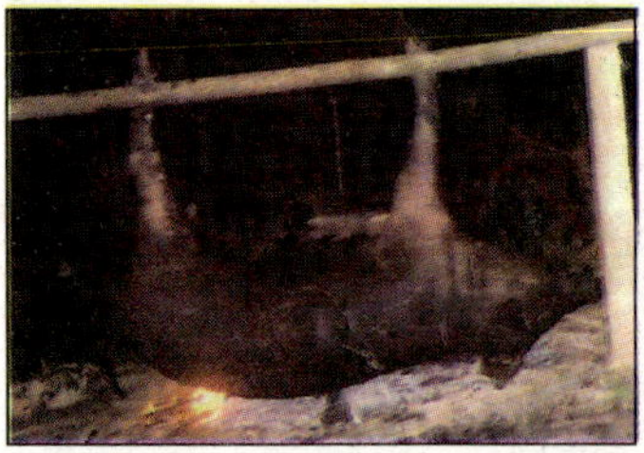

A Pig is being burnt for a feast

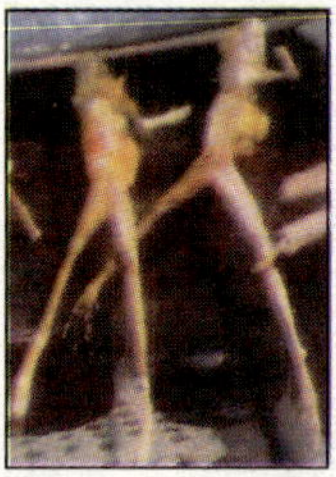

Roasted frog

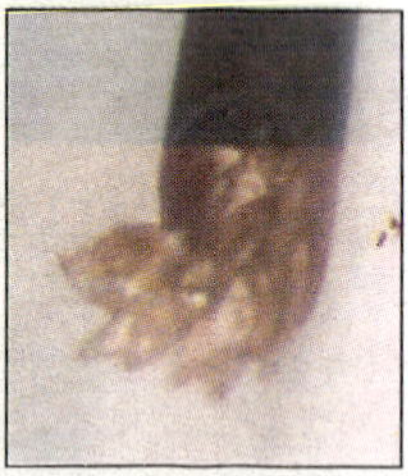

Dry fish

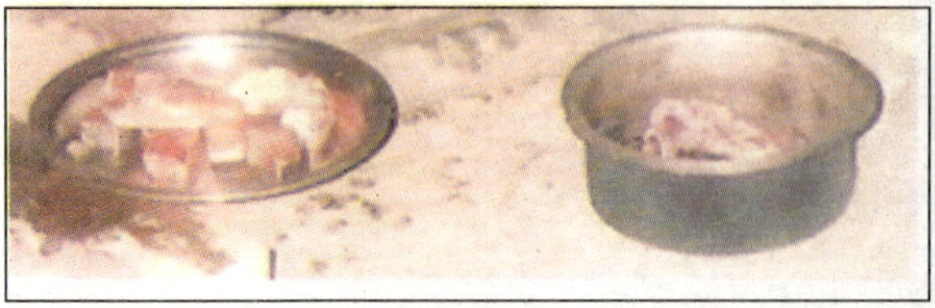

Fish

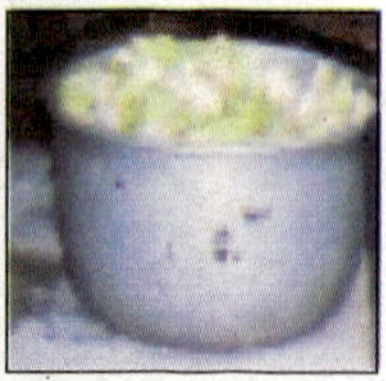

Bamboo shoot

next year are stored in rice bags. The paddies which are used for daily consumption are kept in a big bamboo and cane made basket in the granary.

For preservation, the hearth plays the most important role. As noted earlier, the food items preserved for the future consumption are placed on a bamboo platform above the hearth. In this platform they generally keep the things in the bamboo pipes which is corked by a leaf (like banana leaf) to air tight. The items which are kept in these bamboo pipes are dry fish, seeds of bitter gourd, seeds of different crops etc. Besides, these they also keep brinjal, lady's finger, kidney bean and corn as open on the bamboo platform for future use in the jhum fields. Even the meat of animals killed in a hunting expedition or brought from market is not immediately consumed, a portion is smoked over the family hearth and preserved on the platform above the hearth for future consumption.

They also keep the excess uncooked pieces of fish for future consumption by slight heating the pieces in the hearth fire and then the pieces are smoked over the family hearth for future consumption.

They store the bamboo shoots in plastic jar and bottle by filling water in it for future consumption and keep it as air-tight.

The other items such as powder milk, tea, sugar, turmeric powder, mustard oil, rice etc. are kept in the airtight plastic jars.

The people store water in the bamboo pipes, as they have to carry it from the water tanks in these bamboo pipes. This water is used for all their household works.

The above discussion thus makes it apparent that their total food intake is by and large insufficient to provide the required nutrient input. It may be due to the fact that most of the people do not attach any importance to the correlation between diet and their proper health. They generally give priority to the quantity rather than the quality of food.

In general, the people do not have the idea of the need of a balanced diet. They have the belief that flesh foods (viz. meat and fish items) contain all the required nutrients for the baby.

On the whole, it seems, ignorance, poverty and negligence play their respective roles in the community to deprive the people of having a proper and balanced diet for maintaining a desirable health.

LIVING CONDITION

The overall living condition of a group of people refers to the housing facilities, availability of drinking water, the quality of personal hygiene, toilet system etc. All these factors do influence the total health scenario of the members of a community to a significant extent.

Housing Condition

Along with food and clothing, shelter is regarded as a basic need for human life. Housing condition refers to house type including the provision of proper light and ventilation etc., average space available to an inmate of the household and the other associated facilities required for a healthy living.

Housing is one of the basic requirements for human survival. For a normal citizen, owning a house means significant economic security and dignity in society (Selvarajan and Elango, 2004). The quality of our home environment has an important bearing on our quality of life and it also has pervasive effect on our health and our relationships with other people.

According to Sharma (2001), "Housing is a major health resource can protect individuals from physical and mental ill health. Alternatively it can increase their vulnerability, depending on the standard, location and type of accommodation they live in. Like food and eating, poor housing affects health directly through physiological processes and indirectly through behavioural and psychological processes. Housing conditions also help or hinder parents, particularly mothers, in their role as careers. For parents living on the breadline, parenting in poor housing becomes an even more arduous task. Homes can be a major source of personal wealth. They can be used for investment or collateral or as a way of passing on wealth. In this sense, housing is a key resource that can meditate a family's access to other health resources, such as leisure, transport and health care facilities. Furthermore, housing is also a marker of social status and a marker of social mobility."

Housing condition is an important determinant of human health. Housing should be given high planning priority. Proper and adequate shelter is a must for healthy life because it enhances the performance of the residents in their domestic and economic duties (Rahman, 1998).

WHO defines a house as the residential environment the physical structure that man uses for shelter and the environment surrounding it, including all necessary services, facilities, equipments and devices needed or desired for physical and mental health and social well-being of a family (cited in Kumar and Kumar, 1987).

The World Health Organization (WHO) in one of its recent publications, summarizes the health implications of housing in the following statements (cited in Tewari, 1991)

> "Housing is intimately related to health. The structure, location, facilities, environment and use of human shelter have a strong impact on the state of physical, mental and social well-being. Poor housing conditions and uses may provide weak defenses against death, disease and injury or even increase vulnerability to them. Adequate and appropriate housing conditions, on the other hand, not only protect people against

health hazards but also help to promote robust physical health, economic productivity, psychological well-being and social vigour."

A document prepared by United Nations Centre for Human Settlements (UNCHS-Habitat) for presentation at the 1998 Healthy Public Policy Conference at Adelaide has emphasized the role of housing in healthy living. As observed in this document, though the relationship between housing and health is both intimate and complex and is compounded by a myriad of factors such as poverty, nutrition, levels of income, literacy etc., which act together to defy the establishment of precise links, even so it can be said that poor housing is always associated with high mortality and morbidity rates (cited in Tewari, 1991).

WHO, in a study to assess the extent of morbidity and mortality resulting from specific pathological conditions which are most obviously related to housing; estimated that 5 million deaths, i.e. 10 per cent of all deaths worldwide, could be prevented if housing conditions everywhere in the world could meet safe standard levels. WHO also estimated that at least two to three million cases of permanent disability could be prevented through improved housing (cited in Tewari, 1991).

With regard to minimum housing requirements, 'National Housing Code in India' recommended the following standards (cited in Kumar and Kumar, 1987) :

(a) *Site:* (i) The site should be elevated from its surroundings so that it is not subject to flooding during rains, (ii) the site should have an independent access to a street of adequate width, (iii) it should be away from the breeding places of mosquitoes and flies, (iv) it should be away from nuisances such as dust, smoke, smell, excessive noise and traffic, (v) it should be in pleasing surroundings, and (vi) the soil should be dry and safe for founding the structure and should be well drained. The sub-soil water should be below 10 feet.

(b) *Set back:* For proper lighting and ventilation, there should be an open space all-round the house this is called "set back".

(c) *Floor:* The floor should be pucca and satisfy the following criteria : (i) it should be impermeable so that it can be easily washed and kept clean and dry, (ii) the floor must be smooth and free from cracks and crevices, (iii) rhe floor should be damp-proof, and (iv) the height of the plinth should be 2 to 3 feet.

(d) *Walls:* The walls should be (i) reasonably strong, (ii) should have a low heat capacity, i.e. should not absorb heat and conduct the same, (iii) weather resistant, (iv) unsuitable for harbourage of rats and vermin, (v) not easily damaged, and (vi) smooth. These standards can be attained by 9 inch brick-wall plastered smooth and coloured cream or white.

(e) *Roof:* The height of the roof should not be less than 10 feet.

(f) *Rooms:* The number of living rooms should not be less than two. The number of area of rooms should be increased according to size of the family.

(g) *Floor area:* The floor area of a living room should be at least 120 sq. ft. for occupancy by more than one person and at least 100 sq. ft. for occupancy by a single person.

(h) *Cubic space:* The height of rooms should be such as to give an air space of at least 500 c.ft. per capita, preferably 1,000 c.ft.

(i) *Windows:* (i) Unless mechanical ventilation and artificial lighting are provided, every living room should be provided with at least 2 windows and at least one of them should open directly on to an open space, (ii) the windows should be placed at a height of not more than 3 feet above the ground in living rooms, and (iii) windows area should be 1/5th of the floor area. Doors and windows combined should have 2/5th of the floor area.

(j) *Lighting:* The day light factor should exceed 1 per cent over half the floor area.

(k) *Kitchen:* Every dwelling house must have a separate kitchen. The kitchen must be protected against dust and smoke; adequately lighted; provided with arrangements for storing food, fuel and provisions; provided with water supply; provided with sink for washing utensils and fitted with arrangements for proper drainage.

(l) *Privy:* A sanitary privy is a must in every house, belonging exclusively to it and readily accessible. In the developed areas, the majority of dwelling units are equipped with water carriage systems.

(m) *Garbage and refuse:* These should be removed from the dwelling at least daily and disposed of in a sanitary manner.

(n) *Bathing and washing:* The house should have facilities for bathing and washing belonging exclusively to it and provided proper privacy.

(o) *Water supply:* The house should have a safe and adequate water supply available at all times.

Therefore, a house having all these facilities is considered to be fit for human habitation. It also helps to maintain good health. Thus, home is to some extent responsible for the status of man's health and well-being. It is difficult, however, to demonstrate the specific cause and effect relationship because housing embraces so many facets of environment. By deductive reasoning, a strong relationship can be established between poor housing and the following conditions (cited in Kumar and Kumar, 1987) :

(a) *Respiratory infection:* Common cold, tuberculosis, influenza, diphtheria, bronchitis, measles, whooping cough, etc.

(b) *Skin infection:* Scabies, ringworm, impetigo, leprosy.

(c) *Rat infection:* Plague.

(d) *Arthropods:* House flies, mosquitoes, fleas and bugs.

(e) *Accidents:* A substantial proportion of house accidents are caused by some defect in the home and its environment.

(f) *Morbidity and mortality:* High morbidity and mortality rates are observed where housing conditions are substandard.

(g) *Psychological effects:* These effects must not be overlooked. The sense of isolation felt by persons living in the upper floors of high buildings is now well known to have harmful effects.

With this background of the ideal requirements, in the following pages, an attempt has been made to have an idea about the ground reality with regard to the housing and other associated facilities, available to the people under investigation.

As the villages under study are situated on the steep slope of the hill, houses are arranged from little below the top of hill to the bottom in a gallery. Except a few houses which are constructed on levelled land in certain parts of the village (constructed on a bamboo frame based on piles on all sides), all the rest have their front portion resting on the hill side and the back portion raised on piles. The height of the piles varies in accordance with the steepness of the slope of the hill in that particular portion. The dwellings of the Aos are situated in clusters of thirty to hundred houses forming what are called settlements. Houses are arranged on both sides of the village path with entrances on sides just from the path or through the courtyards. There is no plan in the arrangements of the houses and also there is no restriction in the facing. The floor space of a house varies with the size of the family. Most of the compound of a house is not demarcated with any fencing and most of the houses are very close to one another. In some case the back of one house faces the front of the other.

General Plan of the House

A typical Ao house for a nuclear family is rectangular in plan and has two main parts; a front room (*surujakdak*) which serves as a parlour and an inner room as bedroom (*ayiptak*). The roofless projection of the platform serves as a verandah (*sunglang*) used for drying up the crops and cleaning the dirty utensils and also for washing cloths. One corner of the platform is also used as bathroom (*metshumushi*) for bathing as well as urinal. There is only one door at the entrance. A wooden ladder (*apo*) is used for climbing up the floor.

The front room is about 13 ft. length and is about 15 ft. in breadth is used by the family for receiving the guests. The rear portion of the room is used for keeping household articles. The fire place (hearth) is also constructed in a corner either right or left side in this room. The hearth is generally plastered with mud and is about 5 sq. ft. About 4 ft. above the hearth a square bamboo rack known as (*chakten*), is kept hanging from the ceiling where spices and other odds and ends are kept. The carrying baskets and straps are also kept on this rack for smoking. Some of the collected firewood is also stored in one side of the hearth. In some houses, in this room, i.e. parlour-cum-kitchen there are some bamboo and wooden racks on the walls to keep the cooking and other utensils. Thus, there is no separate dining room and kitchen; food is taken in this same room. During the winter season most of the hearths are kept lit throughout the whole day and night to keep the room warm. There is no notable furniture in the room, however, some of them possess a few plastic chairs and wooden chairs. There is one door in the entrance of this room and a window in the opposite side of the door. The door is about 3 ft. in breadth and the window is about 2 ft. in breadth.

The inner room or bedroom is partitioned from the front room by a bamboo partition and there is about a 3 ft. door in between the two rooms. There is also a 2 ft. window in the bedroom. Generally, the people use mattress and also the wooden planks for sleeping. On one side of the wall of this room, used cloths of male and female members of the house are kept hang. Some families also possess dressing table in this room.

The open space (roofless) in the side of the front room (which is raised on piles) is known as *sunglang*. It is raised on wooden or bamboo piles and projecting over the slope of the hill. It is about 11 ft. in length and 10 ft. in breadth. The floor of the platform is made of bamboo. The water for domestic use is preserved here in large drums or pitchers and all household works, as for example, cleaning utensils, sunning the paddy, washing cloths, etc., are done here. There is one verandah in the entrance of the house which runs along the axis of the house and is known as *kazutak*. In some families this *kazutak* is guarded with bamboo or wooden railings and is about 26 ft. in length and 6 ft. in breadth. Depending on the plan of the house the place of construction of the *sunglang* also varies. In some families this *sunglang* is constructed in the back side of the front room. On the whole, this *sunglang* most ingeniously secured, meet up to a certain extent the demand of domestic space on such a steep hill. Towards the extreme end of the *sunglang*, there is a small enclosure (*metsumushi*) of 5 sq. ft. which is used by the inmates as lavatory and for bathing.

Very few exceptions do not have separate granary and the crops are stored within the household. The paddy is stored in huge baskets made of plaited bamboo which is kept in a corner of the verandah. Most of the families possess a separate granary which is very near to the house. There is no provision of latrine within the house and latrines are constructed outside the house at a little distance. The people do not take milk except a little with tea and a few of them keep cows mainly for the supply of bullock to be used in ploughing the paddy fields. Outside the house the people construct the fowl pen and the pig sty. In some families the latrine, fowl pen and the pig sty are constructed in the same row and all these are constructed on the steep slope of the hill.

Thus, there is no plan in the arrangement of the houses and also there is no restriction in the facing. But an uniformity is observed in one respect; all the houses including the fowl pen, pig sty and latrines are constructed on the steep slope of the hill by resting the front portion on the hills and the back portion raised on the piles.

As the houses are constructed on the steep slope of the hill, courtyards are not generally met with. House on certain portions where the land is a bit levelled, have courtyards or open sandy pitches in front or on sides, without any boundary wall. A temporary shed is constructed at the back or side of the houses for keeping firewood to be used during the rainy season. Sometimes firewood is stored beneath the house which is raised on piles. Most of the houses have gardens of betel nut or other fruit trees twisted with the betel leaf creepers. There is no boundary or compound wall of the houses (except a few houses with loose bamboo fencing). The boundaries of the gardens are identified with rows of trees.

Material use for Construction

Though the construction of a typical house is same, variations in respect of construction and materials used in the same is observed in a few cases depending on their economic condition.

They have their own cultural beliefs and traditional customs in the construction of house.

A typical Ao house is rectangular in shape and it is built on stilts and above the ground. As noted earlier, the height of the piles varies in accordance with the steepness of the slope of the hill in that particular portion. Generally, in construction of a house, use of bamboo is very important. They use bamboo for all purposes in a house such as in the construction of platform, side walls, roof etc. There are two types of bamboo which are found in their locality; one is light known as *ani* and the other is heavy known as *longmi*. The light (*ani*) is used in the construction of the side walls (*jara*) of the house while the heavy (*longni*) is used in the construction of the floor (*atam*). The floor of a house space varies with the size of the family.

The roof is generally two-sloped and *toko* leaves are used for thatching the roof. Tying material is cane. The *toko* leaves for the roof are tied with bamboo strips. The partitions, which are made of bamboo in between two rooms, do not reach the roof. All the side walls, partitions and the floors are made of reed or plaited bamboo. The only difference is the type of bamboo use in the making of side walls and partitions and in the making of floor.

The two most important articles in house construction are bamboo and *toko* (*sara*) leaves which are available in their forest. The villagers go to the forest and cut bamboo and *toko* leaves from their respective land as they require for construction. Usually in the months of December to March before the approach of monsoon, the new construction, repairing and re-thatching of roof are done. They have the belief that if they cut bamboo in the monsoon season, the bamboo does not last for long period and it might be damaged by insect within one week. So, every year in this period (December-March), the villagers repair their houses and re-thatch their roofs. In this process, the clan members help each other. Generally, after constructing a new house, the owner of that particular house whether married or unmarried invites the village council members and church members on a auspicious day as a house warming ceremony before taking the new house. The suitable day is selected by owner on a week day and not on Sunday as they do not work on Sunday. Then all the invitees are entertained with a feast. Depending on their economic condition they arrange this feast and sometimes only tea and biscuits are given.

Construction of a house is not very expensive in hilly areas in comparison to valley, as the materials are found in the forest that requires only physical labour. They are also very fond of constructing traditional types of small hut whenever needed and wherever they go, for cultivation or in any farming area to take rest, eat and sleep whenever necessary in order to be protected from sun, rain, cold and wild animals etc. In the traditional practices the roofs of the houses are slanting downward with less number of windows making it so steep that rainwater easily falls down. But now, these traditional types of roofing of the houses are not seen among the people under study. In the past, the walls of the houses were decorated with heads of the animals like wild pig, buffaloes, tigers, etc. and beautiful birds' feather, which indicates the degree of expertise and brevity in hunting animal. During the present investigation, in a few houses, similar decorations are observed. However, in all bamboo made dwelling houses, they cover walls with newspaper. In some houses one can also witness different means of embellishment in which things like posters, clocks, etc. are employed to fill up the empty looking walls.

As a sign of improved economic condition with better educational knowledge variations are seen in few families and they start making completely modern type of houses with improved building, materials and bricks. However, it is very less in number and in the present investigation, two such types of houses are found in Lirmen village. A few families also have C.I. sheet as roofing and few of them also use wood both for the platform and floor as well as for side walls of the house.

But in some houses roofs are still covered by thatch and all other parts are made by bamboo, which in reality indicates traditional old customary type.

Personal Hygiene

The quality of personal hygiene is also an important factor that has tremendous influence on the overall health scenario of a cultural group. The term personal hygiene includes the habits and practices of day-to-day life, with regard to bathing, washing of clothes, cleaning of teeth, trimming of nails, sleeping habit and practices of abolution etc. Any disruption of these activities may impair health. For example, neglect of oral hygiene may predispose to tooth and gum ailments, neglect of personal cleanliness may predispose to scabies, eczema and fungal infection etc. (Kumar and Kumar, 1987). Thus, all these influences the overall health scenario of a person in particular and a community in general.

During the present investigation all efforts have been made to collect as much as data possible, on different aspects of day to day life of the people with regard to their maintenance of personal cleanliness.

The houses do not seem to be very clean. In most of the houses, there are no proper windows and other means of light and ventilation. Because of scarcity of light and air, at any time of the day the inner side of a house always remains dark and stuffy. The situation worsens because of the smoke that is generated from the hearths that remain lit for almost 24 hours at least in winter season. The floor in most of the houses is dirty. The people sit and sleep on the floor without putting anything on it. After meal they wash their mouths and hands where they sit and the interspaces allow the water go down. In case home delivery, it has been observed that discharges come out from the delivery mother also go down between the interspaces of the floor.

Bathing is one of the most important aspects of the people's life and is reflected of the level of their personal cleanliness. The people use one corner of the bamboo platform as both for urinal and for bathing. These enclosures are made of bamboo and none of these has any roof. They never pour water after urine and there is always a smell of urine in the enclosure and as such the enclosure does not provide a hygienic environment for taking bath.

With regard to bathing habit, however, it has been observed that both menfolk and womenfolk take bath only one time after returning home from the jhum field. Non-working persons usually take their bath in the mid-day after completing the household works. All the people take bath only one time whether summer or winter. Generally during the winter many of them do not take bath regularly.

Use of toilet soap has been found to be reasonably infrequent among the people under investigation. Though the toilet soap or shampoo is not an unknown item for them but use of these items depends on the economic condition of the people. However, a few elite members do use the same while bathing.

Regarding the washing of clothes it has been observed that the people use to wash their clothes on Sunday as they get free time. The children as well as the elderly members are very often found to be in dirty clothes. However, the youths and the educated members have been found to relatively more conscious with regard to cleanliness of their dress as well as body. Generally on Sunday everyone looks very neat and clean with proper dress while going to Church.

With regard to the cleaning of teeth, it has been observed that most of the people under investigation do not clean their teeth regularly. Majority of them use to brush their teeth with charcoal, betel nut peel and a few use tooth paste and tooth brush. However, all the educated young boys and girls have been found to use tooth paste and tooth brush.

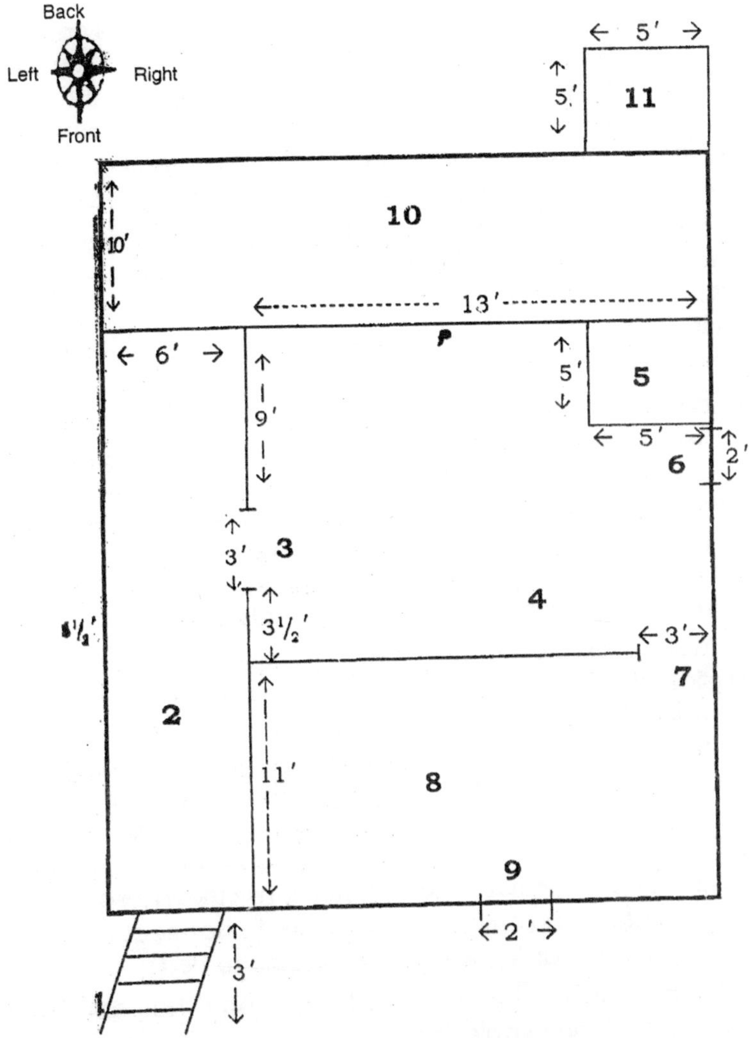

1. Ladder (apo)
2. Open front platform (kazutak)
3. Front door
4. Front room (*Surjakdak*)
5. Hearth
6. Wiondow
7. Door to inner room
8. Sleeping room (*ayiptuk)*
9. Window
10. Open back platform (*sungtang*)
11. Bathroom cum Urinal (metsumushi)

Fig. 6.1 : House Plan of a typical Ao Dwelling (Showing internal arrangements)

Trimming of nails is not done at regular intervals and they do it whenever they find nails conspicuously long. They use a blade or a knife for this purpose. Children and infant depend upon their mothers for this purpose. Sometimes these become very long and dirt accumulates under the same and they generally do not wash their hands before taking meals.

On the other hand shaving of beards and hair cuts are not their regular practice. Menfolk rarely go to the nearest hair cutting shop (saloon) for the purpose and mostly they cut each other in the village. The women and girls also cut hair by helping each other.

Habit of sleeping is another one important factor, intimately connected with issues of health and disease. Though all the people under investigation possess pile dwelling house but most of the houses have only two rooms. Thus, for a bigger family (where the numbers of children are more) the accommodation becomes relatively overcrowded and as such the sleeping arrangement becomes congested and unhealthy.

In summer, most of them are seen to sleep on the floor by the side of the hearth. The children also sleep on the floor. They do not use any cot. During winter, they feel very cold due to bamboo construction which may be considered as an important factor contributing towards the frequent incidence of cough, cold, pneumonia etc. Very frequently they use blankets, shawls etc. Use of mosquito net is also found to be irregular and in the day time they never use this mosquito net for their infant and children. They also do not seem to have the habit of face or leg wash before going to bed.

With regard to the practice of abolution it has also been observed that the people are not very conscious. Use of toilet soap has not been found even after abolution. They do not use separate cloth and go with bare foot.

Environmental Sanitation

Environmental sanitation is also one important indicator of

health status of a community. It refers to the totality of physical environmental of any community's habitat. Generally, environmental sanitation includes the sources of water, the habit of defecation and toilet system, drainage system etc. The following pages deal with the nature of some of the relevant aspects of environmental sanitation as observed among the people under investigation.

Sources of Water

Water is one of the basic needs of our life. Besides drinking, water is required virtually for all tasks like cleaning, washing, cooking etc. It constitutes— 79 per cent of blood, 80 per cent of brain and muscles and 10 per cent of bones, i.e. two-third of the total weight of the body is water. Every person requires about 30 gallons (136.3% litres) of water per day for all purposes (cited in Rongmei and Kapoor, 2005).

The availability of water varies from place to place and also from village to village depending on geographical location and developmental status. Since the people under study are widely distributed in the hills in rural settings, they totally depend on the river and spring water for drinking as well as for other purposes. This water is carried through the pipe or canal system towards the village area, where they usually have a big tank to store. There are also some open tanks in the study villages and all the people carry water in bamboo pipes from these tanks. Due to scarcity of water and as the tanks are far away from their individual houses, they also store water in iron drums and in the bamboo pipes for 3-4 days and these are not properly washed. In rainy season, they also store the rain water and it is seen only in the tin roofed houses. The preserved water, however, mostly remains uncovered. Generally, they use boil water for drinking and cooking.

Storing of water properly is the best way to be away from water contamination. Most of the households under study have medium income and as such they store water in open containers. So, these households are at the high risk due to water pollution because when the water is left open, a large number of micro-organisms from their surroundings get mixed with water causing water borne diseases. Most of them store water in buckets. Some households also possess overhead cemented tanks where they store the rain water. The only problem with the overhead tanks is that they do not clean the tank regularly so microbes get developed in these tanks. The households are not aware of this type of pollution and this resulted in some diseases. In this regard, Mohan (1977) opined that polluted drinking water act as vehicle for disease transmission is a knowledge perhaps required by the scientific world recent centuries. Enteric fever, bacillary dysentery and cholera form the classic triad of water borne diseases. The other common water borne diseases are typhoid, paratyphoid, amoebic dysentery and hemorrhagic jaundice. In recent years infectious hepatitis has also become well established as a deadly disease. As the people under investigations are not getting satisfactory quality of water and as they keep water in open containers inside the house, all these factors together contribute to diarrhoea, cholera, typhoid, jaundice, malaria and gastro-enteritis to these poor households.

Toilet System and Drainage System

Toilets are considered an indicator of the social status and the economic background of the society. Proper toilet facilities are very important health factors as most of the diseases are borne from open field or *kachcha* type of toilets. Among the people under investigations, it has been observed that except two households in Lirmen village who possess sanitary latrine, all the other households have *kachcha* type of toilets.

The people go to these latrines with bare foot and they do not use a separate cloth for it. They are also not conscious about the use of toilet soap after defecation.

There is no drainage system in the villages. All the garbage accumulated below the floor on the ground. After washing cloths, bathing, washing utensils the house sullage water is not properly disposed of. In the backyard of the house, silage water accumulates and a very offensive smell is generated and it becomes the breeding ground for various germs and bacteria. As the latrines and pig sties and poultry are very near to the house and also for accumulated spots, heaps of debris etc., emit striking odour at any time of the year, particularly during the monsoon. The people are seemed to consider all these as 'given condition' for their day-to-day life and no one seems to think of the necessity of betterment in the sphere of personal cleanliness, hygiene and sanitation practices.

Thus it has been observed that the people by and large are not very particular and conscious about personal hygiene and cleanliness. Their overall living condition and their ignorance about the need of having proper personal hygiene and environmental sanitation do contribute towards the incidence of a number of diseases among the people.

7

HEALTH SCENARIO AMONG THE PEOPLE

The concept of health, disease and treatment is as varied as culture. Health does not mean merely the absence of disease, but complete adjustment of individual to external environment, both physical and social.

Health is the general condition of the body or mind with reference to soundness and vigour. It also means freedom from disease or ailments. Disease is usually known as a condition of the body in which there is incorrect function resulting from the effect of heredity, infection, diet or environment.

Health status is a valid indicator of human development. Good health, by itself improves the quality of life. It is also the basic necessity to ensure participation in economic activities. Health status therefore has multi-dimensional impact, both on the individual and the community as a whole. Health is an essential input for the development of human resources and the quality of life and in turn social and economic development of the nation.

Health is regarded a priority for sustained development at the individual, community and national levels. Improved health is a part of total socio-economic development and is regarded as an index of social development (Kanungo and Mahanta, 2004).

Provision of basic health care services to community is the primary objective of the Government as well as Non-

Governmental Organizations in the context of national development. Health services, safe drinking water, sanitation, nutrition etc. have therefore, been brought together in the form of an integral package to improve the social, economic and health conditions of the people. Therefore, the primary goal of any health care delivery system is to organize the health services in such a manner as to optimally utilize the available resource, knowledge and technology, with a view to preventing and alleviating diseases, disabilities and suffering of the people.

Thus, it is also a fact that the health of a particular group of people depends, along with the other parameters, on the health resources available at their door and in their immediate neighbourhood.

Therefore, in order to have a proper understanding of the prevailing health scenario of the people under investigation, the discussion has conveniently been confined to their health care practices, considering the health resources available in and around the study area and their utilization depending upon the pattern of morbidity prevalent among the people. Maternal and child health are the indices of health status of the population in any society. Information regarding maternal and child health care practice among the people has also been included here. Brief discussions have also been incorporated on causes of child mortality among the people.

Health Care Practice

Health care covers not merely medical care but also all aspects of preventive care too. Nor can it be limited to care rendered by or financed out of public expenditure within the government sector alone but must include incentives and disincentives for self care and care of citizens to get over ill health.

Broadly health care may be divided into three categories i.e. (a) Informal health care; (b) Interface health care; and (c) Formal health care (Babu, 1998).

(a) Informal Health Care

Informal health care is provided by non-professionals such as family members for whom these activities do not constitute an occupation, at least not a paid one. At the functional level, illness provides an occasion for reinforcing solidarity amongst relatives, friends and all others concerned. Treatment is mediated through cultural mechanisms which interact with biological factors. In this form of health care, the important elements are self-care, family, and the community.

Self-care is one major aspect that involves self-diagnosis and self-treatment in the face of perceived symptoms. Self-treatment can take many forms, occasionally bizarre, but more frequently mundane such as rest, dietary change (local customary foods) or the use of drugs, both previously prescribed and over the counter. Another form of self-care, not usually identified as such, is doing nothing, just letting nature take its course without interference, often the best form of "treatment" for self-limiting conditions. Another type of informal care is that provided by a family member, which may indeed be intertwined with self-care for sick adults.

(b) Interface Health Care

Some occupations are on the border line. These are traditional healers, pharmacists in drug stores etc. They work for pay, but are not scientifically trained, although they may have a wealth of experience and shrewd perceptions of what treatment will work.

(c) Formal Health Care

Formal health care can be provided by several professionals like (from various systems of medicine)—nurses, physical therapists, physicians etc.

Therefore, sickness is perceived in biological, social and cultural and psychological terms in a holistic framework.

Health practices in any country are the sum total of people's reactions, through personal practical experience, to the health services operating in a community and the way these experiences fit in their frame of reference. This, in turn, is dependent on the prevailing cultural factors in that community. Any assessment (diagnosis) regarding the effectiveness of measures taken to provide health service in a community will have to take this aspect into consideration. The diagnosis or assessment, thus arrived at, provides a clue to the people's behaviour related to the acceptance or rejection of a service (Pokarna, 1994).

Tribal concept of health is as varied as culture. They have their own system of beliefs and practices concerning health, ill-health and treatment of diseases which they consider more as functional one than clinical. Their health care system is a unique culture-bound constellation. To become healthy and disease free, generally the tribals maintain a three way relationship, viz. man-man, man-nature and man-supernature (Paul, 2006).

To lead a healthy life one has to understand and discriminate between good and bad practices. Preservation of good health depends on the understanding of the function conducive to good health and factors causing ill health. Individuals have selected perceptions and in functioning as members of the society they conform to social norms and groups sanctions.

Thus, the nature and extent of acceptance of any health care system by a cultural group, as a matter of fact, depends on a number of factors. The importance of socio-religious beliefs practices and attitudes as well as the economic background and availability of medicare services in the neighbourhood etc. play a significant role in this regard.

Before taking up a specific discussion on the medicare system/health care practice of the study group, it would probably be prudent to have an idea about the different types of health services available in and around the area under investigation. Thus, the following pages are devoted to have an idea about the different types of health resources available in and around the study area and to have an understanding as to the extent of utilization of the same by the people under investigation.

Health Resources

The health of a nation depends on health of the people who inhabit it. And the responsibility of a Government is to provide adequate health services to the people.

The health system can be broadly defined as the coherent whole of many interrelated component parts, both sectoral and intersectoral as well as the community itself, which produces a combined effect on the health of a population (Prakash, 2001).

The health system is usually organized in levels. Primary health care pays particular attention to the point of initial contact between members of the community and health services.

Primary Health Care is essential health care based on practical, scientifically sound and socially acceptable methods and technology made universally accessible to individuals and families in the community through their full participation and at a cost that the community and country can afford to maintain at every stage of their development in the spirit of self-reliance and self-determination. WHO defined Primary Health Care as "essential health care and universally accessible to all citizens and acceptable to them through their full participation and at a cost that the community and country can afford" (cited in Kanungo and Mahanta, 2004). It addresses the main health problems in the community through preventive, curative, promotive and rehabilitative medical and health services. Thus, the delivery of primary health care is the foundation of health care system and forms an integral part of the National Health System.

Efficient and effective delivery of primary health care is considered to be the core activity of any health care system. The primary health care strategy as outlined in the Alma Ata declaration of 1978 envisaged a revolutionary strategy which recognized that health for the majority of the people could not be achieved through the conventional hospital star-based health system on the assumption that benefits would eventually ' trickle down' to reach the poor. The Alma Ata strategy of primary health care upholds that health care would not only be available but it should be accessible, affordable, acceptable and appropriate to the needs of the people (cited in Kanungo and Mahanta, 2004).

Health Resources Available in the Micro-field

The prevailing health resources in the micro-field under investigation may be divided into two broad categories: modern resources and traditional resources. The traditional resources can again be divided into two types: magico-religious and herbal medicines. The people of Yajang-A and Yajang-B villages by and large, take the services from both the resources depending on the nature and severity of the diseases. But the people of Lirmen village, mostly, take the service from modern resources. However, in some preliminary health problem, they take some indigenous herbal medicines.

Health Resources in Lirmen Village

In Lirmen village, there is a Government dispensary with a pharmacist, one nurse and one midwife. The dispensary is a katcha type and where facilities of treatment for minor diseases are available.

The people of this village first consult the pharmacist or nurse for their diseases and depending on the nature and severity of the disease they give medicines and if it is not curable by them, the people then go to Morioni, Dimapur or Mokokchung for better treatment. However, in initial stages of some diseases they try to cure by taking some indigenous herbal medicines.

There is not any reputed traditional medicine man and magico-religious medicine man in this village.

Health resources in Yajang-A Village

In Yajang-A village, there is one health sub-centre with one nurse and one midwife. The sub-centre is also katcha type and not in regular service. During the investigation it has been observed that most of the time, the nurse is not available in the health sub-centre and she uses to get transfer within a short duration. The people of this village, therefore, have to depend on health resources available in the nearest town for allopathic treatment.

But there is a reputed herbal medicine man and a magico-religious man in Yajang-A village. People of this village mostly depend on these two experts, depending on their nature of the diseases. In case of, harm of evil spirit and snake bite they approach the magico-religious man. For all other diseases, they first approach the herbal medicine man, as they believe that he can diagnose the actual disease and cure it. It has been reported that the medicine man cures some diseases which are not cured by the modern medicines. Their economic condition is a factor, for which they approach the medicine man. They have their own view that if they go to modern practitioners they need money and the disease is also not cured. The traditional medicine man never demand them and most of the time, he gives free checkup.

The medicine man diagnoses the case first and depending on the nature of the disease, he gives his prepared medicine. In case, the disease is not curable by him, he advises the particular case to take help from modern resources. Sometimes, in some minor cases, he prescribes the medicines to be taken from the pharmacy nearest to them. Thus, the medicine man serves both traditional herbal practices as well as modern allopathic practices.

An overall idea about the magico-religious man and the herbal medicine man as well as the nature of their treatment etc. can be understood from the following two cases.

Magico-religious Treatment

Case 7.1

Akomba Aier (65 years) of Yajang-A village hails from a nuclear family. He is the head of the family and lives with his wife. He has read up to class two. He acquired the knowledge of magico-religious treatment from his father.

He generally treats the patient whose ailments are the result of the wrath of some malevolent spirit (*mojing*). The disease is known as *tamanem eice apu*. The patient normally develops a symptom of fear psychosis. It becomes so acute and intense that sometimes he behaves like an insane person. Occasionally, the patient may fall unconscious too.

Mr. Aier also cures snake bitten people, poison affected people and magical harm by others. While attending the patient first he diagnoses the disease by taking recourse to divination. If he finds that the disease has been caused by the wrath of some spirit (*mojing*), he starts his treatment which is known locally as *imtuksa*. He chants some hymns (*nemnem*) and simultaneously beats the patient with a bunch of wild leaves on his body. Sometimes, he makes two dolls, one for the spirit and the other for the patient and with hymns he tries to fight each other. After all these are done properly, as reported by him, the patient starts feeling better and gets fully cured in one day. For poison affected person and magical harm by others, he cures with the hymns.

In case of snake biting, the affected area of the patient is tied with a reed and simultaneously beat the area with another reed by chanting some hymns and within a short time the patient gets relief.

Herbal Treatment

Case 7.2

R. Temen Lamtor (71 years) is a reputed herbal medicine man of the Yajang-A village. Most of the people in and around the village avail of his services. He is the head of a nuclear family and lives only with his wife. Presently, he is a retired school teacher and has read up to class VII. In 1978, he took a government training course on First Aid (Diploma course, one year) in Kohima. After coming to his own place, he got busy with the herbal medicines, and used to treat the village people. Now, he has become expert to render his treatment in some diseases which are caused by natural factors. He treats the diseases like jaundice, diarrhoea, dysentery, diabetes, high blood pressure, cold, cough, chest pain, pneumonia, asthma, urinary problem etc. and more others. He prepares the medicines from locally available herbs and most of these herbs are available in his garden.

While attending a patient, he first listens to the symptoms as narrated by the patient himself/herself or by some one else. He then examines the patient by feeling the pulse and the affected part/organ, by measuring the temperature with a thermometer and also by a total observation of the patient. Depending on the diagnosis, made by him on the basis of these exercises, he prepares the appropriate medicine from the locally available herbs and provides the patient with necessary instructions. Sometimes, he makes these medicines in capsule form. He collects the expired capsules from pharmacies and cleans these and filled up his own compositions. He never demands money from the patient for his treatment.

Thus, for example, for case of jaundice he prepares a medicine from the root of a plant (no equivalent name in English) in the form of a powder. The effectiveness of this powder does not expire before 5 years. He advises the patient to take this medicine for 5-7 days on an empty stomach.

For the patient of diabetics and high blood pressure he prepares a medicine from the leaves of tamarind, neem (*Melia india*), bitter gourd (*Momordica charatia*), curry leaves and from the roots of a wild creeper. The medicine is not a curative one completely, but in severe condition it normalizes the patient. The patient is advised to take one spoonful of the medicines in half cup of lukewarm water.

He treats diarrhoea and dysentery also. For the purpose, he prepares medicine from periwinkle leaves (*leper naro*), grapes leaves and *titaphool* leaves (no specific name, a kind of red and bitter flower plant) and the *longer* (complete plant, locally available in jhum field after harvesting) and also mix the peel of pomegranate. The patient can take one spoonful of this mixture in a half cup of lukewarm water before/after meal. The adult patient can take it directly, without mixing in lukewarm water.

He also gives the treatment of the patient suffering from cough, chest pain, pneumonia early stage, typhoid early stage, gastritis, constipation, asthma and kidney stone by providing a mixture, namely honey mixture. He prepares the mixture from honey, tulsi juice (*Ocimum sanctum*), tamarind juice, lemon juice (*Citrus medica*), and ginger juice. He prescribes the medicine, 10 ml. three times a day for four days for the adults and 5 ml. for children, three times a day for four days.

For scabies (*musakar*) he prepares a medicine from Indian eucalyptus leaves and little quantity of lime. The patient is advised to apply the paste on the affected portion. He prepares another paste from the leaves of one wild plant *Ajunaro* for ring worm. He also treats high blood pressure patient by providing him the leaves of a wild plant (no specific name) to chew with a glass of water. The patient can take it any time as required.

As claimed by him, he can even cure the initial stage of kidney stone (*tazung poktsutam*), gall bladder stone (*tasu*) and the problem of urinary tract (*tezungjang*). For that purpose, he prepares a medicine as powder from *phylanthus* plant. The patient is to take one teaspoonful of the powder before meal two times a day till not cured. Generally, it takes 2-10 days, depending on the intensity of the disease.

For the patient of skin burn from fire and hot water, he gives gum of the leaves of *aloe vera* plant to apply on the affected areas. He also uses this *aloe vera* plant for the patients suffering from gastric ulcer. The patients are advised to take the gum of the leaves directly. For smoothing skin and to prevent pimples, he suggests to use the gum of the leaves of *aloe vera* plant in face.

Health Resources in Yajang-B Village

In the village Yajang-B, there is no health sub-centre or dispensary. So, the people of this village go to the nearest town Haluwating and Amguri for allopathic treatment. As the people of this village originally came from Yajang-A village and from same clan, therefore, they by and large depend on the medicare man (*Temen*) of Yajang-A village. The people first approach the herbal medicine man in time of their diseases. If the disease is not curable by him then according to his suggestion they take the help of other modern (allopathic) health resources where available.

For snake biting, and wrath of malevolent spirit they take the help of magico-religious man of Yajang-A village.

Utilisation of Health Resources

Health care and utilization of health and family welfare services is one of the most important of all human endeavour to improve the quality of life. To utilize proper medical and health services is one of the main fundamental rights of every individual (Dwivedi and Sharma, 2005).

Disease or ill health has been one of the fundamental concerns of man since his appearance on the earth. Every society has developed its own responses and methods of coping up with disease and ailments; and eventually a body of its own medical system. Medical system refers to all scientific knowledge, beliefs, actions and skills, which are utilized for health promotion, treatment and disease cure. While discussing about the utilisation of health care, Majumder (2006) gave the following conceptual framework.

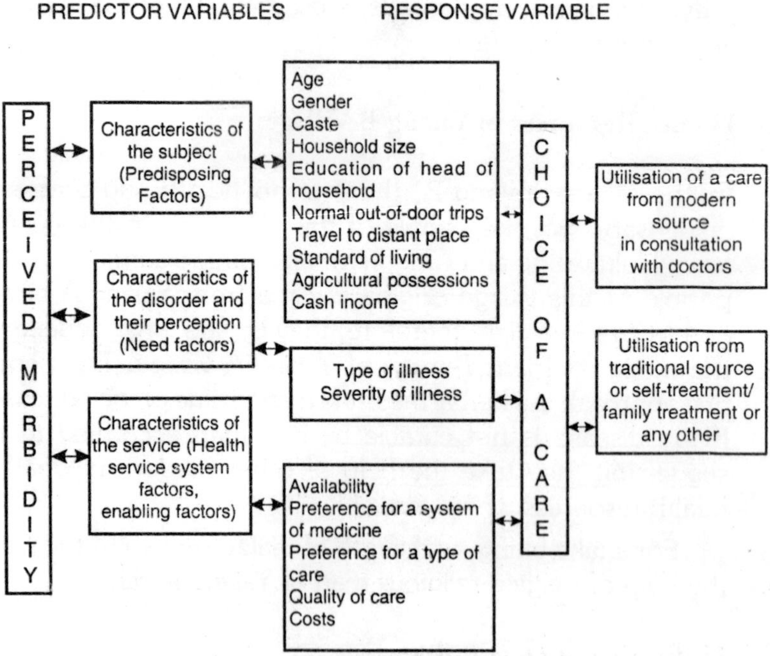

Fig. 7. 1 : Conceptual Framework

Source : Majumder, 2006.

Intensity of illness and number of spells significantly affect utilisation of health care services. Higher the severity or number of spells the higher the degree of utilisation of services.

There are predisposing factors which are supposed to make an individual susceptible to a specific action or behaviour or experience. Different factors in this category are: family characteristics (age, gender, household size, and marital status), social structure (education, employment, and ethnicity) and assets/affordability (land, livestock, cash income).

Though illness is a random event, it has a fair degree of predictability with respect to demographic factors like age, gender, family size, marital status, etc. As the need for health care changes with age, gender, and marital status utilisation of services also conforms accordingly. Size of the household may work positively or negatively. In a large family per capita income may be less and so also ability to pay for health care. It may reduce chances of utilising a care from modern source. On the contrary in larger families interaction among the members or with the neighbours may be more intensive and that may increase chances of utilising a care.

Impact of education, employment and ethnicity towards utilisation of services is universally acceptable. There is a significant positive relationship between education and utilisation of maternal and child health care services. Employment status or occupation and ethnicity have also been found important determinants of utilisation of care.

The relationship between family income or wealth and utilisation of health care is quite unexplored in India. Studies in general found positive relationship between household income and utilisation of services.

Besides, there are some ennobling factors such as availability of health facilities, accessibility to health care, quality of care and costs which play an important role in utilisation of health care.

The hospital output increases with the inputs. The

availability of drugs and dressing, pharmaceuticals, beds, are important service related determinants. Increased distance between residents and health care providers decreases the utilisation of health care.

The notion of quality of care, which has been characterised as a social construct, takes different meaning. These meanings vary with professionals, managers, governments, users, and among others in relation to the type of care under consideration as well as the social and technological context in which the care is delivered. Among these approaches, the analysis of user perception of quality offers a useful complement to those evaluations conducted from the point of view of professionals or public health authorities.

Keeping all these realities and possibilities in mind, the following pages have been devoted to have an understanding of the degree and extent of utilization of different available and accessible health care systems of the people under study.

To start with, let us first discuss the morbidity scenario of the people under investigation. In the process, both quantitative as well as analytical picture has been given.

Morbidity Among the People

Generally, the people are apparently seemed to possess a good health. It has been observed that the people are quite laborious and work hard throughout the day in the jhum field without any observable restriction. Besides these, womenfolk perform their domestic works very efficiently.

Though the people are physically strong yet a good number of them very frequently suffer from a variety of diseases; some of these being fatal and some being endemic in nature.

Disease/ailment of any kind in local term is generally called *yimra*. Each *yimra* has, however, a specific name. The most common diseases among the people are parasitic infections, diarrhoea, dysentery, skin disease, respiratory infections, cough etc. Serious diseases such as tuberculosis, malaria, jaundice, typhoid are also common. Health facilities do not reach them because the norms prescribed by the State Government for establishing Primary Health Centres and Health Sub-Centres are inappropriate in their localities.

As mentioned earlier, the data on morbidity has been collected through house-to-house investigation in the villages under study. All the reported disease episodes during the period July 2005 to June 2006 have been recorded. It is seen that during the period there have been at least 52 different diseases/ ailments from which the people have suffered. The total number of people, reportedly fallen sick during the period (July 2005 to June 2006) is 494 (42.29%) out of the total population 1168. It may be relevantly noted here that while collecting the local terms for the various ailments, it has been found that for some diseases, like anaemia, high blood pressure, beriberi, haemoglobin deficiency, appendicitis, scabies, pneumonia, paralysis etc., they do not have any local nomenclature. The exact reason for the same could not be gathered from the people. It is, however, possible that the ailments were either non-existent or were clubbed with some other ailments in the remote past.

The data (quantitative in nature) have been presented in five consecutive tables (Tables 7.1, 7.2, 7.3, 7.4 and 7.5). The first table (7.1) shows the village-wise distribution of the diseases and their frequencies. It also contains the available local terms of the respective diseases. The second table (7.2) incorporates the overall morbidity data of the villages under study by age and sex. The rest three tables (7.3, 7.4 and 7.5) show the age and sex-wise distribution of the morbidity data in the village Lirmen, Yajang-A and Yajang-B respectively.

The table (7.1) shows that the incidence of the disease like malaria (13.36%), fever (9.10%), gastritis (8.70%), intestinal problem (5.26%), liver problem (5.06%), dysentery (4.65%), typhoid (4.04%) etc., are more frequent among the people under study. These are followed by kidney and urinary tract problem (3.84%), cough (3.84%), stomach pain (3.03%), sinusitis (2.63%), respiratory problem (2.42%), jaundice (2.42%) and others. The data further reveal that the people, very frequently become the victims of skin diseases as well as infectious or communicable diseases. They also suffer from the ailments caused due to deficiency of minerals and vitamins (viz., eye problem, rheumatism, headache etc.).

If we make a comparative analysis of the disease episodes in the three study villages, it will be seen from the table (7.1) that out of the total of 494; 308 (62.34%) cases have been reported from the Lirmen village. The corresponding figure for village Yajang-A and Yajang-B is 158 (31.98%) and 28 (5.66%). Similarly, when we consider the percentage of the reported ailments out of the total population of a village, it will be seen that 49.35 per cent of the total population in Lirmen village were inflicted with various diseases during the period under discussion. The corresponding figure for the village Yajang-A and Yajang-B is 38.16 per cent and 21.53 per cent.

An overall idea about the distribution of the different diseases among the people by age and sex can be had from Table 7.2. For the purpose of the classification, the life span of a person has conveniently been divided into four stages, namely the infancy (0 to 4 yrs.), childhood (5-17 yrs.), adulthood (18-60 yrs) and old age (60 yrs. onwards).

A cursory glance of the table makes it apparent that, the various diseases show an observable correlation with specific age and sex group. For instance, the infancy and childhood have relatively limited number of (20.63 %) diseases, whereas the highest frequency (68.42%) of the morbidity is associated with the adults and the lowest is with the olderly people (10.93%).

With regard to the sex-wise distribution, the table reveals that the disease infliction is relatively more (57.08%) with males than with the females (42.91%).

Table 7.1: Distribution of the diseases/ailments episodes among the people under investigation (2005-2006)

Sl. No.	*Name of the Disease/ailment (Local term, if available)*	*No. of afflicted Person (%)*			
		Lirmen	*Yajang-A*	*Yajang-B*	*Total*
1	*2*	*3*	*4*	*5*	*6*
1.	Malaria *(Ramen)*	16 (3.23)	36 (7.28)	14 (2.83)	66 (13.36)
2.	Fever *(Yimra)*	6 (1.21)	38 (7.69)	1 (0.20)	45 (9.10)
3.	Gastritis *(Tar tipen)*	40 (8.09)	–	3 (0.60)	43 (8.70)
4.	Intestinal problem *(Tar tashi tak)*	25 (5.06)	1 (0.20)	–	26 (5.26)
5.	Liver problem *(Temesen angoba)*	19 (3.84)	6 (1.21)	–	25 (5.06)
6.	Dysentery *(Pokchi)*	6 (1.21)	16 (3.23)	1 (0.20)	23 (4.65)
7.	Typhoid *(Tuku tashi tak)*	10 (2.02)	10 (2.02)	–	20 (4.04)
8.	Kidney & unrinary tract problem *(Tezungjang)*	15 (3.03)	4 (0.80)	–	19 (3.84)
9.	Cough *(Akutba)*	11 (2.22)	8 (1.61)	–	19 (3.84)
10.	Stomach pain *(Pokcha)*	5 (1.01)	10 (2.02)	–	15 (3.03)
11.	Sinusitis *(Teni tangpangba)*	13 (2.63)	–	–	13 (2.63)
12.	Respiratory problem *(Kurik)*	11 (2.22)	–	1 (0.20)	12 (2.42)
13.	Jaundice *(Tasu)*	–	11 (2.22)	1 (0.20)	12 (2.42)
14.	Mensturation problem (*)	10 (2.02)	–	–	10 (2.02)
15.	Eye problem *(Tanuk angba)*	9 (1.82)	1 (0.20)	–	10 (2.02)
16.	Anemia (*)	9 (1.82)	–	–	9 (1.82)
17.	High blood pressure (*)	5 (1.01)	–	–	9 (1.82)
18.	Gall bladder stone *(Backtsutem)*	8 (1.61)	4 (0.80)	–	9 (1.82)
19.	Tonsilitis *(Tekong tezu tem)*	6 (1.21)	–	–	8 (1.61)
20.	Asthma (Teku tepangba)	6 (1.21)	–	2 (0.40)	8 (1.61)

(Contd.)

Table 7.1 : *(Contd.)*

21. Back pain (Terem chain)	6 (1.21)	–	–	6 (1.21)
22. Rheumatism (Teli chain)	6 (1.21)	–	–	6 (1.21)
23. White discharge (Temesung aoba)	6 (1.21)	–	–	6 (1.21)
24. Dental problem (Tuba angaba)	5 (1.01)	1 (0.20)	–	6 (1.21)
25. Beri-beri (*)	5 (1.01)	–	–	5 (1.01)
26. Neurological Problem *(Tezu tashidak)*	5 (1.01)	–	–	5 (1.01)
27. Haemoglobin Deficiency (*)	5 (1.01)	–	–	5 (1.01)
28. Tuberculosis (*)	2 (0.40)	3 (0.60)	–	5 (1.01)
29. Headache *(Takolak angaba)*	3 (0.60)	1 (0.20)	–	4 (0.80)
30. Diabatics *(Chini tashitak)*	3 (0.60)	1 (0.20)	–	4 (0.80)
31. Lungs Problem *(Tebokbok)*	3 (0.60)	–	–	3 (0.60)
32. Bodyache (*)	3 (0.60)	–	–	3 (0.60)
33. External injury (*)	3 (0.60)	–	–	3 (0.60)
34. Appendisitis (*)	2 (0.40)	–	1 (0.20)	3 (0.60)
35. Scabis (*)	3 (0.60)	–	–	3 (0.60)
36. Ear problem *(Tun oarong angoba)*	1 (0.20)	2 (0.40)	–	3 (0.60)
37. Diarrhoea *(Tupakeaa)*	–	3 (0.60)	–	3 (0.60)
38. Leprosy *(Temangnang)*	2 (0.40)	–	–	2 (0.40)
39. Mouth ulcer *(Tepang komu)*	2 (0.40)	–	–	2 (0.40)
40. Boil *(Komu)*	1 (0.20)	1 (0.20)	–	2 (0.40)
41. Worms *(Tapzen)*	–	–	2 (0.40)	2 (0.40)
42. Neck gland enlarge (*)	2 (0.40)	–	–	2 (0.40)
43. Ring worm (*)	1 (0.20)	–	–	1 (0.20)

(Contd.)

Table 7.1 : *(Contd.)*

44.	General weakness (*)	1 (0.20)	–	–	1 (0.20)
45.	Hair fall *(Ku tsukba)*	1 (0.20)	–	–	1 (0.20)
46.	Mumps (*)	1 (0.20)	–	–	1 (0.20)
47.	Vinereal disease	1 (0.20)	–	–	1 (0.20)
48.	Nasal bleeding (*)	1 (0.20)	–	–	1 (0.20)
49.	Low blood pressure (*)	1 (0.20)	–	–	1 (0.20)
50.	Vomiting *(Saktsuba)*	–	1 (0.20)	–	1 (0.20)
51.	Pneumonia (*)	–	–	1 (0.20)	1 (0.20)
52.	Paralysis (*)	–	–	1 (0.20)	1 (0.20)
	Grand Total (%)	308 (62.34)	158 (31.98)	28 (5.66)	494 (100)

Note : The local term are not availabale.

Further, the table shows that, with regard to the nature of diseases, infancy and childhood are characterised by the incidence of diseases, like malaria, viral fever, dysentery, cough, etc. However, the adult age seems to be prone to all types of diseases in varying degrees.

Regarding the sex-wise distribution of the diseases, it is apparent from the table that the highest numbers of males suffer from malaria (10.72%), gastritis (5.87%), fever (5.66%), intestinal problem (2.83%) etc. And in case of females these are recorded as follows: fever (3.44%), intestinal problem (2.83%), malaria (2.63%), stomach pain (2.63%) etc. Thus, it seems, both the sexes are equally affected by a few common diseases like fever, malaria, intestinal problem, gastritis etc.

Tables 7.3, 7.4 and 7.5 show the independent distribution morbidity data of the three villages under study according to age and sex. The tables show that the general trend of distribution of the different diseases is by and large similar.

While putting more emphasis on the morbidity scenario, it seems, the incidence of a good number of diseases among the people can be explained in terms of living condition as well as environmental sanitation, food habit and overall lifestyle of the people.

As discussed earlier (*Chapter 6*), many of the prevalent diseases among the people are probably due to their nutritional deficiency and poor living condition.

The food habit and food contents of the people have been briefly discussed in Chapter 6. It may be emphasised here that the people more or less are not aware of the relation between food and nutrition and between nutrition and health. They do not have any idea about the necessity of a balanced diet. Due to the nutritional deficiency, because of the poverty, a number of diseases may originate among them. Anaemia, general weakness and eye problem etc., are some of the frequently incident nutrition related diseases among the people.

With regard to their drinking habits, it may be recollected that purity of water is a non-issue among the people and the contaminated water could result in a number of water borne diseases among them.

The environmental sanitation seems to be one of the responsible factors for various frequent diseases that are prevalent among the people. The prevailing system of their environmental sanitation as a whole is much below the desired level. The poor unhealthy surroundings also help to increase the germs of different bacterial diseases like diarrhoea, dysentery and gastro-enteritis etc. On the whole, their unhygienic surroundings seem to contribute a lot towards the high incidence of a good number of diseases among the people.

The housing condition of the people also does not seem to be adequate. Most of the residential quarters are deficient in proper light and ventilation, besides being overcrowded. As a result the smoke that billows from the hearth accumulate within different rooms and the inmates do not get the required

Table 7.2 : Age and Sex-wise distribution of disease/ailments among the people of study villages (2005-2006)

Sl. No	Name of the Disease	Sex	Age Group				Sub-Total	Total
			0-4 Yrs Infancy (%)	5-17 Yrs Child (%)	18-60 Yrs Adult (%)	60 Yrs+ Old (%)		
1	2	3	4	5	6	7	8	9
1.	Malaria	M	3 (0.60)	9 (1.82)	37 (7.48)	4 (0.80)	53 (10.72)	66 (13.36)
		F	–	2 (0.40)	11 (2.22)	–	13 (2.63)	
2.	Fever	M	7 (1.41)	10 (2.02)	11 (2.22)	–	28 (5.66)	45 (9.10)
		F	3 (0.60)	7 (1.41)	6 (1..21)	1 (0.20)	17 (3.44)	
3.	Gastritis	M	–	2 (0.40)	23 (4.56)	4 (0.80)	29 (5.87)	43 (8.70)
		F	–	1 (0.20)	10 (2.02)	3 (0.60)	14 (2.83)	
4.	Intestinal problem	M	–	–	13 (2.63)	1 (0.20)	14 (2.83)	26 (5.26)
		F	–	1 (0.20)	10 (2.02)	1 (0.20)	12 (2.42)	
5.	Liver problem	M	–	–	13 (2.63)	2 (0.40)	15 (3.03)	25 (5.06)
		F	–	1 (0.20)	7 (1.41)	2 (0.40)	10 (2.02)	
6.	Dysentery	M	3 (0.60)	3 (0.60)	4 (0.80)	2 (0.40)	12 (2.42)	23 (4.65)
		F	–	5 (1.01)	6 (1.21)	–	11 (2.22)	
7.	Typhoid	M	1 (0.20)	3 (0.60)	9 (1.82)	–	13 (2.63)	20 (4.04)
		F	–	1 (0.20)	4 (0.80)	2 (0.40)	7 (1.41)	
8.	Kidney & urinary tract problem	M	–	–	12 (2.42)	–	12 (2.42)	19 (3.84)
		F	–	7 (1.41)	7 (1.41)			
9.	Cough	M	1 (0.20)	3 (0.60)	6 (1.21)	1 (0.20)	11 (2.22)	19 (3.84)
		F	2 (0.40)	3 (0.60)	3 (0.60)	–	8 (1.61)	
10.	Stomach pain	M	–	–	1 (0.20)	1 (0.20)	2 (0.40)	15 (3.03)
		F	–	2 (0.40)	10 (2.02)	1 (0.20)	13 (0.63)	
11.	Sinusitis	M	–	1 (0.20)	2 (0.40)	2 (0.40)	5 (1.01)	13 (2.63)
		F	2 (0.40)	2 (0.40)	4 (0.80)	–	8 (1.61)	
12.	Rerspiratory problem	M	–	–	4 (0.80)	2 (0.40)	6 (1.21)	12 (2.42)
		F	–	–	5 (1..01)	1 (0.20)	6 (1.21)	
13.	Jaundice	M	1 (0.20)	1 (0.20)	5 (1.01)	1 (0.20)	8 (1.61)	12 (2.42)
		F	–	2 (0.40)	2 (0.40)	–	4 (0.80)	

(Contd...)

Table 7.2 : (Contd..)

14.	Mensturation problem	M	–	–	–	–	–	10 (2.02)
		F	–	1 (0.20)	9 (1.82)	–	10 (2.02)	
15.	Eye problem	M	–	1 (0.20)	1 (0.20)	–	2 (0.40)	10 (2.02)
		F	–	1 (0.20)	4 (0.80)	3 (0.60)	8 (1.61)	
16.	Anaemia	M	–	1 (0.20)	5 (1.01)	1 (0.20)	7 (1.41)	9 (1.82)
		F	–	1 (0.20)	1 (0.20)	–	2 (0.20)	
17.	High blood pressure	M	–	–	3 (0.60)	2 (0.40)	5 (1.01)	9 (1.82)
		F	–	–	3 (0.60)	1 (0.20)	4 (0.80)	
18.	Gall bladder stone	M	–	–	3 (0.60)	–	3 (0.60)	9 (1.82)
		F	–	–	6 (1.21)	–	6 (1.21)	
19.	Tonsilitis	M	–	–	7 (1.41)	1 (0.20)	7 (1.41)	8 (1.61)
		F	–	–	1 (0.20)	–	1 (0.20)	
20.	Asthma	M	–	–	3 (0.60)	1 (0.20)	4 (0.80)	8 (1.61)
		F	–	1 (0.20)	3 (0.60)	–	4 (0.80)	
21.	Back pain	M	–	–	2 (0.40)	1 (0.20)	3 (0.60)	6 (1.21)
		F	–	–	3 (0.60)	–	3 (0.60)	
22.	Rheumatism	M	–	1 (0.20)	2 (0.40)	–	3 (0.60)	6 (1.21)
		F	–	–	3 (0.60)	–	3 (0.60)	
23.	White discharge	M	–	–	–	–	–	6 (1.21)
		F	–	–	6 (1.21)	–	6 (1.21)	
24.	Dental problem	M	–	–	2 (0.40)	1 (0.20)	3 (0.60)	6 (1.21)
		F	–	–	3 (0.60)	–	3 (0.60)	
25.	Beri-beri	M	1 (0.20)	–	2 (0.40)	–	3 (0.60)	5 (1.01)
		F	–	1 (0.20)	1 (0.20)	–	2 (0.40)	
26.	Neurological problem	M	–	–	3 (0.60)	1 (0.20)	4 (0.80)	5 (1.01)
		F	–	–	1 (0.20)	–	1 (0.20)	
27.	Haemoglobin deficiency	M	–	–	1 (0.20)	2 (0.40)	3 (0.60)	5 (1.01)
		F	–	–	1 (0.20)	1 (0.20)	2 (0.40)	
28.	Tuberculosis	M	–	–	3 (0.60)	–	3 (0.60)	5 (1.01)
		F	–	–	2 (0.40)	–	2 (0.40)	
29.	Headache	M	–	–	2 (0.40)	–	2 (0.40)	4 (0.80)
		F	–	–	2 (0.40)	–	2 (0.40)	

(Contd...)

Table 7.2 : (Contd..)

30.	Diabetes	M	–	–	1 (0.20)	1 (0.20)	2 (0.40)	4 (0.80)
		F	–	–	–	2 (0.40)	2 (0.40)	
31.	Lungs problem	M	–	–	3 (0.60)	–	3 (0.60)	3 (0.60)
		F	–	–	–	–	–	
32.	Bodyache	M	1 (0.20)	–	–	–	1 (0.20)	3 (0.60)
		F	–	–	1 (0.20)	1 (0.20)	2 (0.40)	
33.	External injury	M	–	1 (0.20)	1 (0.20)	1 (0.20)	3 (0.60)	3 (0.60)
		F	–	–	–	–	–	
34.	Appendicitis	M	–	–	2 (0.40)	1 (0.20)	3 (0.60)	3 (0.60)
		F	–	–	–	–	–	
35.	Scabis	M	–	–	–	–	–	3 (0.60)
		F	–	1 (0.20)	2 (0.40)	–	3 (0.60)	
36.	Ear problem	M	–	–	3 (0.60)	–	3 (0.60)	3 (0.60)
		F	–	–	–	–	–	
37.	Diarrhoea	M	1 (0.20)	–	–	–	1 (0.20)	3 (0.60)
		F	–	–	2 (0.40)	–	2 (0.40)	
38.	Leprosy	M	–	–	–	–	–	2 (0.40)
		F	–	–	–	2 (0.40)	2 (0.40)	
39.	Mouth ulcer	M	–	–	1 (0.20)	–	1 (0.20)	2 (0.40)
		F	–	–	1 (0.20)	–	1 (0.20)	
40.	Boil	M	–	–	–	–	–	2 (0.40)
		F	–	–	1 (0.20)	1 (0.20)	2 (0.40)	
41.	Worms	M	–	–	–	–	–	2 (0.40)
		F	2 (0.40)	–	–	–	2 (0.40)	
42.	Neck gland	M	–	–	1 (0.20)	–	1 (0.20)	2 (0.40)
	enlarge	F	–	–	1 (0.20)	–	1 (0.20)	
43.	Ring worm	M	–	1 (0.20)	–	–	1 (0.20)	1 (0.20)
		F	–	–	–	–	–	
44.	General	M	–	–	1 (0.20)	–	1 (0.20)	1 (0.20)
	weakness	F	–	–	–	–	–	

(Contd...)

Table 7.2 : (Contd..)

45.	Hair fall	M	–	–	–	–	–	1 (0.20)
		F	–	1 (0.20)	–	–	1 (0.20)	
46.	Mumps	M	–	–	1 (0.20)	–	1 (0.20)	1 (0.20)
		F	–	–	–	–	–	
47.	Vinereal disease	M	–	–	–	–	–	1 (0.20)
		F	–	1 (0.20)	–	–	1 (0.20)	
48.	Nasal bleeding	M	–	–	–	–	–	1 (0.20)
		F	–	1 (0.20)	–	–	1 (0.20)	
49.	Low blood pressure	M	–	–	–	–	–	1 (0.20)
		F	–	–	1 (0.20)	–	1 (0.20)	
50.	Vomiting	M	–	–	–	–	–	1 (0.20)
		F	–	1 (0.20)	–	–	1 (0.20)	
51.	Pneumonia	M	–	–	–	–	–	1 (0.20)
		F	–	–	1 (0.20)	–	1 (0.20)	
52.	Paralysis	M	–	–	1 (0.20)	–	1 (0.20)	1 (0.20)
		F	–	–	–	–	–	
	Grand Total (%)		28 (5.66)	74 (14.97)	338 (68.42)	54 (10.93)		494 (100)

Table 7.3 : Age and Sex-wise distribution of disease/ailments among the people of Lirmen village (2005-2006)

Sl. No	*Name of the Disease*	*Sex*	*Age Group*				*Sub-Total*	*Total*
			0-4 Yrs Infancy (%)	*5-17 Yrs Child (%)*	*18-60 Yrs Adult (%)*	*60 Yrs+ Old (%)*		
1	*2*	*3*	*4*	*5*	*6*	*7*	*8*	*9*
1	Gastritis	M	–	2 (0.64)	22 (7.14)	3 (0.97)	27 (8.76)	40 (12.98)
		F	–	1 (0.32)	9 (2.92)	3 (0.97)	13 (4.22)	
2.	Intestinal problem	M	–	–	13 (4.22)	1 (0.32)	14 (4.54)	25 (8.11)
		F	–	1 (0.32)	10 (3.24)	–	11 (3.57)	
3.	Liver problem	M	–	–	9 (2.92)	2 (0.64)	11 (3.57)	19 (6.16)
		F	–	1 (0.32)	5 (1.62)	2 (0.64)	8 (2.59)	
4.	Malaria	M	–	–	10 (3.24)	–	10 (3.24)	16 (5.19)
		F	–	2 (0.64)	4 (1.29)	–	6 (1.94)	
5.	Kidney & urinary tract problem	M	–	–	10 (3.24)	–	10 (3.24)	15 (4.87)
		F	–	–	5 (1.62)	–	5 (1.62)	
6.	Sinusitis	M	–	1 (0.32)	2 (0.64)	2 (0.64)	5 (1.62)	13 (4.22)
		F	2 (0.64)	2 (0.64)	4 (1.29)	–	8 (2.59)	
7.	Respiratory problem	M	–	–	4 (1.29)	1 (0.32)	5 (1.62)	11 (3.57)
		F	–	–	5 (1.62)	1 (0.32)	6 (1.94)	
8.	Cough	M	–	3 (0.97)	6 (1.94)	1 (0.32)	10 (3.24)	11 (3.57)
		F	–	1 (0.32)	–	–	1 (0.32)	
9.	Mensturation problem	M	–	–	–	–	–	10 (3.24)
		F	–	1 (0.32)	9 (2.92)	–	10 (3.24)	
10.	Typhoid	M	–	1 (0.32)	4 (1.29)	–	5 (1.62)	10 (3.24))
		F	–	1 (0.32)	3 (0.97)	1 (0.32)	5 (1.62)	
11	Anaemia	M	–	1 (0.32)	5 (1.62)	1 (0.32)	7 (2.27)	9 (2.92)
		F	–	1 (0.32)	1 (0.32)	–	2 (0.64)	
12.	Eye problem	M	–	1 (0.32)	1 (0.32)	–	2 (0.64)	9 (2.92)
		F	–	–	4 (1.29)	3 (0.97)	7 (2.27)	
13	High blood pressure	M	–	–	3 (0.97)	2 (0.64)	5 (1.62)	9 (2.92)
		F	–	–	3 (0.97)	1 (0.32)	4 (1.29)	
14	Tonsilitis	M	–	–	7 (2.27)	–	7 (2.27)	8 (2.59)
		F	–	–	1 (0.32)	–	1 (0.32)	

(Contd...)

Table 7.3 : *(Contd...)*

15	Fever	M	-	1 (0.32)	3 (0.97)	–	4 (1.29)	6 (1.94)
		F	–	–	1 (0.32)	1 (0.32)	2 (0.64)	
16	Dysentery	M	-	-	-	1 (0.32)	1 (0.32)	6 (1.94)
		F	-	1 (0.32)	4 (1.29)	-	5 (1.62)	
17	Back pain	M	–	–	2 (0.64)	1 (0.32)	3 (0.97)	6 (1.94)
		F	–	–	3 (0.97)	–	3 (0.97)	
18	Rheumatism	M	-	1 (0.32)	2 (0.64)	–	3 (0.97)	6 (1.94)
		F	–	–	3 (0.97)	–	3 (0.97)	
19	White discharge	M	–	–	–	-	—	6 (1.94)
		F	–	–	6 (1.94)	–	6 (1.94)	
20.	Asthma	M	–	–	3 (0.97)	1 (0.32)	4 (1.29)	6 (1.94)
		F	–	–	2 (0.64)	–	2 (0.64)	
21.	Beriberi	M	1 (0.32)	–	2 (0.64)	–	3 (0.97)	5 (1.62)
		F	–	1 (0.32)	1 (0.32)	–	2 (0.64)	
22	Dental problem	M	–	-	2 (0.64)	1 (0.32)	3 (0.97)	5 (1.62)
		F	–	–	2 (0.64)	–	2 (0.64)	
23	Gall bladder stone	M	–	–	1 (0.32)	–	1 (0.32)	5 (1.62)
		F	–	–	4 (1.29)	–	4 (1.29)	
24	Neurological problem	M	–	–	3 (0.97)	1 (0.32)	4 (1.29)	5 (1.62)
		F	–	–	1 (0.32)	–	1 (0.32)	
25	Stomach pain	M	–	–	1 (0.32)	–	1 (0.32)	5 (1.62)
		F	–	1 (0.32)	3 (0.97)	–	4 (1.29)	
26	Haemoglobin deficiency	M	–	–	1 (0.32)	2 (0.64)	3 (0.97)	5 (1.62)
		F	–	–	1 (0.32)	1 (0.32)	2 (0.64)	
27	Lungs problem	M	–	–	3 (0.97)	–	3 (0.97)	3 (0.97)
		F	–	–	–	–	–	
28	Bodyache	M	1 (0.32)	-	–	-	1 (0.32)	3 (0.97)
		F	–	–	1 (0.32)	1 (0.32)	2 (0.64)	
29	Headache	M	-	-	2 (0.64)	-	2 (0.64)	3 (0.97)
		F	-	-	1 (0.32)	-	1 (0.32)	
30	Diabeties	M	–	–	1 (0.32)	1 (0.32)	2 (0.64)	3 (0.97)
		F	–	–	–	1 (0.32)	1 (0.32)	

(Contd...)

Table 7.3 : *(Contd...)*

31	Scabies	M	–	–	1 (0.32)	–	–	3 (0.97)
		F	–	1 (0.32)	2 (0.64)	–	3 (0.97)	
32.	External injury	M	–	1 (0.32)	1 (0.32)	1 (0.32)	3 (0.97)	3 (0.97)
		F	–	–	–	–	–	
33	Tuberculosis	M	–	–	1 (0.32)	–	1 (0.32)	2 (0.64)
		F	–	–	1 (0.32)	–	1 (0.32)	
34	Appendicitis	M	–	–	2 (0.64)	–	2 (0.64)	2 (0.64)
		F	–	–	–	–	–	
35	Leprosy	M	–	–		–	–	2 (0.64)
		F	–	–	–	2 (0.64)	2 (0.64)	
36	Mouth ulcer	M	–	–	1 (0.32)	–	1 (0.32)	2 (0.64)
		F	–	–	1 (0.32)	–	1 (0.32)	
37	Neck gland enlarge	M	–	–	1 (0.32)	–	1 (0.32)	2 (0.64)
		F	–	–	1 (0.32)	–	1 (0.32)	
38	Ring worm	M	–	1 (0.32)	–	–	1 (0.32)	1 (0.32)
		F	–	–	–	–	–	
39	General weakness	M	–	–	1 (0.32)	–	1 (0.32)	1 (0.32)
		F	–	–	–	–	–	
40	Boil	M	–	–	–	–	–	1 (0.32)
		F	–	–	1 (0.32)	–	1 (0.32)	
41	Hair fall	M	–	–	–	–	–	1 (0.32)
		F	–	1 (0.32)	–	–	1 (0.32)	
42	Mumps	M	–	–	1 (0.32)	–	1 (0.32)	1 (0.32)
		F	–	–	–	–	–	
43	Ear problem	M	–	–	1 (0.32)	–	1 (0.32)	1 (0.32)
		F	–	–	–	–	–	
44	Venereal disease	M	–	–	–	–	–	1 (0.32)
		F	–	1 (0.32)	–	–	1 (0.32)	
45	Nasal bleeding	M	–	–	–	–	–	1 (0.32)
		F	–	1 (0.32)	–	–	1 (0.32)	
46	Low blood pressure	M	–	–	–	–	–	1 (0.32)
		F	–	–	1 (0.32)	–	1 (0.32)	
	Grand Total (%)		4 (1.29)	31 (10.06)	234 (75.97)	39 (12.66)		308 (100)

Table 7.4 : Age and Sex-wise distribution of disease/ailments among the people of Yajang-A village (2005-2006)

Sl. No	Name of the Disease	Sex	Age Group				Sub-Total	Total
			0-4 Yrs Infancy (%)	5-17 Yrs Child (%)	18-60 Yrs Adult (%)	60 Yrs+ Old (%)		
1	2	3	4	5	6	7	8	9
1.	Fever	M	6 (3.79)	9 (5.69)	8 (5.06)	–	23 (14.55)	38 (24.05)
		F	3 (1.89)	7 (4.43)	5 (3.16)	–	15 (9.49)	
2.	Malaria	M	–	3 (1.89)	26 (16.45)	2 (1.26)	31 (19.62)	36 (22.78)
		F	–	–	5 (3.16)	–	5 (3.16)	
3.	Dysentery	M	3 (1.89)	3 (1.89)	3 (1.89)	1 (0.63)	10 (6.32)	16 (10.12)
		F	–	4 (2.53)	2 (1.26)	–	6 (3.79)	
4.	Jaundice	M	1 (0.63)	–	5 (3.16)	1 (0.63)	7 (4.43)	11 (6.96)
		F	–	2 (1.26)	2 (1.26)	–	4 (2.53)	
5.	Typhoid	M	1 (0.63)	2 (1.26)	5 (3.16)	–	8 (5.06)	10 (6.32)
		F	–	–	1 (0.63)	1 (0.63)	2 (1.26)	
6.	Stomach pain	M	–	–	–	1 (0.63)	1 (0.63)	10 (6.32)
		F	–	1 (0.63)	7 (4.43)	1 (0.63)	9 (5.69)	
7.	Cough	M	1 (0.63)	–	–	–	1 (0.63)	8 (5.06)
		F	2 (1.26)	2 (1.26)	3 (1.89)	–	7 (4.43)	
8.	Liver disorder	M	–	–	4 (2.53)	–	4 (2.53)	6 (3.79)
		F	–	–	2 (1.26)	–	2 (1.26)	
9.	Kidney & urinary tract problem	M	–	–	2 (1.26)	–	2 (1.26)	4 (2.53)
		F	–	–	2 (1.26)	–	2 (1.26)	
10.	Gall bladder stone	M	–	–	2 (1.26)	–	2 (1.26)	4 (2.53)
		F	–	–	2 (1.26)	–	2 (1.26)	
11.	Tuberculosis	M	–	–	2 (1.26)	–	2 (1.26)	3 (1.89)
		F	–	–	1 (0.63)	–	1 (0.63)	
12.	Diarrhoea	M	1 (0.63)	–	–	–	1 (0.63)	3 (1.89)
		F	–	–	2 (1.26)	–	2 (1.26)	
13.	Ear problem	M	–	–	2 (1.26)	–	2 (1.26)	2 (1.26)
		F	–	–	–	–	–	

(Contd...)

Table 7.4 : *(Contd...)*

14.	Boil	M	–	–	–	–	–	1 (0.63)
		F	–	–	–	1 (0.63)	1 (0.63)	
15.	Headache	M	–	–	–	–	–	1 (0.63)
		F	–	–	1 (0.63)	–	1 (0.63)	
16.	Vomiting	M	–	–	–	–	–	1 (0.63)
		F	–	1 (0.63)	–	–	1 (0.63)	
17.	Eye problem	M	–	–	–	–	–	1 (0.63)
		F	–	1 (0 63)	–	–	1 (0.63)	
18.	Intestinal	M	–	–	–	–	–	1 (0.63)
	problem	F	–	–	–	1 (0.63)	1 (0.63)	
19.	Dental problem	M	–	–	–	–	–	1 (0.63)
		F	–	–	1 (0.63)	–	1 (0.63)	
20.	Diabetes	M	–	–	–	–	–	1 (0.63)
		F	–	–	–	1 (0.63)	1 (0.63)	
	Grand Total (%)		18 (11.39)	35 (22.15)	95 (60.12)	10 (6.32)		158 (100)

Table 7.5 : Age and sex-wise distribution of disease/ailments among the people of Yajang-B village (2005-2006)

Sl. No	*Name of the Disease*	*Sex*	*Age Group*				*Sub-Total*	*Total*
			0-4 Yrs Infancy (%)	*5-17 Yrs Child (%)*	*18-60 Yrs Adult (%)*	*60 Yrs+ Old (%)*		
1	*2*	*3*	*4*	*5*	*6*	*7*	*8*	*9*
1	Malaria	M	3 (10.71)	6 (21.42)	1 (3.57)	2 (7.14)	12 (42.85)	14 (50)
		F	–	–	2 (7.14)	–	2 (7.14)	
2.	Gastritis	M	–	–	1 (3.57)	1 (3.57)	2 (7.14)	3 (10.71)
		F	–	–	1 (3.57)	–	1 (3.57)	
3.	Asthma	M	–	–	–	–	–	2 (7.14)
		F	–	1 (3.57)	1 (3.57)	–	2 (7.14)	
4.	Worm	M	–	–	–	–	–	2 (7.14)
		F	2 (7.14)	–	–	–	2 (7.14)	
5.	Desentary	M	–	–	1 (3.57)	–	1 (3.57)	1 (3.57)
		F	–	–	–	–	–	
6.	Jaundice	M	–	1 (3.57)	–	–	1 (3.57)	1 (3.57)
		F	–	–	–	–	–	
7.	Pneumonia	M	–	–	–	–	–	1 (3.57)
		F	–	–	1 (3.57)	–	1 (3.57)	
8.	Fever	M	1 (3.57)	-	–	–	1 (3.57)	1 (3.57)
		F	–	–	–	–	–	
9.	Respiratory problem	M	–	–	–	1 (3.57)	1 (3.57)	1 (3.57)
		F	–	–	–	–	–	
10.	Appendicities	M	–	–	–	1 (3.57)	1 (3.57)	1 (3.57)
		F	–	–	–	–	–	
11.	Paralysis	M	–	–	1 (3.57)	–	1 (3.57)	1 (3.57)
		F	–	–	–	–	–	
	Grand Total (%)		6 (21.42)	8 (28.57)	9 (32.14)	5 (17.85)		28 (100)

free air and light. All these are believed to be detrimental for health; and are likely to herald a number of diseases such as respiratory problem, lungs problem, asthma etc. The poor lighting inside the houses due to lack of proper ventilation also affect their eyes and as a result they also suffer from eye problems.

Frequent affliction by various types of skin diseases such as scabies, boil, ring worm etc. can also probably be explained in terms of their unhygienic living condition as well as lack of personal cleanliness. Use of toilet soap has also not been found even after ablution. The habit of going outdoor for defecation in barefoot may be one of the important causes of worm infestation. All these factors contribute towards the high incidence of the same.

To sum up, it may be highlighted that the overall morbidity scenario among the Aos under investigation is characterized by the high incidence of cough, fever, gastritis, jaundice, malaria, diarrhoea, typhoid, skin diseases, respiratory problem etc. Anaemia and tuberculosis are another important health problems that affect the overall health scenario of the group.

In fact, the overall living condition of the people and food habits along with illiteracy and ignorance seem to be mainly responsible for a great deal of their suffering.

People's Views about Health and Disease

During the present study a good number of respondents have been interviewed to have a first-hand understanding of their views with regard to health and disease and available health care services. The responses have shown some expected variation according to age, sex, level of education and economic background etc.

The meaning of the word 'Healthy Person' is not clearly understood by many of the villagers. Some respondents defined healthy person as those who are not having any kind of disease and have the ability to carry on his/her daily duties properly. Majority are not aware of the concept of a sick person. They assume that a person who sleeps on a cot/bed throughout the day is unhealthy/sick person. The concept of reason of one falling sick is also not clear. They also believe that sickness is caused of intake of unrich food and impure water, polluted atmosphere or due to attack of ghost or spirit. Some of them also consider sickness as caused due to hard industrious and also due to the affect of divine punishment.

Health Seeking Behaviour

As noted earlier, the health care services utilized by the people may broadly be divided into two categories: the modern and the traditional one. The traditional medicare system may again be conveniently divided into two types: the herbal and the magico-religious ones. The people of Lirmen village mostly depend on the modern health resources available in their village. The people first consult with the pharmacist or nurse of the dispensary of the village for their diseases and depending on the nature and condition of the disease they give medicines and if it is not curable by them, the people then go to Mariani, Dimapur, Mokokchung for better treatment. However, in some initial stage for some minor diseases they try to cure by taking some indigenous herbal medicines.

But the people of Yajang-A and Yajang-B villages mostly depend on the traditional health resources available in their village. It is due to the fact that though there is a health sub-centre in Yajang-A village, it is not in regular service. As noted earlier that there is only one nurse and one midwife in this sub-centre and most of the time the nurse is not available and gets transfer very frequently. Besides it has been reported by the villagers that most of the medicines available in the sub-centre have crossed the expiry date and so these are not usable for them.

For modern health resources, they have to come Haluwating and Amguri and in this regard their transportation facility is not good. They have to come on foot or have to hire taxi from Haluwating to reach these modern resources at the cost of rupees 300-400.

Again they have the views on modern health resources that the quality of care is not good and modern health professional cannot predict the actual disease. The cost of care is also high and in most of the cases they have to pay a high cost but in result they do not get much relief from the disease.

Thus, the people of Yajang-A and Yajang-B villages first approach the traditional herbal medicine man or healer for their health problems and treatment. They prefer the services of the traditional healer, because he is not required to pay immediately in cash but could be remunerated in kind. He never asks for cash and in most of the time he gives free check-up.

It may also be noted here that according to the people's beliefs, the traditional healer can detect the actual disease and he can cure it within a short period of time.

Generally, the traditional healer diagnoses the patient by touching his/her pulse. If he considers the disease as curable, he gives herbal medicines prepared by him and if he finds that the disease is not curable by his medicine, he advises the patient to consult a physician. Thus, the cases which are not curable by the traditional healer are taken to the nearest town hospital/ health centre to have a better treatment.

However, the traditional healer is also expert to some extent in modern allopathic medicines. Thus, sometimes he also prescribes some medicines for the patients to take from their nearest available pharmacy.

For snake biting and wrath of malevolent spirit they take the help of magico-religious man as the traditional healer cannot cure such diseases. From time immemorial, they have been seeking the treatment of magico-religious man for such diseases.

On the whole, the nature and the course of treatment depend on the nature of disease as well as the disease etiology diagnosed by the traditional healer.

In order to have a quantitative idea, information as to the nature of treatment has been collected with regard to 494 reported morbidity episodes (2005-2006). Table 7.6 presents the village-wise break up of the data. It will be seen from Table 7.6 that out of a total of 494 disease episodes (2005-2006), 370 (74.89%) people have resorted to modern medicare system whereas, 115 (23.27%) have taken up traditional one and 9 (1.82%) have gone for both the systems.

Table 7.6 : Village-wise distribution of the people according to acceptance of different medicare systems

Sl. No.	*Name of the village (%)*	*No. of ailment episodes (%)*	*Type of medicare system*		
			Modern (%)	*Traditional (%)*	*Both (%)*
1	*2*	*3*	*4*	*5*	*6*
1	Lirmen	308 (62.34)	308 (62.34)	–	–
2	Yajang-A	158 (31.98)	45 (9.10)	113 (22.87)	–
3	Yajang-B	28 (5.66)	17 (3.44)	2 (0.40)	9 (1.82)
Grand Total (%)		494 (100)	370 (74.89)	115 (23.27)	9 (1.82)

While comparing the rates of acceptance of different medicare systems in the three villages under study, it will be seen from Table 7.6 that in Lirmen village utilisation of modern medicare system is more than the Yajang-A and Yajang-B village. But, in Yajang-A and Yajang-B villages both traditional and modern medicare systems are used simultaneously.

A fairly detailed village-wise break-up of the data on the acceptance or utilisations of different curative measures for different disease/ailments have been presented in Tables 7.7, 7.8 and 7.9.

Table 7.7 shows that in Lirmen village people depend mostly on modern system of treatment for any disease/ailment.

Table 7.7 : Distribution of the disease/ailments by use of different medicare systems by the people of Lirmen village

Sl. No.	Name of the Disease	Total morbidity Episodes	Age Group			No Treatment
			Modern	Traditional	Both	
1	2	3	4	5	6	7
1.	Gastritis	40	40 (100)	–	–	–
2.	Intestinal problem	25	25 (100)	–	–	–
3.	Liver problem	19	19 (100)	–	–	–
4.	Malaria	16	16 (100)	–	–	–
5.	Kidney & urinary tract problem	15	15 (100)	–	–	–
6.	Sinusitis	13	13 (100)	–	–	–
7.	Respiratory problem	11	11 (100)	–	–	–
8.	Cough	11	11 (100)	–	–	–
9.	Mensturation problem	10	10 (100)	–	–	–
10.	Typhoid	10	10 (100)	–	–	–
11.	Anaemia	9	9 (100)	–	–	–
12.	Eye problem	9	9 (100)	–	–	–
13.	High blood pressure	9	9 (100)	–	–	–
14.	Tonsilitis	8	8 (100)	–	–	–
15.	Fever	6	6 (100)	–	–	–
16.	Dysentery	6	6 (100)	–	–	–
17.	Backpain	6	6 (100)	–	–	–
18.	Rheumatism	6	6 (100)	–	–	–
19.	White discharge	6	6 (100)	–	–	–
20.	Asthma	6	6 (100)	–	–	–
21.	Beriberi	5	5 (100)	–	–	–
22.	Dental problem	5	5 (100)	–	–	–
23.	Gall bladder stone	5	5 (100)	–	–	–
24.	Neurological problem	5	5 (100)	–	–	–
25.	Stomach pain	5	5 (100)	–	–	–
26.	Haemoglobin deficiency	5	5 (100)	–	–	–
27.	Lungs problem	3	3 (100)	–	–	–
28.	Body ache	3	3 (100)	–	–	–
29.	Head ache	3	3 (100)	–	–	–
30.	Diabeties	3	3 (100)	–	–	–
31.	Scabises	3	3 (100)	–	–	–
32.	External injury	3	3 (100)	–	–	–
33.	Tuberculosis	2	2 (100)	–	–	–
34.	Appendicitis	2	2100)	–	–	–
35.	Leprosy	2	2 (100)	–	–	–
36.	Mouth ulcer	2	2 (100)	–	–	–
37.	Neck gland enlarge	2	2 (100)	–	–	–
38.	Ring worm	1	1 (100))	–	–	–
39.	General weakness	1	1 (100)	–	–	–

(Contd...)

Table 7.7 : *(Contd...)*

40.	Boil	1	1 (100)	–	–	–
41.	Hair fall	1	1 (100)	–	–	–
42.	Mums	1	1 (100)	–	–	–
43.	Ear problem	1	1 (100)	–	–	–
44.	Venereal disease	1	1 (100)	–	–	–
45.	Nasal bleeding	1	1 (100)	–	–	–
46.	Low blood pressure	1	1 (100)	–	–	–
	Grand Total	308	308 (100)			

Table 7.8 : Distribution of the disease/ailments by use of different medicare systems by the people of Yajang-A village

Sl. No.	*Name of the Disease*	*Total morbidity Episodes*	*Age Group*			*No Treatment*
			Modern	*Traditional*	*Both*	
1	*2*	*3*	*4*	*5*	*6*	*7*
1	Fever	38	4 (10.52)	34 (89.47)	–	–
2.	Malaria	36	20 (55.55)	16 (44.44)	–	–
3.	Dysentery	16	–	16 (100)	–	–
4.	Jaundice	11	4 (36.36)	7 (63.63)	–	–
5.	Typhoid	10	3 (30)	7 (70)	–	–
6.	Stomach pain	10	1 (10)	9 (90)	–	–
7.	Cough	8	3 (37.5)	5 (62.5)	–	–
8.	Liver problem	6	–	6 (100)	–	–
9.	Kidney & urinary tract problem	4	1 (25)	3 (75)	–	–
10.	Gall bladder stone	4	–	4 (100)	–	–
11.	Tuberculosis	3	3 (100)	–	–	–
12.	Diarrhoea	3	–	3 (100)	–	–
13.	Ear problem	2	2 (100)	–	–	–
14.	Boil	1	1 (100.00)	–	–	–
15.	Headache	1	–	1 (100)	–	–
16.	Vomiting	1	–	1 (100)	–	–
17.	Eye problem	1	1 (100)	–	–	–
18.	Intestinal problem	1	1 (100)	–	–	–
19.	Dental problem	1	–	1 (100)	–	–
20.	Diabetes	1	1 (100)	–	–	–
	Grand Total	158	45 (28.48)	113 (71.51)	–	

Table 7.9 : Distribution of the disease/ailments by use of different medicare systems by the people of Yajang-B village

Sl. No.	*Name of the Disease*	*Total morbidity Episodes*	*Age Group*			*No Treatment*
			Modern	*Traditional*	*Both*	
1	*2*	*3*	*4*	*5*	*6*	*7*
1	Malaria	14	12 (85.71)	–	2 (14.28)	–
2.	Gastritis	3	–	–	3 (100)	–
3.	Asthma	2	1 (50)	–	1 (50)	–
4.	Worm	2	2 (100)	–	–	–
5.	Dysentery	1	1 (100)	–	–	–
6.	Jaundice	1	–	1 (100)	–	–
7.	Pneumonia	1	1 (100)	–	–	–
8.	Fever	1	–	1 (100)	–	–
9.	Respiratory problem	1	–	–	1 (100)	–
10.	Appendicitis	1	–	–	1 (100)	–
11.	Paralysis	1	–	–	1 (100)	–
	Grand Total	28	17 (60.71)	2 (7.14)	9 (32.14)	–

On the other hand, Table 7.8 shows that in Yajang-A village people mostly depend on traditional system of treatment. However, there are some diseases, namely tuberculosis, ear problem, diabetes etc., for which the people generally depend on the modern system of treatment. Table 7.9 shows that the people of Yajang-B village depend both on modern and traditional system of treatment.

The following few concrete cases by way of illustration have been recorded below—

Case 7.3

W. Jamir of Yajang-B village is a 18 years old boy. He is a student of class X. His father I. Tali Jamir is a cultivator by occupation. He had been suffering from lower abdominal pain in right side. Then his father brought him to the traditional medicine man, Temen. The medicine man through divination diagnosed the disease and told that it was due to appendix form. He prescribed two medicines to bring it from Haluwating pharmacy. After giving the medicine as prescribed by him, he was cured within 1 week.

Case 7.4

Achangla Aier (25 years) hails from Yajang-B village. She is a housewife and her husband is a cultivator. She has also two children. Suddenly she had been suffering from jaundice. The symptoms were loss of appetite, pain on the joints, the colour became yellow and difficulty in breathing. She then went with her husband to the medicine man, Temen. Based on the symptoms the medicine man gave her a few capsules and advised to eat a banana after taking the capsule to get relief from irritation which is caused by the medicine (capsule). The course continued three days and she was cured within three days.

Case 7.5

Miren Longkomer (20 years) of Yajang-B village is from a nuclear family and read up to class VI. His father is a cultivator and read up to class V. One day, he went with his friend to cut a tree. After returning from the jungle, he started behaving like an insane person. Then his father called the magico-religious man to attend Miren. The magico-religious man with his indigenous methods diagnosed the ailment to be the outcome of the wrath of some spirit (*mojing*). He chanted some hymns and he became cured. But he warned Miren not to go out at 12.00 in noon and night for two days. Miren did obey his advice, but had to come out at 12.00 a.m. in the next day for urinate. Suddenly, the spirit again attacked him and he started to behave as insane. The magico-religious man was again called and with the hymns he again cured Miren. This time Miren did not go out for two days at 12.00 am/pm.

Case 7.6

Aiengla Aier (40 years) of Yajang-B village has read up to class VI and has eight children. Her husband was a cultivator by occupation. One of her sons had been suffered from jaundice and gall bladder stone and she took him to physician of Amguri twice but no positive effect was found. Then she took him to the traditional medicine man of Yajang-A village and with the medicine prescribed by him, her son cured within three-four days.

Case 7.7

M. Mansen Jamir, (35 yeare aged) hails from Yajang-B village and by occupation he is a cultivator. He read up to class V and a member of a nuclear family. His youngest son had been suffered from liver disease and he took him to the medicine man, Temen. The medicine man prescribed him a medicine to buy from the Haluwating pharmacy and by taking it, he was cured within one week.

Case 8.8

Mr. T.C. Jamir (54 years) hails from Yajang-A village. He is the head of a nuclear family and lives with his wife and unmarried children. By occupation he is a cultivator and the village headman of Yajang-A village. He has read up to class IX. One day, he was cutting bamboo in forest. Suddenly, one snake bit him in his hand four times. He then informed another person to call the magico-religious man. The Kabiraj came there and tied a reed (azo) in his hand and with another reed he rubbed the area by chanting some hymns. After doing that, he got relief from the pain. In the fourth day he was cured totally.

Case 7.9

Pandang Wapang Aier (33 years) of Yajang-A village lives with his wife and six children. He is a cultivator and level of education is up to class VII. One day all of his sons went to forest to cut tree and suddenly his third son behaved like an insane person. Then his wife called the magico-religious man and he cured his son by chanting some hymns.

Case 7.10

Imkobchiba Aier (70 years) of Yajang-A village lives with his wife. He is a cultivator and read up to class VI. One day he went to cut bamboo in the forest and after returning from the forest, on the way a snake bit him in his leg three times. His son was also accompanied with him and he took him to the magico-religious man. The magico-religious man chanted some hymns and tied a reed in the affected area. But this time it took more time as the patient approached the magico-religious man in the later stage.

Case 7.11

Likok Jamir (46 years) hails from Yajang-A village, lives with his mother, wife and children. He is a cultivator by occupation and read only up to class X. Once he had been suffered from jaundice. He did not like to eat for a few days and his colour became yellow. Then he went to the herbal medicine man, Temen, for treatment. Temen gave him medicine for that and as per his advice and medicine he was cured in three days.

Case 7.12

Manen Longkomer (58 years) lives with his wife and children in Yajang-A village. He is a cultivator and read up to class VII.

Once he had been suffered from severe fever. The herbal man diagnosed and told that he had been suffering from malaria. Then the herbal man prescribed him to bring one injection from Haluwating pharmacy. Accordingly, the injection was brought and the medicine man gave three doses of that injection and after taking that he was cured in one week.

The foregoing cases thus make it apparent that the people of Yajang-A and Yajang-B villages by and large, prefer to consult the traditional medicine-man and the magico-religious man first, for curative measures, considering the symptoms of the diseases.

Sometimes, it so happen that the patient does not have the expected progress from the traditional medicare system and takes the help of modern medicare system.

Case 7.13

Tenla Aier (20 years) of Yajang-B village hails from a nuclear family. She read up to class VIII. She had been suffering from asthma for last three years. At first, she went to the traditional medicine man of Yajang-A village. The medicine man after diagnosing the disease, gave her the herbal medicine prepared by him. But she did not get much relief. She then did not go to the herbal medicine-man again, but consulted the physician of Haluwating town. The physician gave her injection and it has been reported that she got cured by taking that injection. However, she used to take that injection whenever needed.

Case 7.14

Pandangla Aier (70 years) of Yajang-B village hails from a joint family. He read up to class IV. He had been suffering from chest pain for last three years. He first approached the traditional medicine man of Yajang-A village. But he did not get cure from the treatment of the traditional medicine man and then consulted with the physician of Mokokchung hospital. The physician prescribed a course for one month and it has been reported that he got cured by the medicine.

It has, however, been observed in the field that on many occasions, residential proximity to the hospital as well as educational background of the family do influence their decision in utilising a particular system as a curative measure. It has also been stated earlier that in most of the time the traditional medicine man gives free check-up. But this is not applicable for all types of diseases. The health sub-centre is generally equipped with medicines of very common diseases like cough and cold, fever, diarrhoea, dysentery, any minor injuries etc. For other diseases the nurse generally prescribes the medicines that are to be purchased from the market. Sometimes, expenditure on the prescribed medicines becomes a stumbling block for many poor families to sustain an allopathic course for a longer period. As an alternative resort, they, therefore, fall back on the traditional medicare system. Besides, unavailability of the nurse in most of the time as transferred very frequently also influence the people to utilise the traditional one without having any alternative means in times of need.

However, during the present investigation it has also been noted that for some particular diseases, the people depend only on the traditional resource as a curative measure.

Thus it is apparent that the people utilise both the traditional as well as the modern medicare systems. Depending on a number of factors, in some cases the people use the modern medicare system, whereas in some other cases they depend on the traditional one. There are still other circumstances when they take recourse to both the systems. However, the use of both the systems in any form is generally made when a particular system does not show the expected results in curing the disease.

To conclude, it would probably be appropriate to have an overall idea as to the different herbal medicines that are used by the people for various types of diseases. In this regard the data generated from the field have been presented in Table 7.10. It will be seen from the table that in some diseases they use the same herbal medicine. Some plants are wild one and can be identified by the traditional medicine man only and the English equivalent and scientific name could not be made available for these.

Table 7.10 : List of herbal medicines used among the people under investigation

Sl. No.	*Disease*	*Herbal*	*Preparation*	*Administration*
1	*2*	*3*	*4*	*5*
1	Jaundice	A kind of arum plant, no specific name	Dry tubers of the plant are ground to make powder	200 mg of the powder for children and 500 mg or adult with a banana once daily for three days in empty stomach
2	Diabetes	Tamarind, neem (*Melia indica*), bitter gourd (*Momordica charatia*), curry leaves and wild creeper (no specific name)	Dry leaves of these plants and roots of the creeper are ground to make a mixture	One tea spoonful of the mixture with half cup of lukewarm water to be taken twice daily for three days.
3	Dysentery	Periwinkle (*Lepernaro*), grapes, *titaphool* (a kind of red and bitter flower plant; no specific name, *Phlogacanthus thyrsiflorus*), *longer* (locally available), pomegranate	Dry leaves of periwinkle, grapes, titaphool and complete plant of longer (dry) and peel of pomegranate (dry) are ground to make a mixture.	One tea spoonful of the mixture with half cup of lukewarm water to be taken once daily for four days.
4	Diarrhoea	- do-	- do-	- do-
5	Cough	Tulsi (*Ocimum sanctum*), tamarind, lemon (*Citrus medica*), ginger (*Zingber officinale*), honey	The juice of these herbs is mixed with honey to make a mixture.	10 ml of the mixture for adult and 5 ml for the children to be taken thrice daily for four days.
6	Chest pain	- do-	- do-	- do-
7	Pneumonia	- do-	- do-	- do-
8	Typhoid	- do-	- do-	- do-
9	Gastritis	- do-	- do-	- do-
10	Constipation	- do-	- do-	- do-
11	Asthma	- do-	- do-	- do-
12	Kidney stone	- do-	- do-	- do-
13	Scabies	Indian Eucalyptus, lime	The leaves of the plant are ground with a little quantity of lime to make a paste.	The paste is to be smeared on the affected area.
14	Ringworm	*Ajunaro* (no specific name)	The leaves of the plant are ground to make a paste.	The paste is to be smeared on the affected area

(Contd...)

Table 7.10 : *(Contd...)*

15	Small pox	Neem (*Meiia indica*)	The dry leaves of the plant are ground to make powder	The powder is to be rub on the affected area
16	High blood pressure	A wild plant (no specific name)	The leaves of the plant	A few leaves to be chewed with a glass of wateras required
17	Kidney stone	*Phylanthus*	Complete dry plant is ground to make powder	One tea spoonful of the powder is to be taken twice daily till not cured.
18	Gall bladder stone		-do-	-do-
19	Urinary tract problem		-do-	-do-
20	Stomach pain	Tulsi (*Ocimum sanctum*)	The leaves of the plant	A few leaves to be chewed as required
21	Skin burn	Aloe vera	The gum of the leaves of the plant	The gum of the leaves to be smeared on the affected area as required
22	Urine problem	*Dopor tenga* (An acid plant)	The leaves of the plant	A few leaves to be chewed as required with a glass of water.

MATERNAL AND CHILD HEALTH CARE PRACTICE

Maternal and child health is the index of health status of the population in any society. Both mother and child health care ought to begin right from the beginning of conception, i.e. the mothers should be properly protected against disease and have proper nutrition or balanced diet which is necessary for maintaining good health both for the mother and for the fetus. Both tradition and culture determine the attitudes, beliefs and practices in regard to mother and child health care. Mother and child health status among the tribal becomes a victim of their ignorance, economic deprivation and inaccessibility to medical facilities.

Almost all tribal communities have their own traditional belief in mother and child health care system and practices. Presently an attempt has been made to understand the mother and child health care practices prevailing among the people under study.

Pregnancy Diagnosis and Restrictions

Conception is a good sign among the Aos after marriage and they think that it is a natural process. Due to the absence of proper health resources, women usually rely on their own diagnosis for knowing about pregnancy, in which the absence of periods, vomiting, feeling of hotness, nausea, greedy for sour are the key factors. Though there is no specific restriction for a pregnant woman but there are some moral restrictions and superstitious beliefs at the stage of pregnancy which a conceived woman should observe. Thus, a pregnant woman is not allowed to go alone to the river side and outside in the evening. There is a strict prohibition that she should not go to the burial ground. It is believed that if they go to such places during pregnancy period, the evil spirit (*mojing*) may harm the woman and the baby. The woman (pregnant) is advised to cover the body with a *chadar* to avoid from evil spirit. As the people are jhum cultivators, both men and women are bound to go to the jhum field. In this regard, the pregnant woman also compelled to go to the jhum fields in the advance stage. On seeing a snake, by a pregnant woman directly is believed to be harmful for the baby, as snake is poisonous. So, the pregnant woman is advised to go always in middle with others and not in the first and in the last so that she cannot see any poisonous thing and also to get rid of from evil spirit. When the pregnant women go out, they take a few leaves of tulsi in their basket (*khung*) and also rub the leaves of tulsi on their whole body to avoid the evil spirit. The husbands of pregnant women are to follow certain restrictions. Such as, a husband is not allowed to kill any living animals during this period and should not stay together with his wife in the forest. They believe that if they do so something wrong may happen. Such as if anyone kills a lame or a blind animal then the new born will be lame or blind.

Food Habit During Pregnancy

There is no restriction on food during pregnancy period and no specific or special diet is prescribed for the pregnant women. As they are mostly depended on nature, they like to consume the available foods and wild animal's and bird's meat of the forest. Generally, the husband of the pregnant woman brings these items and these are the crab, prawn, local fish, meat of wild birds, animals etc. They believe that these food items increase the growth of the embryo and the baby becomes healthy and strong. They are not concerned about maintaining a balanced diet during pregnancy and they take normal diet as other members of the family. No special preparation is made for her. However, as reported by a few elderly women, they do not take too much bitter things, like chilli, lemon etc. during pregnancy as it may harm the fetus.

Daily Activities of Pregnant Women

The people usually lead a busy daily routine of work. As the people are mostly jhum cultivators, most of the inhabitants belonging to both the sexes except the old persons and children are engaged in their jhum field for the entire year. Besides, nuclear family is predominant among them. They have the traditional custom that after marriage the newly married couple is to live separately in a new house constructed by the husband. Due to survival in the new family both husband and wife have to do hard work. However, the womenfolk remain relatively busier as compared to their men counterpart. The women leave their bed early in the morning and get busy with their day-to-day activities such as preparation of morning meal, take care of children, splitting firewood, and then go to the jhum field and work there for the whole day. On their way back, they collect firewood in their baskets and the edible roots and leaves also. After reaching home they again get busy for the dinner. Besides, they collect water by going down a steep hill for thousand feet or more to fetch water from local pits and ponds and they draw water in their big bamboo tubes. The Ao women do not get much leisure in the midst of their multifarious pre-occupation. From early morning till night women generally remain busy with their work at home as well as in jhum field in addition to the child bearing and child rearing exercises. The pregnant women are also to continue these daily works till the time of delivery. Some elderly women commented that there are some cases where women delivered a baby immediately after returning from the jhum field. They believe that if they do hard work, the delivery will be normal. As nuclear family predominates among the Ao Nagas, the pregnant women are bound to perform their daily activities for their consumption.

Mode of Delivery

During the present investigation it has been observed that most of the deliveries are carried out at home by traditional midwives. Sometimes, a trained midwife or nurse is called if available. A woman is likely to be taken to a clinic or hospital when she has serious complications.

The traditional midwives are self-trained and provide variety of services, such as antenatal care, abdominal massage, foetal positioning, prescribing herbal medicine and delivery services etc. At the time of home delivery, the labouring woman is associated with the midwives and other women who stay throughout. However, involvement of male members is avoided even the husband of the woman.

When severe pains begin, the labouring woman lies on a bed or on the floor. Her head is raised on a pillow, her knees bent and heels pressed against the side of the bed or floor. The midwife (*taapara*) plays the vital role to complete the child birth process.

As the baby is born, the *dai* holds the baby and cut the umbilical cord by either a blade or a sharp piece of bamboo split with her own measurement. Then the baby is taken to clean by the experience lady and the *taapara* again concentrates on the new mother and press or massage the belly to deliver the placenta. For cleaning the new born baby they use lukewarm water. After cleaning they tie the cord with thread and sometimes use Johnson powder and mustard oil. Then the baby is wrapped-up with warm cloths.

After releasing the placenta (*menden/nusem*) the husband of the delivered woman buries it in a specific area where nobody moves. There is also a belief associated with the burying of the placenta. While going for burying the placenta, the husband should not move his hand (the hand carrying the placenta) too much. If they do so, the baby will get shock in sleeping time. After burying the placenta, husband should not press the particular area with his feet. If they do so, the baby will get trouble in breathing. The husbands are also warned not to bury any wooden/bamboo post in that area as it also cause problem in breathing of the baby. If by chance, someone does this mistake, then the alternative is either to dig out the post or may put a straw in that area. They believe, if a straw is put in that area, without withdrawal of the post, the baby can relief from the breathing problem.

Activities after Birth

After cleaning the mother and child, the mother feed her baby. They considered the first drop of breast milk as medicine and for that they try to give it to her baby. To increase the flow of breast milk of the mother, they prefer to eat papaya after delivery.

Among the Aos, no pollution is observed after child birth like the others. They are not concerned with the care of the umbilical cord. However, for easy removal of the umbilical cord, they use mustard oil and powder both talcum and

Johnson. Until the naval is removed or fall the mother is advised to do not take spicy food, chilli, black peper etc. They prefer to take boiled food items including the meat items during that period.

After delivery, the delivered woman is given rest and the period of rest is compulsory for 15 days. In case of joint family a woman is expected to get more time for rest because of availability of other family members, who are always ready to offer their helping hand. In case of nuclear family the woman does not get much rest and in that period, generally, her husband or the clan members give support. After the delivery, the delivered woman is strictly prohibited to have intercourse for one month. All the people maintain this rule.

In the room of new mother and child, they keep a bunch of tulsi (*nangphara*) with a belief that evil spirit cannot harm the mother and the newly born baby. People from outside are prohibited to go directly to the newly born child as they believe that evil spirit can come with them. Therefore, the persons coming from outside first go to the fire place and after warming their bodies they come to the new born baby's room.

On the day of birth of the new born, the family members and attended persons pray to God (Jesus Christ) for giving the baby and then the people (family members and the attendant members) together have a feast with the meat of chicken or pig whatever available.On the third day (from birth), they observe the naming ceremony (*tenung ajaba* in chongli and *tening chuba* in mongsen) of the new born. On that day, they invite their clan members from both father and mother sides. The eldest member generally takes the major role in this ceremony. Presence of the Pastor of the Church on that day is also essential and therefore, they also invite the Pastor. The eldest person gives a few names and they call with these names to the baby. Out of these names, they give that particular name which is seen to accept by the baby. After naming the new baby, if the baby gets ill, then again they change the name. If the new born is a girl, then they also perform the ceremony of bering the ears on that day by an elderly man and give red thread to wear in the ear holes. This is known as *tenarong atuba* in chongli and *tenarong tuba* in mongsen. After naming, all the invited people are entertained with a feast. The meats of cow, pig, chicken etc. are the most important items in this feast. Depending on their economic condition they also invite the neighbouring people on that day. This naming ceremony is observed by the people for their every issue.

Reproductive Behaviour

In order to have an idea about the reproductive behaviour of the women, data have been generated on health checkup during pregnancy, place of delivery and reproductive performance.

Generally, it is seen that the reproductive age for woman is 15-50. With this fact, the respondents are considered with an age grade 15-49 married women. The current age of married women in their reproductive years village-wise has been presented in Table 7.11.

Table 7.11 : Current age of married women in their reproductive years village-wise

Sl. No	Name of the Village	Age Group							Total
		15-19	20-24	25-29	30-34	35-39	40-44	45-49	
1	2	3	4	5	6	7	8	9	10
1	Lirmen	0	1 (1.56)	4 (6.25)	17 (26.56)	13 (20.31)	20 (31.25)	9 (14.06)	64 (100.00)
2	Yajang-A	2 (3.22)	9 (14.51)	10 (16.12)	10 (16.12)	10 (16.12)	10 (16.12)	11 (17.74)	62 (100.00)
3	Yajang-B	0	2 (10)	7 (35)	2 (10)	4 (20)	2 (10)	3 (15)	20 (100.00)
Grand Total		2 (1.36)	12 (8.21)	21 (14.38)	29 (19.86)	27 (18.49)	32 (21.91)	23 (15.75)	146 (100.00)

From Table 7.11 it has been observed that in Lirmen village, more number of women are in the age group of 40-44 years (31.25%), and least (1.56%) in the age group of (20-24) years. In Yajang-A village highest is found in the age group of 45-49 years (17.74%) and least is (3.22%) in the age group of 15-19 years. In Yajang-B village, the highest number of married reproductive women was found in the age group of 25-29 years (35%) and least is in the age groups 20-24, 30-34 and 40-44 years, where the percentages are same, i.e. (10%).

Health check-up during Pregnancy (Antenatal Check-up)

The health of a mother and her new born child depends not only on the health care she receives during her pregnancy and delivery, but also on the care she and the infant receive during the first weeks after the delivery.

Antenatal care (ANC) refers to pregnancy related health care provided by a doctor or a health worker in a medical facility or at home. The Safe Motherhood Initiative proclaims that all pregnant women must receive basic professional antenatal care. The RCH programme of the Government of India recommends that as part of antenatal care, women should receive two doses of tetanus taxied vaccines, adequate amount of iron and folic acid tablets or syrups to prevent and treat anaemia, and at least three antenatal check-ups that include blood pressure checks and other procedures to detect pregnancy complications (Maiti *et al.*, 2005).

Among the people under investigation it has been observed that from conception to delivery of the child they by and large do not have any idea of medical check-up. They do not seem to be very much concerned about the necessity of some special care of the mothers' health. It is due to the non-availability of adequate health resources and health education among the people. The Ao women carry more of the work burden of the household and therefore have less time to seek out health care services making them disadvantaged relative to men in their access and utilization of health care services. However, a few educated women are found to take health check-up during pregnancy period from the physician of nearest town.

Table 7.12 shows the village-wise distribution of the women attending antenatal check-ups before delivery. From Table 7.12, it is seen that in the villages under study out of 138 women, 7.97 per cent women went for antenatal check-ups before delivery, while 92.02 per cent women did not. Considering the villages independently it is seen from the table that in the village Lirmen, 11.66 per cent women went for antenatal check-ups before delivery, while about 88.33 per cent women did not. Similarly, in the village Yajang-A 6.89 per cent went for antenatal check-ups, while 93.10 per cent women did not. But in the village Yajang-B not a single women went for antenatal check-ups before delivery.

Table 7.12 : Village-wise distribution of the women attending antenatal check-ups

Sl. No	*Name of the village*	*No. of women*	*Yes*		*No*	
			N	*%*	*N*	*%*
1.	Lirmen*	60	7	11.66	53	88.33
2.	Yajang-A*	58	4	6.89	54	93.10
3.	Yajang-B	20	–	–	20	100.00
Total		138	11	7.97	127	92.02

* 4 newly married women of Lirmen village and 4 newly married women of Yajang-A village are excluded from the table.

Place of Delivery and Birth Attendants

Place of delivery and personnel attended the delivery are important indicators that determine the maternal and infant mortality, morbidity and general health status of women. One of the most important major thrust areas of the RCH

Programme in India is to encourage and promote deliveries under proper hygienic conditions under the supervision of trained health professionals (Maiti *et al.*, 2005). Most birth in less developed countries, about 60 per cent occur outside health facilities (Murugan, 2005).

During the present investigation it has been recorded that most of the deliveries are carried out at home by village elderly *dais* and sometimes by the trained nurse if available. A woman is likely to be taken to a clinic or hospital when she has serious complications. Table 7.13 shows the village-wise distribution of place of delivery. From Table 7.13, it is seen that out of 433 births, 93.76 per cent were delivered at home while 6.23 per cent were delivered at hospital. Considering the villages independently, it is seen from the table that in Lirmen village, out of 189 births, 91 per cent were delivered at home while 8.99 per cent were delivered at hospital. In the village Yajang-A, out of 172 births, 96.51 per cent were delivered at home and 3.48 per cent were delivered at hospital. Similarly, in the village Yajang-B, out of 72 births, 94.44 per cent were delivered at home while 5.55 per cent were delivered at hospital. Thus, it is seen that in all the three villages, the percentage of home delivery is maximum than that of hospital delivery.

Table 7.13 : Village-wise distribution of place of delivery

Sl. No	*Name of the village*	*No. of women*	*Place of delivery*		*Total*
			Home (%)	*Hospital (%)*	
1	Lirmen	60	172 (91.00)	17 (8.99)	189 (100)
2	Yajang-A	58	166 (96.51)	6 (3.48)	172 (100)
3	Yajang-B	20	68 (94.44)	4 (5.55)	72 (100)
	Total	138	406 (93.73)	27 (6.23)	433 (100)

Reproductive Performance

Village-wise distribution of the reproductive performance of the women has been given in Table 7.14. The table shows that in the village Lirmen out of 60 women, total number of conception is 192, live birth 179, still birth 1, abortion 3 and post birth death 9. In the village Yajang-A out of 58 women, total number of conception is 172, live birth 164, and post-birth death 8. In the village Yajang-B out of 20 women, total number of conception is 73, live birth 62, still birth 3, abortion 1 and post-birth death 7. It has been observed that in all the three villages post-birth death is very common.

Table 7.14 : Village-wise distribution of the reproductive performance of the women

Sl. No	*Name of the village*	*No. of women*	*Total No. of Conception*	*Live Birth*	*Still Birth*	*Abortion*	*Post-Birth Death*
1	2	3	4	5	6	7	8
1	Lirmen	60	192	179	1	3	9
2	Yajang-A	58	172	164	-	-	8
3	Yajang-B	20	73	62	3	1	7
	Total	138	437	405	4	4	24

Family Planning Practices

Family planning is a scientific designing of the parents to realize maximum health wealth and happiness from the individual family and from the social and national points of view. Women need birth planning to maximize the chances of survival of children while protecting their own health as pregnancy is a serious problem for many women. There is practically no prevalence of traditional birth control measures or practices among the Aos. With regard to the modern family planning methods, it has been reported that from Mokokchung Civil Hospital some AIDS Department N.G.O. visited the villages and some N.G.O. from Mongkolomba came to motivate the people about these contraceptive methods. Thus, now-a-days the people are aware about the various contraceptive methods. Generally awareness of contraception through sterilization is found to be the higher among the women than the contraceptive tablets. However, majority of them are aware of the natural birth control measure and use the self-control method. Though they have some knowledge of condom, yet no one is found to use it.

Child Care

The child care/rearing process generally refers to all the interaction between parents and their children. These interactions include the parents expressions of attitudes, values, interest and beliefs as well as their care taking and behaviour training modes. Hence, this process is a combination of socialization and enculturation (Yadav *et al.*, 2001).

The Government of India is striving hard to reduce the infant mortality rate, by providing a variety of maternal and child health care services. The child care services are mainly focused through the immunization of children against the six major killer diseases and also to educate the mothers regarding diarrhoea and pneumonia which are dangerous for children, all targeted at reduction of infant mortality. Proper breast feeding and weaning practices, complete and timely coverage of immunization of the children are the two prime aspects in child care, as they ensure the health and chance of survival of the child (Babu & Rao, 2006).

Among Aos children are taken care by their parents. However, in the first neo-natal stage, the infants are taken care by the mothers. In absence of a mother or in case of death of a mother in the delivery time, the new born is looked after by the father or the grandparents. As nuclear family predominates among them, both husband and wife are bound to go to the jhum field for their survival. They do not take the new born babies to the jhum field till 3 years and during this period the only alternative is the neighbours residence or clan relatives to look after their children.

The women themselves know the act of breast-feeding. They consider the first drop of breast milk as medicine and so, they try to feed it. They feed their baby immediately after delivery, as a natural process. If required, they also supply bottle feeding. In absence of the mother of a baby, the attending woman feed her breast milk if she has. The women are not concerned about the cleaning of the breast before feeding the child. They continue their breast milk for one year and sometimes till their next pregnancy or delivery. From 9-10 months, they start to give other milk like cow etc. Weaning starts after sixteen to eighteen months of delivery. Generally, the children automatically wean when they begin to take solid food. From three months onward they provide semi-solid food to their babies. They mix rice powder with milk and feed their babies. After one year they start to give solid foods to their babies.

Balanced diet is very important for leading healthy life. Good nutrition is the key of child's optimal growth and intellectual development. The food eaten and the type of nutrition provided during the early years, lays the foundations for short and long term health. Among the Aos except a few educated women, others are not concerned about the balanced diet of their children. The supplementary feeding is not different from the diet of the other family members and they also do not maintain any proper time schedule for feeding their babies.

Approximately 2.5 million infants die every year in India from disease, which can simply be prevented by immunization. Immunization against preventable disease is the central concept of the primary health and reproductive and child health care (Jain & Sharma, 2006). Vaccination is a preventive therapy against various diseases of children. To save a pregnant woman and the child in her womb from Tetanus disease it is necessary to give her two injections of TT vaccine during her pregnancy period. During the present investigation it has been reported that except few educated women, all the rest do not vaccinate their children properly. However, O.P.V. (Oral Polio Vaccine) under compulsory programme is given to all of their issues which are supplied by the government from time to time at free of cost.

As there is no proper health centre and no health professional, the people are not aware about the importance of vaccination. They do not know that to save their children from malignant diseases (Tetanus, T.B., Diptheria, Whooping Cough, Polio, and Measles) vaccination is must. They even do not know about the vaccination schedule for pregnant women and for infant. Most of the children suffer from various diseases such as fever, diarrhoea, cough, measles, jaundice, malaria, typhoid etc. In some cases death episodes are also recorded from these diseases. Though all kinds of necessary vaccination are free supplied by the government but people are deprived from it as, available health centres have got no any scientific equipment to store the vaccines safely. Besides, the health centres where the vaccines are available are far away from their villages and their communication problems do not allow them to receive it.

Moreover, though some of them have got the knowledge of vaccination, but due to their poor economic conditions they cannot get it from the nearest private health resources where these are available. In this context, Babu and Rao (2006) opined, "The problem of child health care of the scheduled tribe is a complex one and is not comparable with the general caste population or even scheduled caste segment. Promotion of modern health care among the tribal societies depends on their capacity to receive it, their stage of socio-cultural evolution, ecological settings and mode of economy and so on."

Causes of Infant and Child Mortality

The mortality of infants and children cannot be isolated from women's health status because most of the causes of infant mortality are related to exogamous factors related to mother such as nutritional and health status of mother followed by utilization of maternal and child health services. Among the Aos infant and child mortality is very common. Thus, an attempt is also made to have a general understanding of the causes of mortality. For the purpose, a few cases have been recorded below.

Case 7.15

Tengla Aier of Yajang-B village is a woman of 20 years having one child. She hails from a nuclear family and read up to class six. Her husband (22 years) is a cultivator and read up to class seven. Her first delivery was a still birth. The delivery was conducted by three local *dais* at home and as reported by her, everything was normal but the baby born was dead and they could not know the exact cause of death. She did not take any health check-up during pregnancy due to lack of adequate health resources in their area.

Case 7.16

Achangla Jamir (36 years) of Lirmen village hails from a nuclear family. She read up to class four. She has six children. When her third issue became of 2 years, he suffered from jaundice. She could not take him for better treatment, due to economic constrains. As a result the child died.

Case 7.17

Ayangla Jamir (46 years) of Yajang-A village hails from a nuclear family. She has three children. She read up to class six. Her second issue died in two years from birth due to dysentery. She took her baby to a physician for treatment in Amguri but it did not give any positive effect and finally the baby died. She did not give the necessary vaccines to her baby except Oral Polio Vaccine (O.P.V.) as these are not available in their health centre.

Case 7.18

Atula Jumir (28 years) of Yajang-B village hails from a nuclear family. She read up to class seven. She has three children. Her first issue suffered from measles/pox. She first took her baby to the traditional medicine man of Yajang-A village but the medicine man could not cure her baby and then she approached one physician in Amguri. But no positive effect was found and the baby died when it was just of 5 months. As reported by her, she also lost her third issue in the same way in six months from birth.

Case 7.19

Arenla Ozukum (28 years) of Yajang-B village hails from a nuclear family. She has three children and read up to class four. However, her third issue was suffered from jaundice in three years from birth. She took her baby first to the traditional medicine man of Yajang-A village. The medicine man tried to cure her baby with his medicines but the baby did not get any relief. Then she approached the physician of private hospital at Amguri. The physician tried to cure her baby, but it was already very late and finally the baby died in the private hospital at Amguri.

The foregoing cases thus make it apparent that due to lack of proper health resources they cannot give proper health check-up to their children. As a result, the children die without getting timely proper health check-up. It is also a fact that the mother's education and the general socio-economic condition have a very high relationship on infant and child mortality.

Plate No. 9

Interior Views of a Typical Ao Naga Kitchen

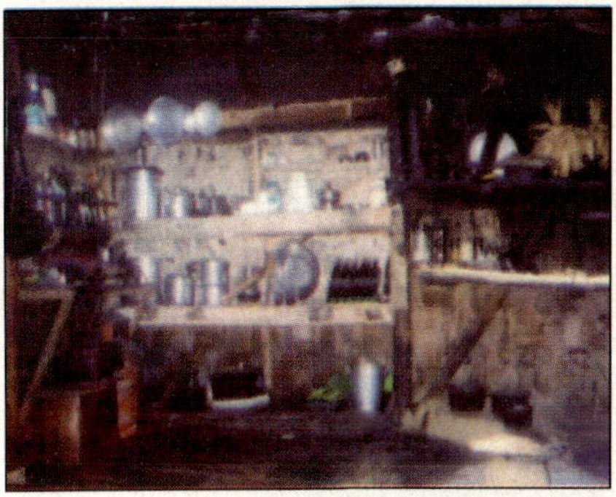

Showing utensils used in the kitchen

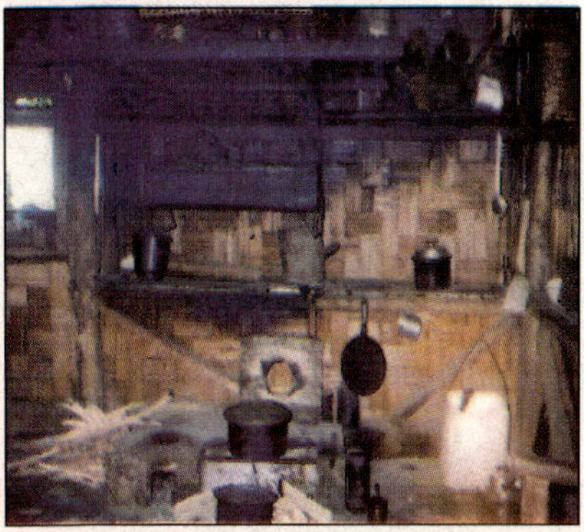

Close view of a hearth

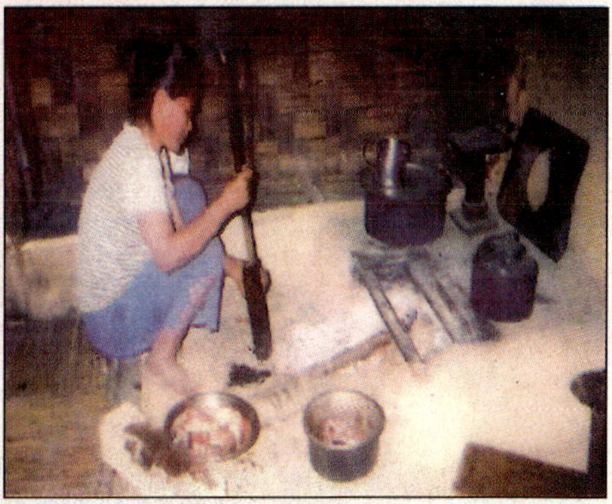

A woman attending her kitchen

Plate No. 10

Food Storing and Preservation

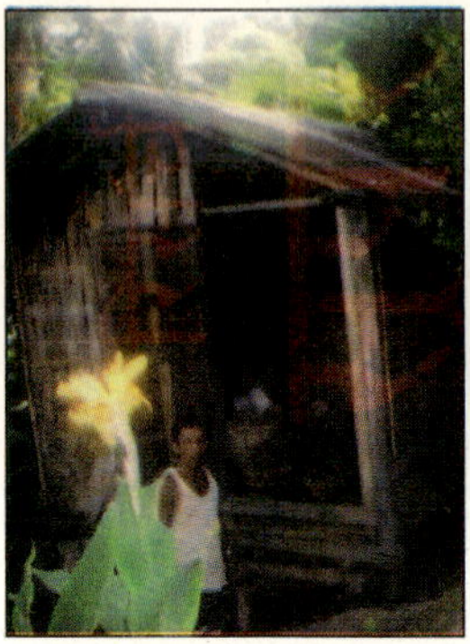

A granary

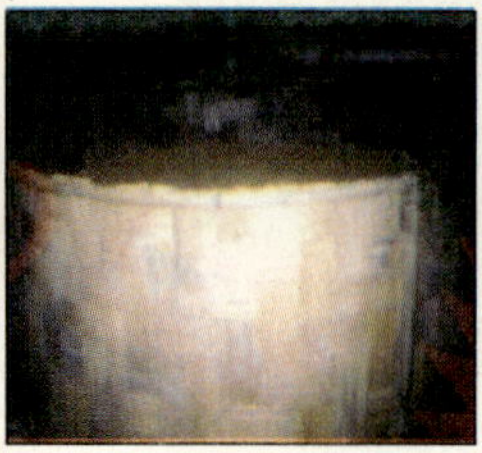

Stored paddy grains

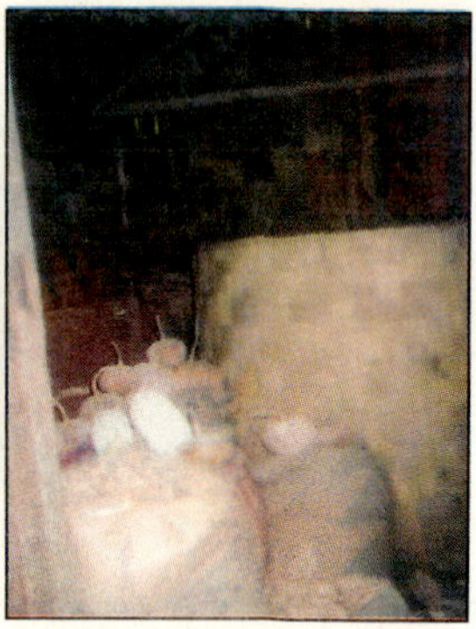

Inside of a granary

A portion of meat is smoked over the family hearth for future consumption

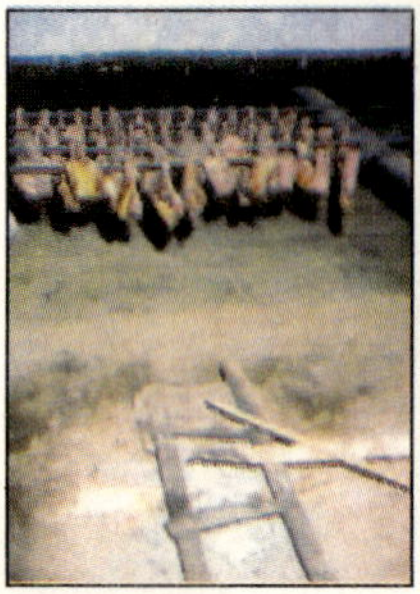

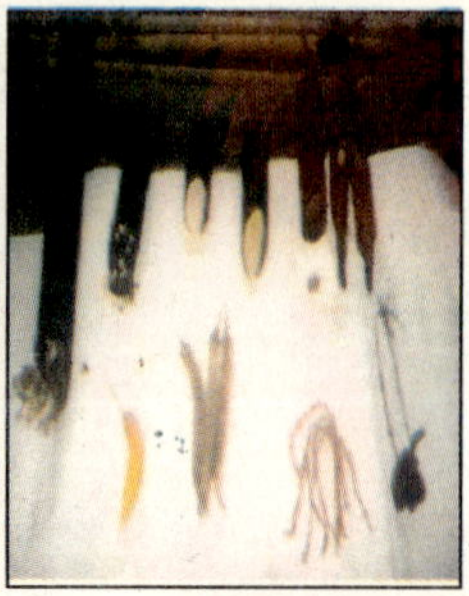

Preservation of seeds and dry fish for future use

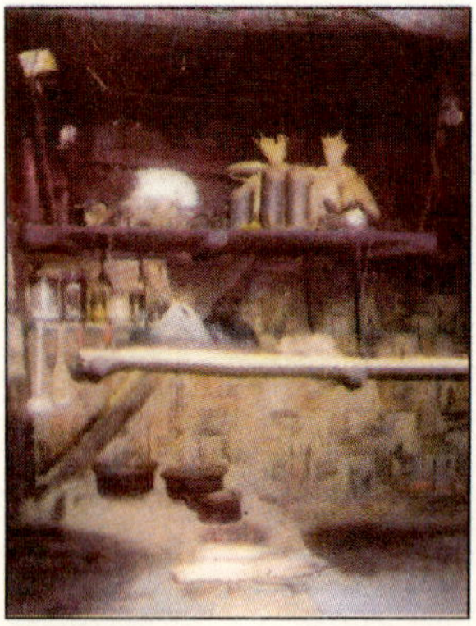

A fumigation shelf over the kitchen hearth use for storing and preserving food materials

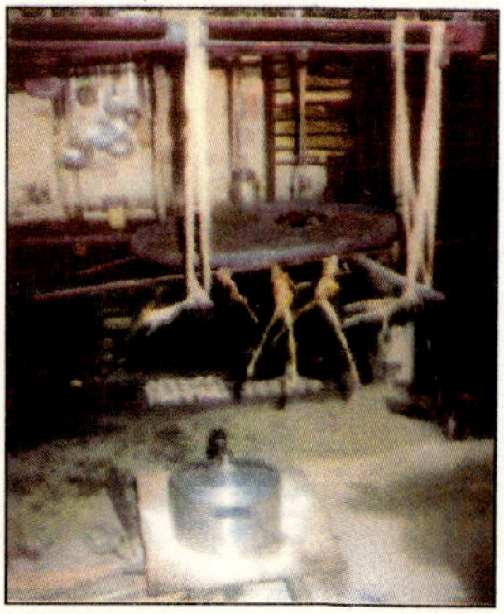

Plate No. 11

Reflecting Housing Condition

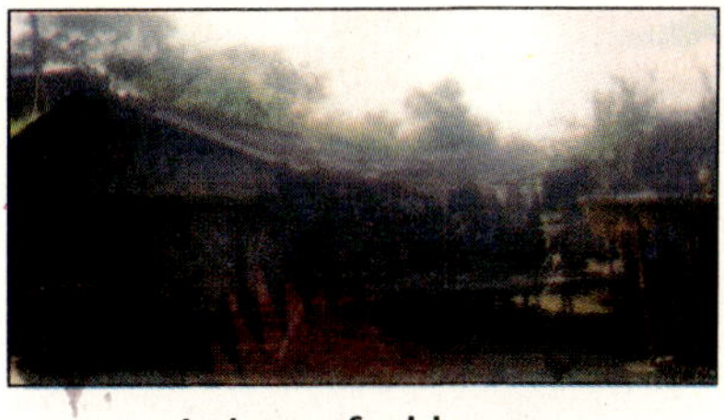

A tin roofed house

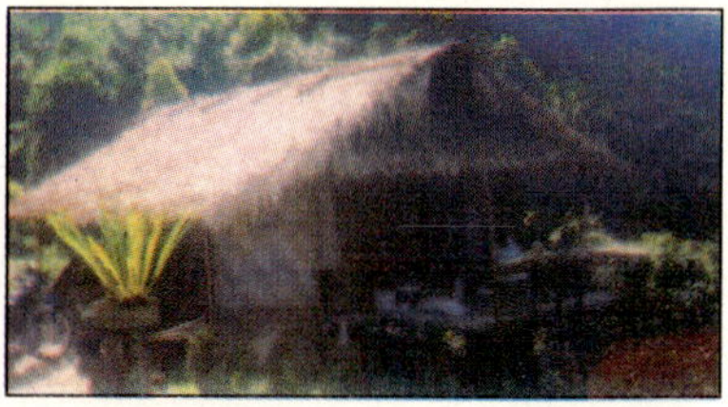

Side view of a house

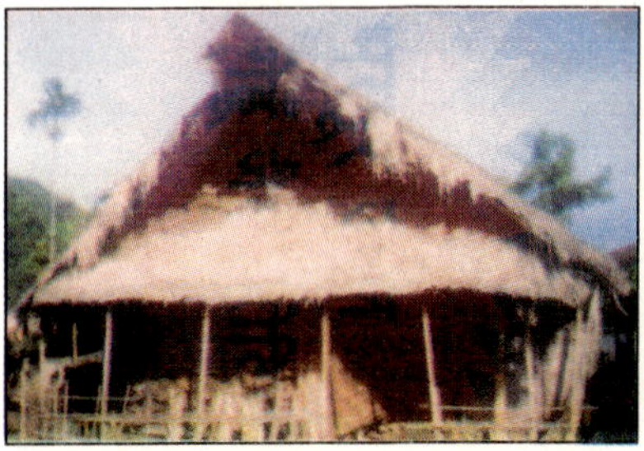

Front view of a house

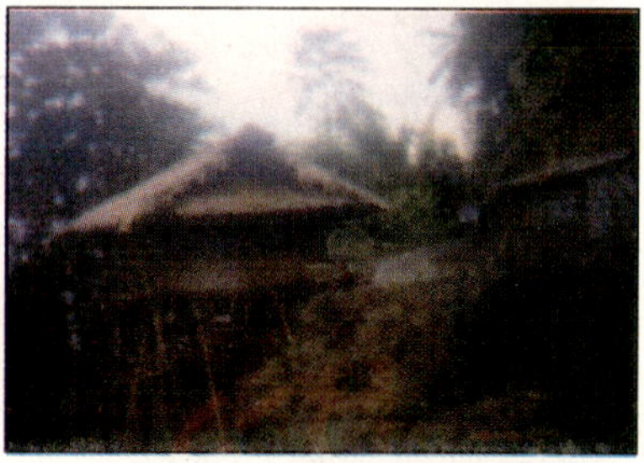

Back view of a house

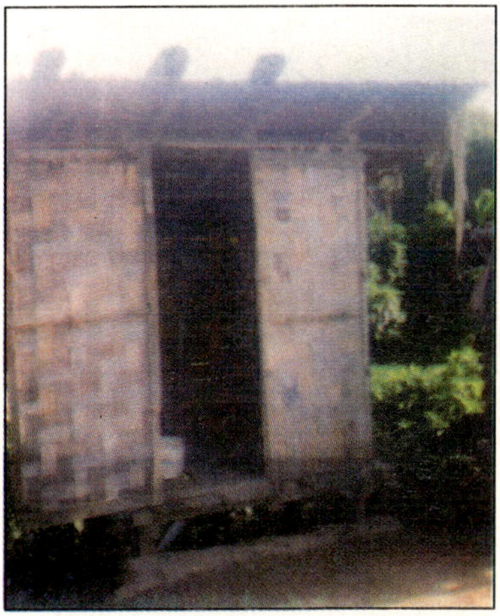

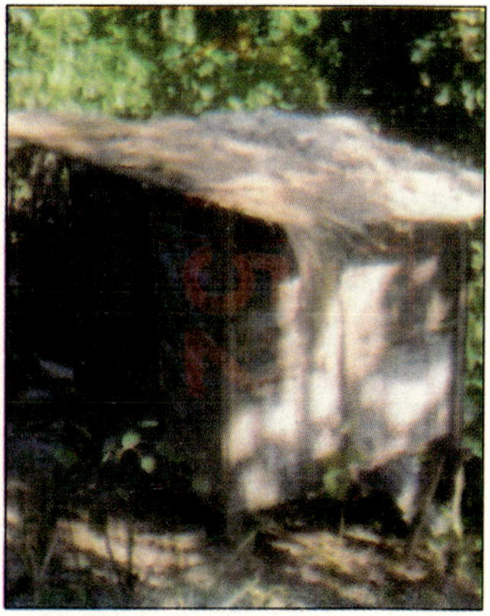

Views of latrines

Plate No. 12

Drinking water source and means of transportation

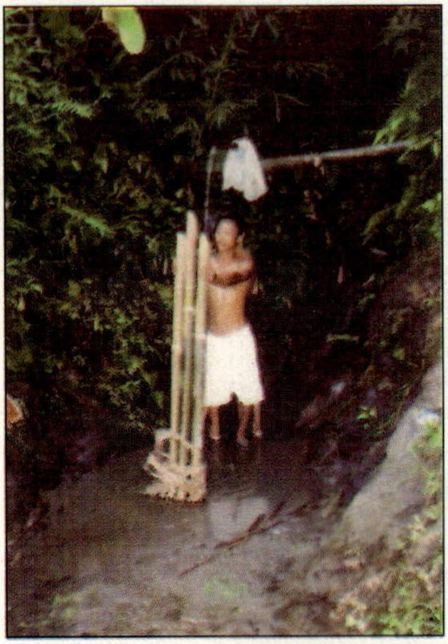

A boy filled up bamboo tubes with drinking water

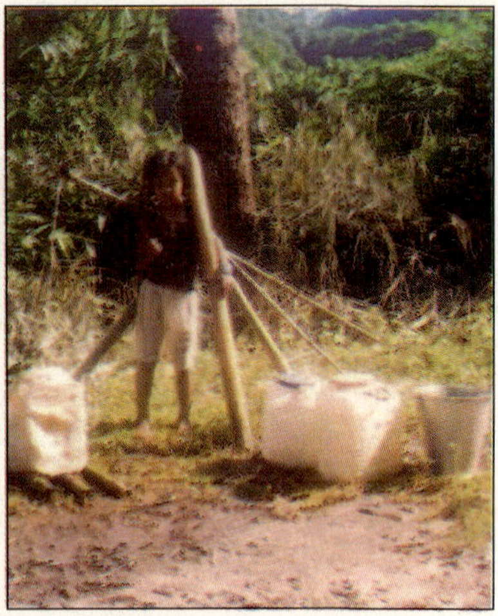

A little girl fetching water

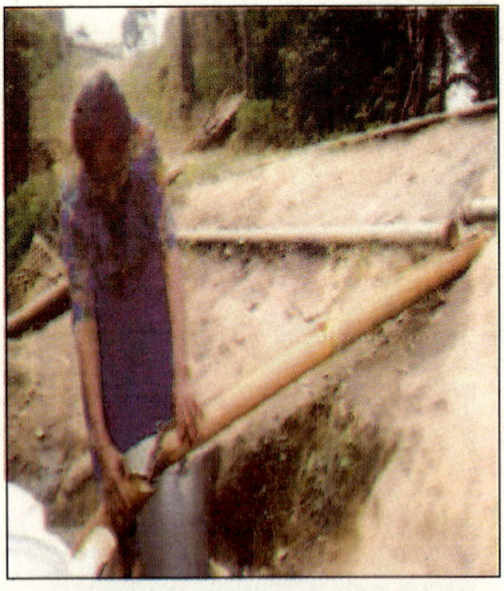

An elderly woman fetching water from a broken water supply pipe

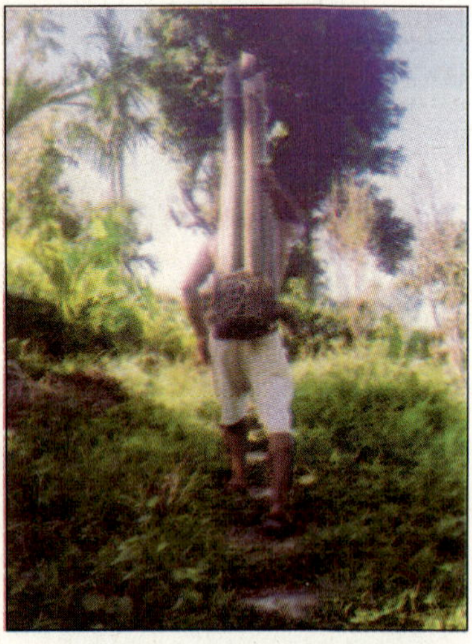

A boy carrying water filled bamboo tubes on his back

Plate No. 13

Health Scenario among the People

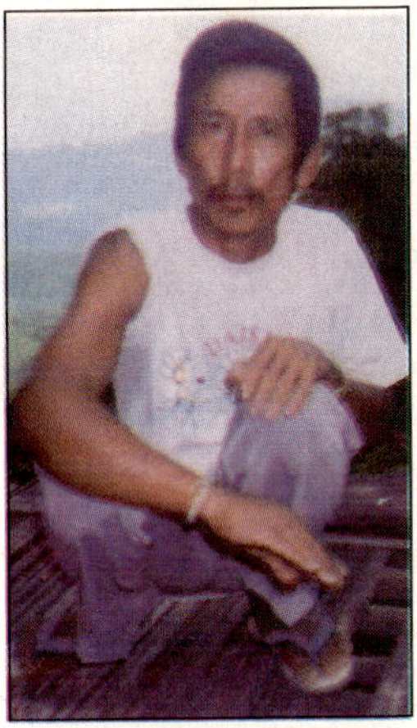

A man showing his wrist tied with enchanted reed given by magico-religious man to cure him from snake bite

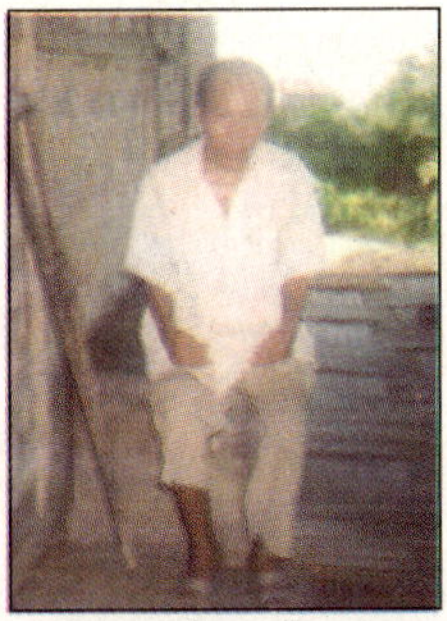

A paralysed man

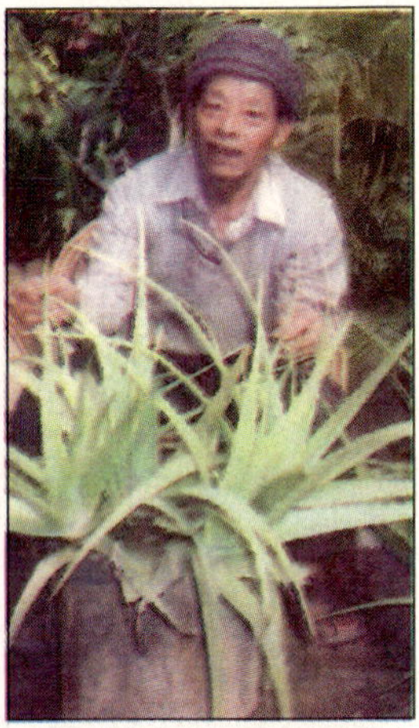

The traditional herbal medicine man of Yajang-A village

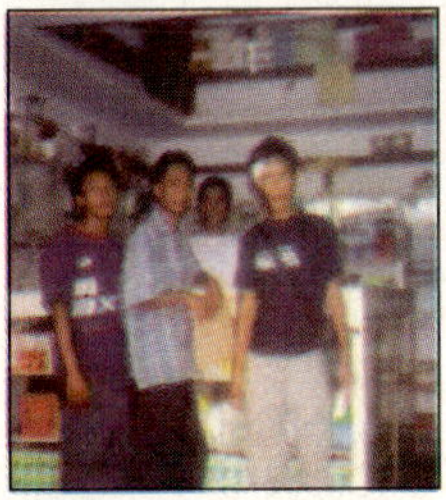

Village boys buying medicines from Haluwating pharmacy

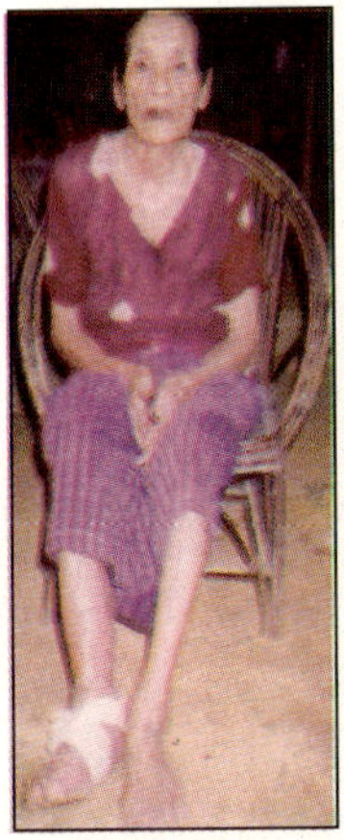

An old woman is suffering from skin disease

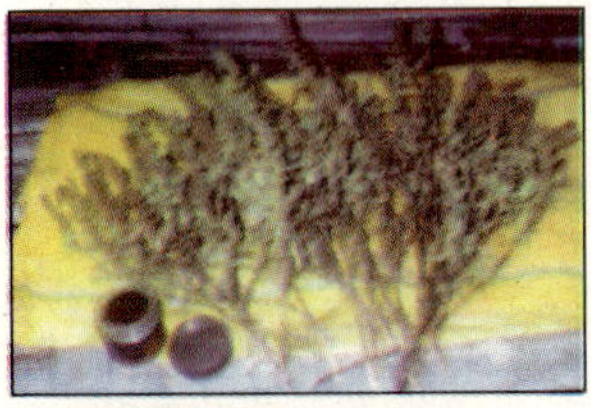

Nangphara (Tulsi), A popular herbal medicine

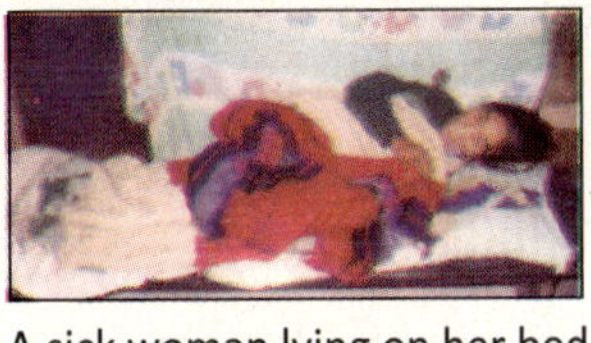

A sick woman lying on her bed

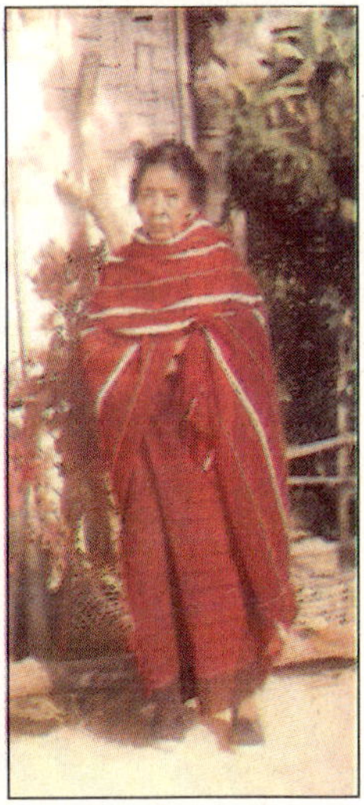

A traditional *dai* of Yajang-A village

Plate No. 14

Ao Naga Women in their Day-to-Day Life

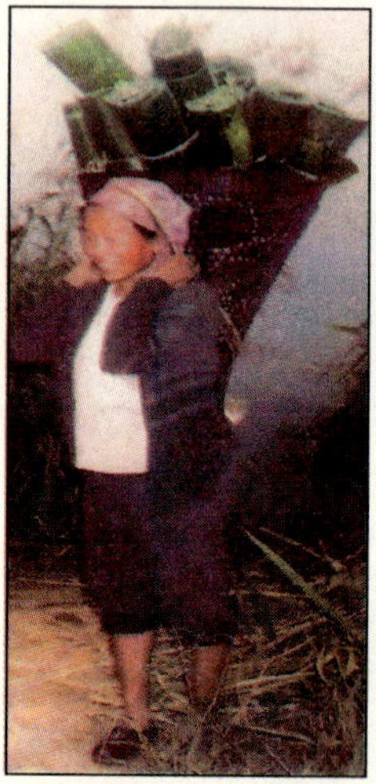

A woman carrying betel leaves

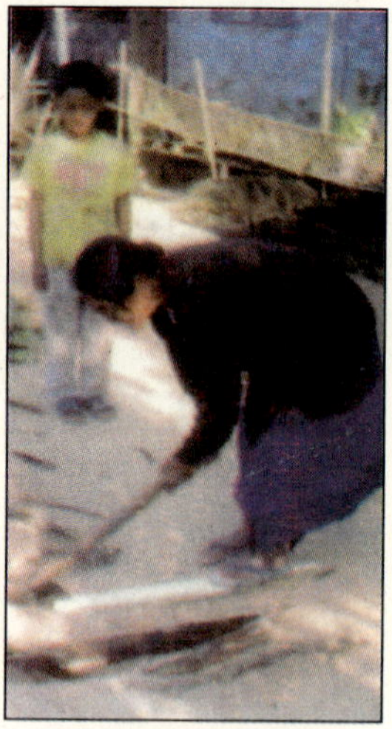

A woman splitting firewood

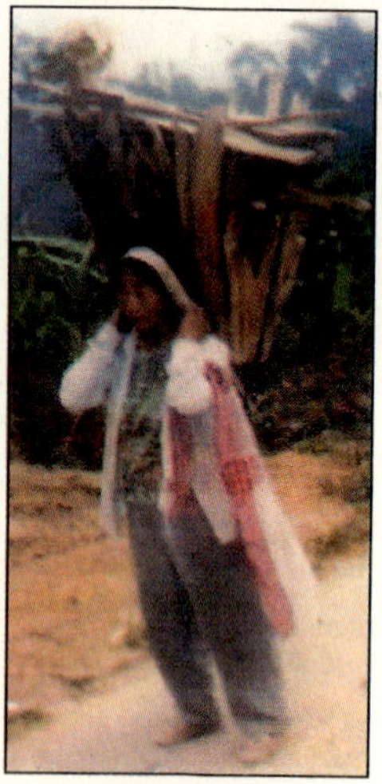

A woman carrying firewood

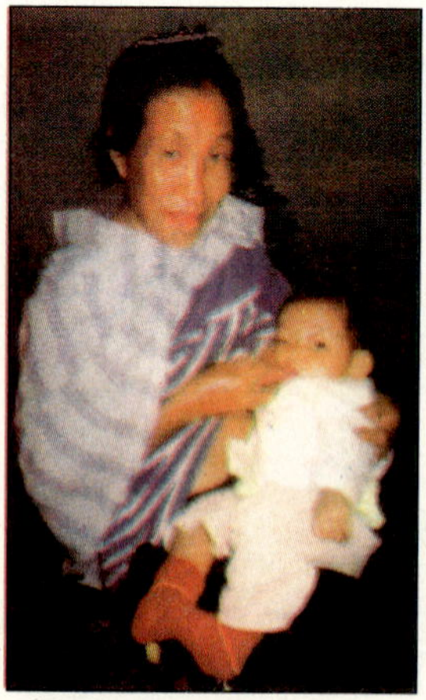

A mother suckling her baby

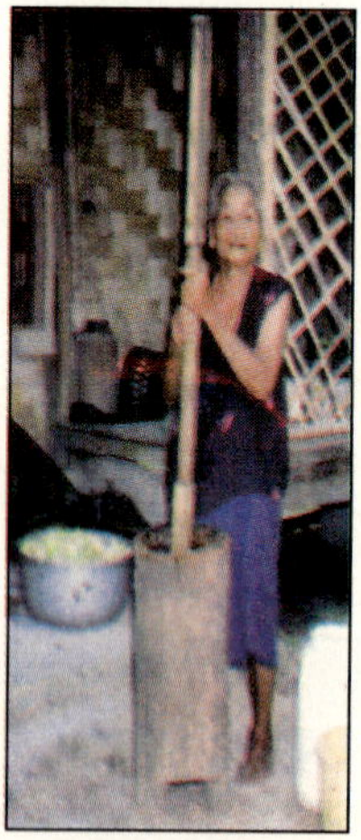

A woman pounding bamboo shoots in a log mortar

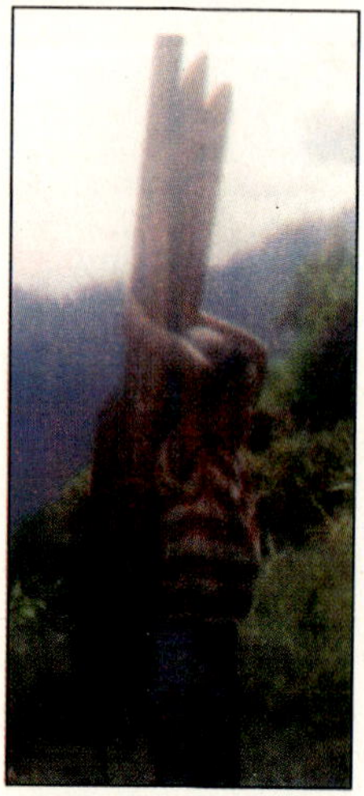

A woman fetching water in bamboo tubes

Plate No. 15

Reflecting Home Delivery

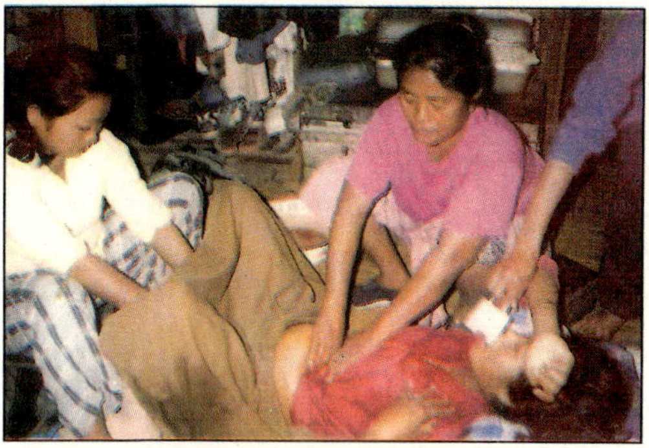

A nurse (ANM) attending a home delivery

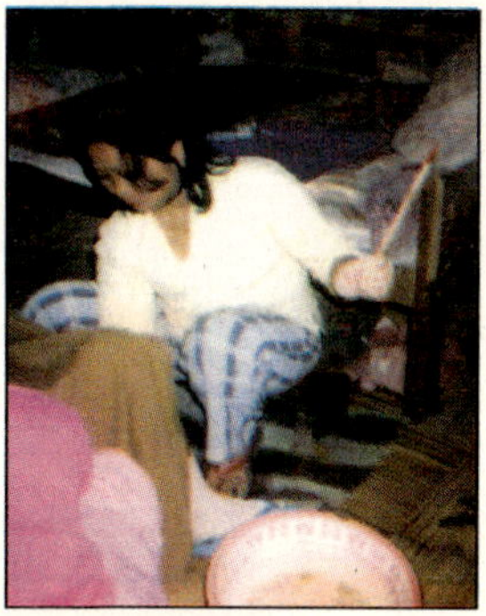

A bamboo split is being used to cut the naval cord

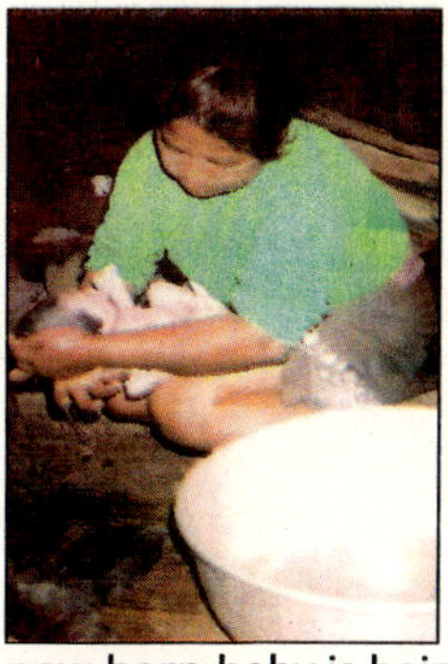

A new born baby is being given a bath

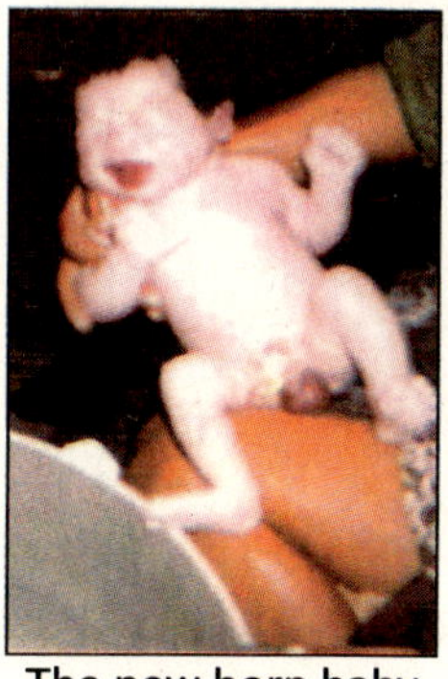

The new born baby after bath

Plate No. 16

Researcher in Action

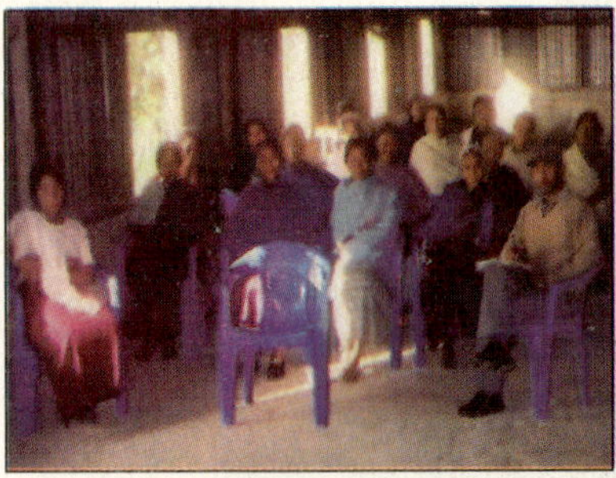

Group interview with women

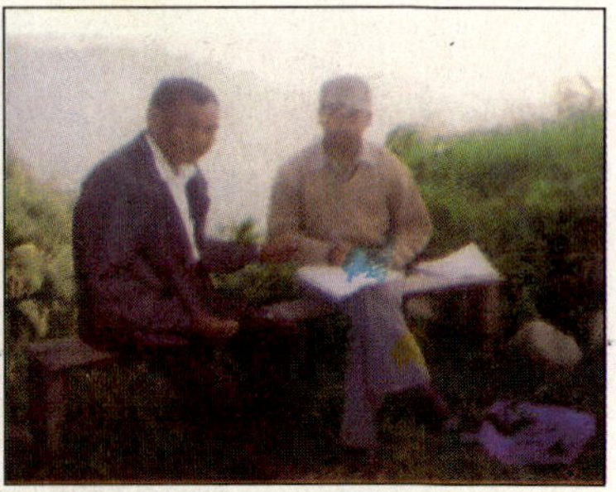

Interviewing with magico-religious man

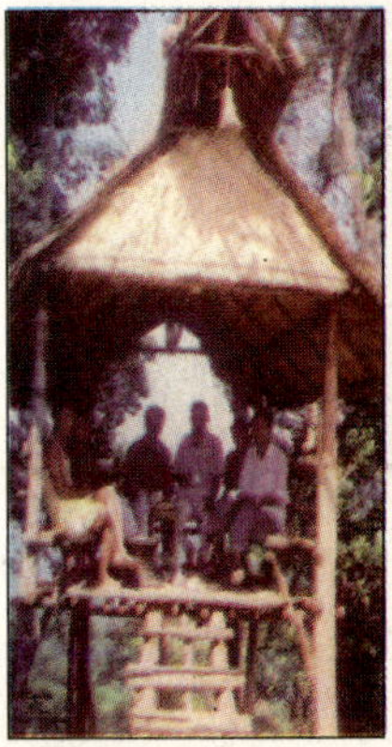

Discussing with elder people

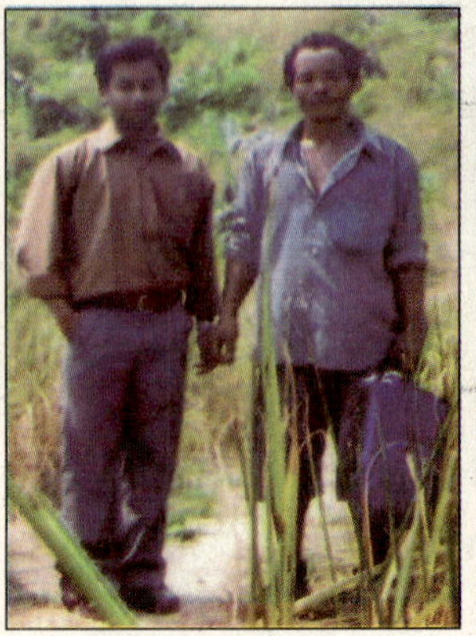

Researcher with jhum cultivator

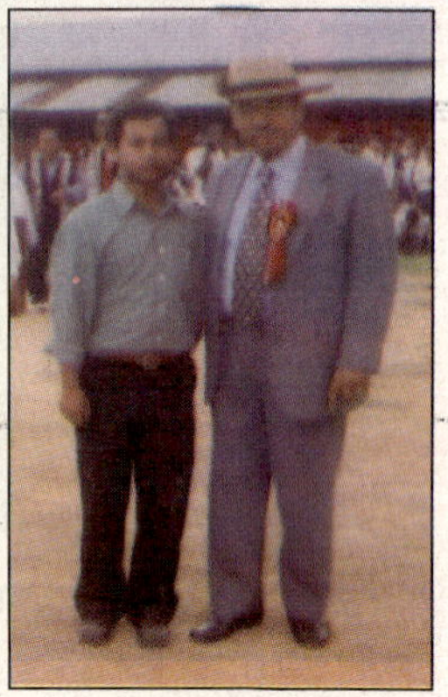

Researcher with Governor of Nagaland

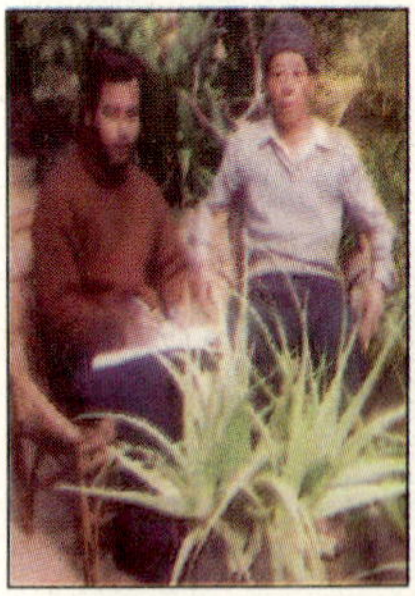

Researcher with herbal medicine man

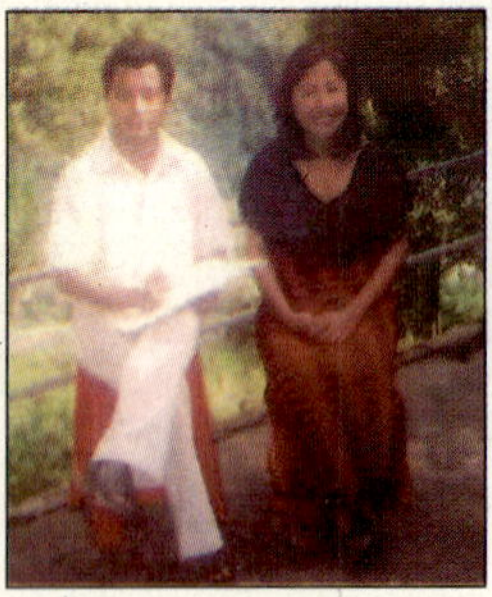

Interviewing with school teacher

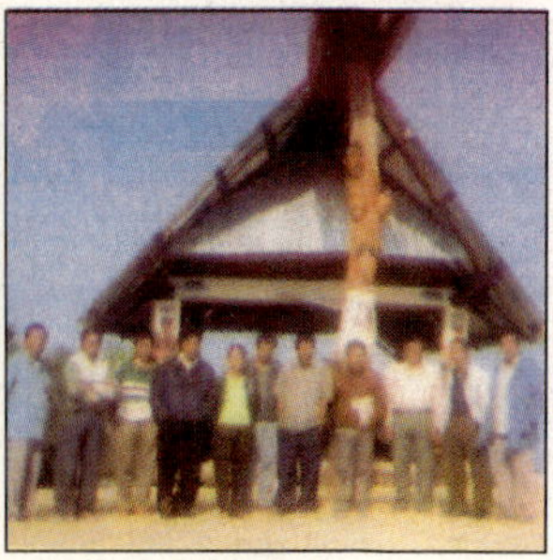

Researcher with Villagers

8

SUMMARY AND CONCLUSION

The chapter has been devoted to recapitulate and summarize the data presented and discussed in the preceding chapters. In the process some concluding remarks have also been incorporated here and there. An endeavour has been made to highlight the salient findings with regard to the socio-cultural dimension of health and health care practices of the Aos under investigation.

Health of an individual as well as the community is largely influenced by social and cultural factors which are deeply interwoven with the social fabric of life. These factors have wide variation from one community to another and within the community itself.

Health and hygiene are a set of biological needs that are common to all human beings. In a community it is directly related to the interaction between socio-cultural life and environment. The socio-economic status of a community has tremendous impact on morbidity pattern, which is largely dependent on social customs, cultural beliefs and health seeking behaviour.

Social, economic and cultural inequality is detrimental to health of any society. Tribal society in this context provides unique opportunity to study socio-cultural dimension of health as the tribal people have distinguished themselves by their unique social, cultural, economic and ethnic identity. The health status of the tribal is mostly affected by insufficient diet, lack of personal hygiene, living conditions, under availability of potable water, socio-cultural practices and inappropriate health care services. Thus, it is apparent that socio-cultural perspectives invariably affect the health care practices and it is, therefore, necessary to understand the community in its socio-cultural context before any health programme is implemented or evaluated.

The health problems need special attention in the context of tribal communities in India because of their settlements in difficult areas and circumstances. The health, nutrition and medico-genetic problems of diverse tribal groups present a formidable challenge for effective health care delivery. Similarly, the common beliefs, customs and practices connected with health and disease are intimately connected with the treatment of disease.

Despite gradual expansion of modern education and increasing contact with the outside world, very often it is observed that the social, economic and cultural factors poise as barriers in availing of modern medicare facilities.

Since the health care practices of a community are also prescribed its deep-rooted traditions like beliefs, customs, practices, literacy and prevailing health care facilities, therefore, studies on socio-cultural correlated of the tribe will help to understand their health seeking behaviour which in turn will be helpful to plan interventions to improve their health status.

In the present study, *Health Care Practices among the Ao Nagas*, therefore, an attempt has been made to examine their socio-cultural life and to understand the socio-cultural dimension of health as well as the nature and extent of the interaction between their traditional health care practices and the modern medicare system.

In order to have a detailed holistic understanding of the problem, it has been decided to make the study an intensive one. For that purpose, it is proposed to carry out the study in three homogeneous Ao Naga villages (micro-field), namely

Lirmen, Yajang-A and Yajang-B under rural setting in Mokokchung district, where they are a numerically dominant group.

The intensive investigation has been carried out with the following specific objectives in mind :

(1) To describe the socio-cultural life of the Ao Nagas.
(2) To trace the health care practices and how the socio-cultural life influences the health care practices of the Ao Nagas.

The following parameters have been considered to deal with the above-mentioned objectives :

(i) Some relevant socio-demographic aspects: (a) Type, composition and size of the families, (b) level of education by age and sex of the individuals and (c) economic background of the people.
(ii) To examine the nature of changes in the concept of health, disease and treatment and the causes of disease under the new socio-cultural system.
(iii) To understand the overall living condition, personal hygiene and environmental sanitation that is prevalent among the people *vis-à-vis* their health scenario.
(iv) To collect information about the food habit of the people including food timing, food taboos and the possible distribution of the proximate principles etc.
(v) Access to modern medical services as well as traditional medical services (i.e., available health resources).
(vi) To collect the morbidity history.
(vii) Concept of health, disease (ailment), etiology

(disease causation) and traditional beliefs, customs and practices with regard to treatment (curative measures).

(viii) To get an idea about the traditional preventive, curative and promotive health care practices that is prevalent among the people.

(ix) To identify the factors that contributes towards acceptance/non-acceptance of modern health care practices.

(x) To examine people's view towards both traditional and modern medicare system and the level and the extent of interaction between the two.

(xi) To understand the mother and child health care practices and the changing trends.

The population (i.e. Ao Nagas) has been selected for the purpose of present investigation mainly on the basis of the following considerations :

(i) They are one of the numerically dominant tribe in the Mokokchung district in Nagaland.

(ii) No such intensive study in this spheres has till date been carried out among them.

For choosing the micro-field, in the beginning, a good number of Ao Naga villages have been visited in Mokokchung district in Nagaland. However, explorations have been made as to the prospective convenience with regard to easy accessibility in terms of transport and communication and anticipated co-operation in terms of availability of formal permission etc., from the village authority. Considering all these factors it was finally decided to carry out the intensive investigation among the Ao Nagas under Japokong range in Mokokchung district, Nagaland.

The methods and techniques that have been employed in generating the data from the field are as follows:

(i) Household census schedule.
(ii) Interview; individual and group, structured and unstructured.
(iii) Observation.
(iv) Collection of concrete case histories and life histories.
(v) Informal discussion.

The entire mass of data generated from the field as well as collected from other sources have after proper organisation, analysis and interpretation been arranged systematically and presented conveniently in eight different chapters in the dissertation.

In *Chapter One (Introduction)* an attempt has been made to introduce the theoretical background of the problem in its proper perspective. It incorporates a discussion on the study, review of literatures, the objectives, relevance of the study, the method and techniques followed in the study and an overall plan of the data presentation.

Chapter Two (The Ao Nagas), is devoted to provide a brief historical note on the Nagas including the origin of the word Naga, their migration, racial affinity, geographical distribution, language and cultural commonalities and way of life. A brief ethnographic account of the Ao Nagas including their origin, migration, distribution etc. has also been presented in the chapter.

The micro-field (where the present intensive study has been carried out) in its proper geographical and ethnographic perspectives has been introduced in the *Chapter Three (The Setting).* The discussion begins with a brief geographical historical note on the North East India in general and Nagaland in particular. Then, attempt has been made to introduce

Mokokchung district (where micro-field is located) from geographical, historical and ethno-demographic points of view.

The villages under study (micro-field) have been introduced with some details about their location, social boundary and history of establishment etc. Along with a discussion on the physical features (e.g., climate, flora, fauna, topography and hydrography etc.), some data on the socio-economic infrastructural facilities (e.g. place of worship, educational institutions, transport and communication, important public places, agricultural land and market facilities etc.) have also been incorporated here in brief details.

The chapter also deals with the total number of households and families distributed in the three villages under study.

The chapter concludes with a preliminary analysis of the population under study. The total population of the villages under study is 1168. Out of this, there are 622 (53.25%) male and 546 (46.74%) female. Considering the study villages independently, it is seen that the total population of the study village Lirmen is 624 (53.36% male and 46.63% female). In the village Yajang-A the total population is 414 (53.14% male and 46.85 % female). On the other hand the total population of village Yajang-B is 130 (53.07% male and 46.92% female).

Chapter Four (Social Life) is devoted to provide a brief discussion on the social life of the study group.

The chapter deals with their family life, educational attainment, clan, marriage, inheritance of property and village administration.

Family is the basic unit of the society. With regard to the type and composition of family, it has been found that the nuclear type of family is the numerically dominant (83.78%) one. The Ao mostly live in small families. After the marriage, the newly married couple lives separately in a new house constructed by the husband. Therefore, the nuclear family is the main type that prevails among the Aos, other types which show characteristics of joint or extended family types are very rare. In the villages under study there are only 1.54 per cent joint families and 14.67 per cent broken families. Data on family size shows that, the average size of the family stands at 4.50. The frequent size of family is medium having 4-6 members. However, there are at least 32 (12.35%) families with 7-9 members as inmates.

In view of the fact that, the family life influences the overall health scenario of a group of people, an attempt has been made to have a better understanding of the same. As revealed by the data, it seems, in their daily life, both men and women remain busy in their day-to-day activities. They exert their labour in both their duties in jhum field as well as in the household works, and they keep themselves engaged from early morning to evening. They do not get sufficient leisure and relaxation opportunities in the midst of their daily preoccupations. As a result they do not get sufficient time to check-up their health.

With regard to the level of education, it has been observed that the literacy rate of the people as a whole is 91.01 per cent, consisting of 48.8 per cent males and 42.12 per cent females. However, the highest literacy rate is only up to secondary level (68.92%).

Clan among the Aos is exogamous and patrilineal. Even after the marriage, the title of the wife does not change as in case of other societies. Clan system is the fundamental social fabric of the Aos and every aspect of their customs and culture is normally based on it.

With regard to marriage system it has been observed that a tremendous change has taken place in the system of Ao marriage with the advent of Christianity. The people under investigation are Christians by religion and the most socially accepted marriage among them is the Christian marriage in the Church. But in-spite of the multifarious changes, the people still follow the traditional rules of marriage.

Data on marital status of the people show that, there are 58.30 per cent unmarried and 38.52 per cent married. Among the unmarried ones there are 32.87 per cent males and 25.42 per cent females. Similarly, among the married persons there are 19.26 per cent males and females. Further, there are 3.16 per cent widow (1.11%) and widower (2.05%) in the population.

The Aos are patrilineal in inheritance. The customary laws of Aos define rights and obligations about ownership of various things at the level of community, clan, private and by gender. Under the Ao customary rules of inheritance, property develops upon the heirs by succession and inheritance is always in male line. As the daughters after their marriage come under the care of a different clan and family, they are not entitled to own the properties of their father. However, the father can give the daughter a share of property as a gift if he desires. Regarding succession of property among the sons, all the sons may jointly hold ownership of the ancestral and self-acquired property of their deceased father besides divisions of the property. As a general rule, son whether from the same mother or not get the parental property equally. The eldest son is given the first privilege to select his preferred portion. In the absence of sons, the brother, brother's son, cousins, nearest kinsmen and so on in that order inherit the property of the brother.

With regard to the village administration it has been observed that the *putu menden* or village council is the highest authority in a given Ao village and all the members exercise their supreme power collectively in their village administration.

Generally, in every Ao village there are two village level political organisations, viz. traditional village council and statutory village authority. The existence of these two political organizations should not be understood as a two tier political organisation. In fact, the former represents the continuation of the traditional political organisation and the latter, the introduction of the local self-government by the state. The statutory village authority, i.e. the present village council is made up of a chairman, a secretary and members.

During the present investigation, it has been recorded that the village Lirmen has ten village council members and one secretary. Out of these ten members, one is chairman who also acts as headman. There are also three more headmen from these members. Thus, in Lirmen village, there are in all total four headmen. The village Yajang-A has forty eight members. Out of these one is chairman, two are headmen and one is secretary. The village Yajang-B has eleven members out of these one is chairman, one is headman and one is secretary.

In *Chapter Five (Religious Life),* a detailed description has been made on religious life of the people under investigation. The chapter incorporates some discussion on the traditional religion and Christianity among the Ao Nagas, Church organisation and impact of Christianity on the life of the Ao Nagas.

The Aos are Christians by religion at present but traditionally they were animist. The traditional religion was based on oral doctrine propitiating deities and spirits, but worship of images or idols were not practised. In the past there was no fixed worshipping place and there was no professional priesthood in the Ao villages. The oldest man in the village performed the religious ceremonies. *Gennas* (means something prohibited or taboo) and different ceremonies were observed by them. However, these systems are not observed after the advent of Christianity to their land. Today, the traditional religion is of academic interest only. Christianity has made tremendous advances.

As opined by different authors such as Sangma (1987), Singh (1972), Rev. Miles Bronson was the first Missionary to the Nagas. According to the views of the same authors, after the coming of Christianity many changes have taken place in the indigenous Naga practices and religion which was regarded as animism and it had been replaced by the religion which American missionaries brought during the middle of the nineteenth century.

The American Baptist missionaries were the first among

the missionaries to enter the Naga Hills in 1888 and they worked among the Namsangias. In 1876, Molung was the mission centre for Nagas. However, the mission centre was then shifted to a more central location at Impur, near Mokokchung on 4th October, 1894. Impur became the mission centre not only for the Ao Nagas but also for other tribes of Naga Hills. This marked the beginning of organised Christian missionary work in the Naga Hills. The first Association of the Ao Naga Church was held at Molung on 12th and 13th March, 1897. The missionaries made their impact through evangelistic work, educational work and medical relief work.

With regard to the people under study, it has been recorded that in the village Lirmen the influence of Christianity took place in the year 1885 and in the year 1898, seven members of this village were baptized. These seven members were the founders of this village and they came to this village from Waramong, Tibuya and Yimgemkimong. These seven members who were baptized first were: Imnayongdang, Inobangba, Nukshilemla, Tekatiba, Mayangtemba, Tongpangluba, Intinangpong.

The village Yajang-A was established in the year 1882 and the village was formed by the people who were coming from three different places, namely: Waramong, Molong and Lirmen. At the time of establishment of the village, except Molong, the people from Waramong and Lirmen were not Christians. The people from Molong popularised the Christianity and after that all of them embraced Christianity. In 1885 after 3 years of the establishment of the village, the Church was established there.

The village Yajang-B was established in the year 1970 and from the time of establishment, all the people were Christians as all the people came to this place from Yajang-A village. In other words, the people of Yajang-B are the clan members of the village Yajang-A and they had to come to this place due to the growth of population in the Yajang-A.

With regard to the Church organisation at the village level it has been recorded that each village has one Baptist Church. A Pastor in Baptist Church is a functionary who assumes the role of a priest at the village level. A Pastor conducts Church services every Sunday and in the religious festivals. A Pastor is assisted by deacons. There are 7 deacons in a Church and each deacon has certain specific duties to perform.

A village Church functions under the supervision of a local Church Board which consists of the Pastor, seven deacons, two active Church members; one is secretary and other is treasurer, chairperson of the village women's society and an official from the statutory village authority.

Every village Church has a subsidiary women's organisation. It is called 'Women's Society' and its main work is to organise special Church services for women every Thursday morning. The Christian Youth Endeavour (CYE) is another Church based organisation which carries on duties such as holding discussions among the youths on Christianity and teach them good lessons about Jesus Christ. There is a youth director who conducts this fellowship service, i.e. gathering youth of the village in Church on every Sunday afternoon.

The village level Church is affiliated to a regional organization called Ao Baptist Church Association which was established in 1897 by a few number of local Churches. It is popularly known as the Ao Baptist Arogo Mungdang (ABAM) in Ao which has its headquarters at Impur under Asetkong range in Mokokchung district.

The impact of Christianity on the Ao Naga culture is tremendous on individual, social and religious levels. The people accepted the new religion as the basis of their progress. Conversion to Christianity changed their lives completely and their lives were transformed into a newer and richer life. Evidently, with this the family life and the village life had become different. Christianity has brought about far reaching changes in the field of traditional beliefs and practices as well as in customs, habits and social relations. In many ways, their advancement in education and economy is the outcome of conversion.

With regard to the people under study some notable changes are observed in their socio-religious life after the inception of Christianity.

Before the advent of Christianity Ao Nagas assigned every illness to the wrath of devil or evil spirit. When someone fell ill the Divine (Sacred) man had to be consulted and according to the divine man's prescription pigs, dogs, cows, fowls were sacrificed and offered to God with drinks to propitiate the evil spirit. Now-a-days the Christian Nagas do not perform such sacrifice, as their conceptions about health and disease have undergone much change.

The people (both men and women) are seen to attend Church services in western dresses. Now all the people are seen to wear all modern dresses. They wear their traditional dresses only in the time of festival and in occasional cultural show.

The conversion in Christianity did not lead to abandonment of traditional food except rice beer (*yi*). Now-a-days, instead of rice beer people have switched over to tea drinking.

During the pre-conversion days ritual *kinimong* was observed for six days in case of birth of a male child and in case of female child it was observed for five days. Now-a-days, the new born whether male or female is blessed and given a name by the elder clan member in presence of the Pastor, who also offers prayers on the day in the house of the new born. This ceremony is observed on the third day from the birth of the new born. If the new born is a girl child then, the ritual *tengrong-atuba* is also observed on that day in which the ear hole of the child is done by an elderly man of the clan.

The traditional marriage in Ao society took place because of contact and mutual administration between an adult boy and a grown up girl through free mixing and in this process the female dormitory *tsuki* and male dormitory *ariju* played the most important role. But after Christianity, these dormitory systems no more prevail and Baptist Church does not accept the traditional way of engagement of marriage system of Aos. Today, the most socially accepted marriage among the Aos is the Christian marriage in the Church.

With regard to the disposal of dead, the common feature between the traditional and Christian system is that both the systems provide for disposal by burial. In every village there is a common burial ground. Under the traditional system after the death and before burial, generally a feast with rice and beef are given by the family members of the deceased. A *genna* was observed for few days after death and within this *genna* period the family members did not work in their agricultural field. They erected stone-structures for their respectable person and old and rich deceased in the burial ground. They were buried in such a way so that they may remember the dead members, generation after generation. But now, after Christianity they only follow the Christian procedure in disposal of death.

Though there have been many visible changes in day-to-day behaviour pattern, certain structural rules of social relations have remained same as existed earlier among the people. Thus, the rules of marriage, law of inheritance of property, land holding pattern etc. continues following their traditional rule.

The Ao Nagas had several festivals in year and these festivals and religious ceremonies are usually performed throughout the year according to agricultural calendar. But after Christianity. the Ao Nagas have abandoned most of their traditional festivals. However, they still continue to perform the traditional *moatsu* festival with certain change and modification. Now the people are very much interested to observe the Christian festivals like Christmas and some special days such as Father's Day, Mother's Day, Good Friday, etc.

Chapter Six (Economic Life), deals with the economic

life of the people under investigation. The prevailing food habit of the people has also briefly been introduced in this chapter. A detailed description about the overall living condition of the people including housing condition, personal hygiene and environmental sanitation have also been attempted in this chapter.

With regard to the population under investigation, it may be noted here that the people have predominantly agricultural economy. They are traditionally shifting cultivators. However, since after their settlement in the foothills regions in the recent past, they have acquired plots of land suitable for wet cultivation. Thus they have two types of cultivation—jhum or dry in the hills and wet or permanent in the plains.

The main occupation of the people is cultivation. Nearly all adult members in a household are engaged in agricultural activities in one way or another. Very young children and aged persons are however exempted from tasks in the field. The men and women have specific areas of specialization in economic activities including agriculture. The women are primarily the house keepers in Ao society. However, like other tribes of Nagaland, among the Ao, the women play a very important role in shifting cultivation. Their principal tasks in the field include preparation of the soil, showing, weeding and harvesting. Felling of trees clearing of jungle and firing are masculine tasks.

Agriculture being the primary occupation of the people, under investigation all the people concentrate all their endeavours upon this main economic activity. Now-a-days, however, with the inroad of education as well as because of increase in the population, some of the people have gradually been taking up some other non-traditional occupations. As for instance, for some people service and business are the primary occupations. However, agricultural pursuits are also maintained alongside by some of them. Other categories of occupation are housewife (domestic preoccupation) and students. Individuals who are too young and too old are being conveniently grouped under the category dependants.

Data on the distribution of the population by sex and occupation shows that there are a total of 667 (57.10%) individuals whose primary occupation is agriculture. Out of these, 343 (29.36%) males and 324 (27.73%) females.

There are 10 (0.85%) males whose primary occupation is agriculture and secondary occupation is business. There are in all total 39 (3.33%) people who have service (Government) as their primary occupation. Out of these, 33 (2.82%) males and 6 (0.51%) females. Again there are only 3 (0.25%) males whose primary occupation is service and secondary occupation is agriculture. Only 8 (0.68%) males have business as their primary occupation and 18 (1.54%) males have business as primary and agriculture as secondary occupation. Besides, there are 220 (18.83%) individuals (114; 9.76% males and 106; 9.07% females) who are categorised as student and 38 (3.25%) individuals (22; 1.88% males and 16; 1.36% females) who are primarily students and secondarily involve in agriculture. There are only 23 (1.96%) females which remain only as house-wife. There are 142 (12.15%) individuals (71; 6.07% males and 71; 6.07% females) which are in the dependent category.

Although agriculture is the main occupation of majority of Aos, it does not confine them throughout the year. They are also engaged in other economic activities like raising vegetable gardens, cattle farming, poultry and livestock keeping, basket making, collection of wood both for the purpose of house construction and fuel, hunting and fishing.

With regard to consumption pattern it has been observed that as a matter of tradition the crops produced in a season by the Aos are not consumed instantly. The whole production of paddy in a year is primarily meant to last the whole year. Therefore, everybody feels the necessity of storing it in a secured place, away from fire and various agents of mass destruction. In some of the traditional dwelling houses paddy is stored inside containers made of bamboo which are placed at a corner of the house. Now-a-days, the granaries for storing paddy are built little away from the main dwelling house. They stand on wooden platform and mostly iron sheet roofed. Apart from paddy other seasonal crops like gourd, pumpkin etc. are also stored inside the granary.

Even the meat of animals killed in a hunting expedition or from market is not immediately consumed; a portion is smoked over the family hearth and preserved on a platform above the hearth for future consumption. By continuous exposure to the heat of fire the meat cannot be infected by pests or household flies. Similarly, fish and other food items are also preserved in the same fashion. Apart from paddy, pulses and vegetables, juice of fruit are normally preserved for use throughout the year. In preservation of this item no chemical is used.

Every village has devices to face any dire eventualities like famine and fire. For such occasions the village Church and Church based women's society maintain reserve of paddy. Such reserves are built by way of tithe to be contributed by every household at the rate of one-tenth of its agricultural produce. Similarly, the village women's society also builds up a store of paddy through collection from its members.

The daily expenses in a household are generally met from the cash earned through the sale of forest and jhum products. In a few households nearly all day-to-day expenditure is met with salary of the working members. During November and December, many villagers sell some paddy from their stores to sustain the expenses of Christmas which include buying of new clothes for both young and old at least, if it is not possible to afford new dress for everybody. Majority of the people do not have any savings.

In general, the nature and extent of expenditure varies from household to another depending on the level of income. The majority of the people live at the bare subsistence level economy. Only a handful of the people enjoy a life better than those of the others because of the regular cash income earned in the form of salary. Thus the socio-economic condition of the people as a whole seems to have a negative influence on their overall health and well-being.

With regard to food habit of the people it has been observed that the staple food of the people is rice. They take different varieties of locally available vegetables with rice. The wild roots and shoots as well as the flesh food (viz. pork, chicken, deer, beef, elephant, fish, egg etc.) are their usual delicacies. As a result of the influence of Christianity they have given up the individually prepared rice beer and have switched over to tea drinking. They usually take both black and milk tea. Though rice beer is totally avoided, but they prefer to drink the modern alcohol as available.

The people generally take three major meals a day, i.e. early in the morning, in the mid of the day and in the evening without much restriction of the food items.

With regard to their food habits, an overall idea (qualitative) may be obtained about the distribution of the proximate principles, vitamins and mineral salts etc. in their food items.

Rice is the only cereal used by the people which is the main source of carbohydrate that provides energy. Potato and different edible wild roots also supply them carbohydrate to some extent. The vegetables, wild edible shoots and leaves also provide them some amount of energy.

The food items of the people that contain protein (i.e. the body building nutrient) include fish, pork, chicken, egg, mutton, beef, bean and some other vegetables. However, these items are taken by the people only as delicacies. Normally, these are not included in their usual daily menu. Besides, meat of duck, pigeon and wild birds and animals also sometimes constitute their occasional delicacy. In most of the families fish is taken frequently in all seasons. They also preserve fish and the fleshes of different animals in a fumigation shelf over the kitchen hearth for future consumption. They take the flesh of all wild animals and birds. They also consume some insects (viz. grasshopper, mantis etc.) and the eggs and larvae of some other insects found in the forest. All these substances also fulfil the need of protein and fat in their body.

As most of the food items are boiled without or with minimum oil, whatever fat they get is also derived from fish, meat, egg etc. Vitamins and other nutrients are obtained from green and leafy vegetables, and locally available fruits.

It may be relevantly emphasized here that ignorance of the need of additional nutrients during pregnancy, post-natal period and after prostrated illness etc., seem to be common feature among the people.

In general, the people do not have any idea of the need of a balanced diet. People are fond of the flesh food (viz. meat and fish) and it is believed that these foods contain all the required nutrients for the body. These items are not in regular menu and are taken less frequently than vegetables. However, dry fish are taken very frequently. These seem to fulfil their need of proximate principles, vitamins and minerals in usual state in their health. Poverty and ignorance seem to be playing an important role to deprive the people of having balanced diet in terms of nutrients required for their good health.

With regard to the living condition of the people, it is revealed that, they by and large, are not very particular and conscious regarding the maintenance of a healthy surrounding as well as personal hygiene.

Though all the family possess housing facilities, it seems the standard of the house are far from being adequate. The houses do not seem to be very clean. In most of the houses, there are no proper windows and other means of light and ventilation. Because of scarcity of light and air, at any time of the day the inner side of a house always remains dark and stuffy. The situation worsens because of the smoke that is generated from the hearths that remain lit for almost 24 hours at least in winter season. The floor in most of the houses is dirty. The people sit and sleep on the floor without putting anything on it. After meal they wash their mouths and hands where they sit and the interspaced allow the water go down. In case of home delivery, it has been observed that discharges come out from the delivery mother also go down between the interspaced of the floor. During the winter they feel very cold in the house due to bamboo construction that very often leads to the incidence of cough and cold, pneumonia etc. Similarly accumulation of smokes within the living rooms also results in a number of ailments that could be minimized, if there would have been proper ventilation facilities in the houses.

The people are not very conscious about personal hygiene and cleanliness. It seems they do not have any idea about the correlation between personal hygiene and the overall health scenario. With regard to their bathing habit, it has been observed that both menfolk and womenfolk take bath only one time after returning home from the jhum field. During the winter many of them do not take bath regularly. Use of toilet soap has been found to be reasonably infrequent among the people under investigation. The children as well as the elderly members are very often found to be in dirty clothes.

The prevalent condition of environmental sanitation also does not seem to be very congenial for the maintenance of a proper health. Since the people under study are widely distributed in the hills in rural settings, they totally depend on the river and spring water for drinking as well as for other purposes. This water is carried through the pipe or canal system towards the village area, where they usually have a big tank to store. There are also some open tanks in the villages under study and all the people carry water in bamboo pipes from these tanks. Due to scarcity of water and as the tanks are far away from their individual houses, they also store water in iron drums and in the bamboo pipes for 3-4 days and these are not properly washed. In rainy season, they also store the rain water and it is seen only in the tin roofed houses. The preserved water, however, mostly remains uncovered.

Storing of water properly is the best way to be away from water contamination. Most of the households under study have medium income and as such they store water in open containers. So, these households are at the high risk due to water pollution because when the water is left open, a large number of micro-organisms from their surroundings get mixed with water causing water borne diseases. Most of them store water in buckets. Some households also possess overhead cemented tanks where they store the rain water. The only problem with the overhead tanks is that they do not clean the tank regularly so microbes get developed in these tanks. The households are not aware of this type of pollution and this resulted in some diseases. In this regard, Mohan (1977) opined that polluted drinking water act as vehicle for disease transmission is a knowledge perhaps required by the scientific world recent centuries. Enteric fever, bacillary dysentery and cholera form the classic triad of water borne diseases. The other common water borne diseases are typhoid, paratyphoid, amoebic dysentery and hemorrhage, jaundice. In recent years infectious hepatitis has also become well established as a deadly disease. As the people under investigations are not getting satisfactory quality of water and as they keep water in open containers inside the house, all these factors together contribute to diarrhoea, dysentery, typhoid, jaundice, malaria and gastro-enteritis to these poor households.

Toilets are considered an indicator of the social status and the economic background of the society. Proper toilet facilities are very important health factors as most of the diseases are borne from open field or katcha type of toilets. Among the people under investigations, it has been observed that except two households in Lirmen village who possess sanitary latrine, all the other households have katcha type of toilets.

The people go to these latrines with bare foot and they do not use a separate cloth for it. They are also not conscious about the use of toilet soap after defecation.

On the whole, the overall living condition of the people does not seem to be very favourable to the maintenance of a sound health. Thus, unhealthy living conditions along with their ignorance seem to play a significant role in the incidence of a number of diseases among the people.

In *Chapter Seven (Health Scenario among the People)*, an idea about the available and accessible health care facilities in and around the micro-field have been attempted. A discussion has also been made on the nature and extent of utilization of the different health care systems by the people. Some morbidity and mortality scenario of the people has also been discussed. The chapter also incorporates some discussion on mother and child health care and the nature of interaction between the traditional and modern health care systems and to identify the factors that contribute towards the acceptance/non-acceptance of modern health care practices among the people under investigation.

The prevailing health resources in the micro-field under investigation may conveniently be discussed under two broad categories: modern resources and traditional resources. The traditional resources can again be divided into two types: magico-religious and herbal medicines. The people of Yajang-A and Yajang-B villages by and large, take the services from both the resources depending on the nature and severity of the diseases. But the people of Lirmen village, mostly, take the service from modern resources. However, in some preliminary health problem, they take some indigenous herbal medicines.

In Lirmen village, there is a government dispensary with a pharmacist, one nurse and one midwife. The dispensary is a katcha type and where facilities of treatment for minor diseases are available. But infrastructure of the dispensary is very poor.

The people of this village first consult with the pharmacist or nurse for their diseases and depending on the nature and severity of the disease they give medicines and if they are not cured even after using medicine, the people then go to Morioni, Dimapur, Mokokchung for better treatment. However, in initial stages of some disease they try to cure by taking some indigenous herbal medicines.

There is no any reputed traditional medicine man and magico-religious man in this village.

In Yajang-A village, there is one health sub-centre with one nurse and one midwife. The sub-centre is also katcha type and not in regular service. During the investigation it has been observed that in most of the time, the nurse is not available in the sub-centre and used to get transfer within a short duration. In this regard, the people of this village have to depend on modern health resources available in the nearest town for allopathic treatment.

But there is a reputed herbal medicine man and a magico-religious man in Yajang-A village. People of this village mostly depend on these two experts, depending on their nature of the diseases. In case of, harm of evil spirit and snake bite they approach the magico-religious man. For all other diseases, they first approach the herbal medicine man, as they believe that he can diagnose the actual disease and cure it. It has been reported that the medicine man could cure some diseases which are not cured by the modern medicines. Their economic condition is a factor, for which they approach the traditional medicine man. It is their assumption that if they go to modern practitioners they are to spend a large amount and sometimes even the patient is not cured. The traditional medicine man never demand any amount from them and most of the time, he gives free check-up.

The medicine man diagnoses the case first and depending on the nature of the disease, he gives his prepared medicine. In case, the disease is not curable by him, he advises the particular case to take help from modern resources. Sometimes, in some minor cases, he prescribes the medicines to take from the pharmacy nearest to them. Thus, the medicine man serves both traditional herbal practices as well as modern allopathic practices.

In the village Yajang-B, there is no health sub-centre or dispensary. So, the people of this village go to the nearest town Haluwating and Amguri for Allopathic treatment. As the people of this village originally came from Yajang-A village and from same clan, therefore, they by and large depend on the medicine man (Temen) of Yajang-A. The people first approach to the herbal medicine man in time of their diseases. If the disease is not curable by him then according to his suggestion they take the help of other modern (allopathic) health resources where available.

For snake biting, and wrath of malevolent spirit they take the help of magico-religious man of Yajang-A.

During the present investigation a good number of respondents have been interviewed to have a first-hand understanding of their emic views with regard to health and disease and available health care services. The responses have shown some expected variation according to age, sex, level of education and economic background etc.

The meaning of the word 'Healthy Person' is not clearly understood by many of the villagers. Some respondents defined healthy person as those who are not having any kind of disease and have some ability to carry on his/her daily duties properly. Majority are not aware of the concept of a sick person. Some consider that a person who sleeps on a cot/bed throughout the day is unhealthy/sick person. The concept of reason/ reasons of one falling sick is also not clear. They also believe that sickness is caused due to intake of un-rich food and impure water, polluted atmosphere or due to attack of ghost or spirit. Some of them also consider sickness as caused due to hard industrious and also due to the affect of Devine punishment.

In order to have a quantitative idea, on the overall morbidity pattern and the type of treatment used among the people, primary data have been collected through house to house investigation in the villages under study for the period July 2005—June 2006. The data reveal that people suffered from at least 52 different types of diseases during the period. The frequently incident diseases include fever, malaria, gastritis, dysentery, jaundice, liver problem, cold and cough, kidney problem, intestinal problem etc., and the relatively less frequent diseases include appendix, heart problem, injury, urinal problem etc.

The chapter relevantly incorporates a discussion on the possible correlation between the morbidity scenario and the overall lifestyle of the people. It seems, a good number of frequently incident diseases among the people can be explained in terms of their overall living condition, food habit as well as their ignorance.

With regard to the utilization of different medicare system and the interaction between the traditional and the modern health care system among the people, the data make it apparent that in the Lirmen village people approach the modern medicare system mostly. However, the people of Yajang-A and Yajang-B approach the modern medicare system only when the traditional means fail to yield the desired result. The data, however, show that three different trends prevail among the people with regard the utilization and acceptance of a medicare system. In some cases, the people avail the modern services, whereas in some other cases they depend on the traditional one. Sometimes they take some recourse to both the systems either simultaneously or alternatively.

It has also been observed that the economic background of the patient too plays an important role in utilizing a particular system as a curative measure. Besides, available modern health resources are not in proper physical infrastructure. Health centres are far away from their villages and it is difficult for them to cover a long distance, as their transportation facility is not sound. Most of them are to cover it by walk.

However, the acceptance of a particular type of medicine depends upon the people's beliefs with regard to its causation. Thus, for snake bite and wrath of malevolent sprit they approach the traditional magico-religious man and for other naturally caused diseases they approach the traditional medicine man or the modern ones.

In order to understand the mother and child health care practices and various beliefs and taboos related to it, data have been collected from married women respondents.

For the people, conception is a good sign after marriage and they think that it is a natural process. Women usually rely on their own diagnosis for knowing about pregnancy, in which the absences of periods, vomiting, nausea, greedy for sour are the key factors.

There are no specific restrictions of movement for a pregnant woman. She can move anywhere and is allowed to do all kinds of works as the normal woman. But there are some moral restrictions and superstitious beliefs at the stage of pregnancy which a conceived woman should observe.

There is no restriction on food during pregnancy period and no specific or special diet is prescribed for the pregnant women.

In order to have an idea about the reproductive behaviour, the respondents are considered with an age grade 15-49 married women. Data in this regard shows that there are 64 married women in Lirmen village in this age grade and 62 in Yajang-A village and 20 in Yajang-B village.

With regard to the people under investigation it has been observed that from conception to delivery of the child the Aos by and large do not have any idea of medical check-up. They do not seem to be very much concerned about the necessity of some special care of the mothers' health.

The Ao women carry more of the work burden of the household and therefore have less time to seek out health care services making them disadvantaged relative to men in their access and utilization of health care services.

In the villages under study, most of the deliveries are carried out at home by traditional midwives. Sometimes a trained mid-wife or nurse is called if available. A woman is likely to be taken to a clinic or hospital when she has serious complications.

There is practically no prevalence of traditional birth control measures or practices in the presently studied community. With regard to the modern family planning methods, it has been reported that from Mokokchung Civil Hospital some AIDS Department N.G.O. visited the villages and some N.G.O. from Mongkolomba came to motivate the people about these contraceptive methods. Thus, now-a-days the people are aware about the various contraceptive methods. Generally awareness of contraception through sterilization is found to be the higher among the women than the contraceptive tablets. However, majority of them are aware of the natural birth control measure and use the self-control method. Though they have some knowledge of condom, yet no one is found to use it.

The overall mortality scenario among the people under investigation has also been tried to be understood with the primary data collected from the married women in their reproductive performance. Thus a few cases have been presented to know about the causes of child mortality. Data in this regard reveals that due to unhygienic condition and absence of proper health resources, the infant and child mortality still relatively high.

From the investigation of the present study, it may be understood that the Aos still have to subscribe their traditional medicare system as the modern medicare system is not accessible to them.

In the conclusion, the following few points are again highlighted :

(i) The socio-cultural life of the Aos is quite different at present due to the impact of Christianity. However, along with the changes they still follow their traditional beliefs and customs to a certain extent.

(ii) Socio-cultural factors directly or indirectly influence the overall health scenario of the people. It is a fact that their conversion to Christianity has provided with a better in road of education leading to some observable changes in their traditional outlook with regard to health behaviour. But however, because of economic constraints, the people by and large have not been able to receive more that seventh or eighth standard of education. As a result the changes are not up to the expected extent.

(iii) The socio-religious beliefs and practices do not seem to have any influence on their choice of a particular system of curative measures against a number of diseases in their day-to-day life. However, they believe on evil spirit and in case of harm of evil spirit as well as snake bite they approach the magico-religious man.

(iv) The people's overall living condition (including their food habit and dietary composition) as well as the quality and content of their personal hygiene and environmental sanitation are not very conducive to health for which many incidence are happened.

(v) The economic background plays an important role in utilising the modern medicare system. The people from sound economic background are seemed to utilise the modern medicare system extensively.

(vi) The available modern health resources in their localities are not in proper physical infrastructure.

(vii) Health centres are far away from their villages and it is difficult for them to cover a long distance, as the transportation facility is not sound. Most of them cover it by walk.

(viii) Due to lack of proper health resources, the mother child health is also a problematic one. Among the people, miscarriage, stillbirth and post-birth death are common. It may be due to the improper health check-up during pregnancy and after delivery.

(x) Parental education seems to have an influence on reproductive health. The investigation reveals that the woman level of education has direct affect on her attitude and practices towards family health and welfare.

(xi) Both traditional and modern medicare systems are simultaneously used by the people. However, modernisation seems to have some positive influence (at least in some cases) with regard to the acceptance of modern medicare system.

From the above conclusive study it may be arrived at an opinion that though the development of Christianity highly extended among the people and try to improve their socio-religious-economic aspects but it is seen that the people are still behind in some aspects mainly in case of their health care practices. It has been observed that government health departments have introduced many needful schemes for the well-being of the society but these are yet to reach in rural areas. There is need of proper investigation and inspection to implement the government health schemes in these rural areas. However, to bring an overall development or improvement in health scenario of the people there must be provision of proper free and easy accessible of modern medical facilities. People should be educated and motivated for modern treatment so that they can come out from their traditional habits and practices and can maintain their proper personal hygiene and environmental sanitation. Health education programme for the women is highly needed to promote health awareness among them. This programme should give greater attention to the nutritional aspects as well as regular health check-up for pregnant women. Further, road communication is one of the major problems of the rural people, it should be improved with the help of new technology. To achieve the goal of such a programme, the co-operation of local educated youths has an important role in the society. The government should encourage them in this respect. It is hoped that the combine efforts of all would help to achieve a desired result in the health care practices.

BIBLIOGRAPHY

"A committee of Royal Anthropological Institute of Great Britain and Ireland: 1971. *Notes and Queries in Anthropology* (Reprint, original 1874). London: Routledge and Kegan Paul Ltd.

Ahmed, B.U. 1995. *Socio-Economic Changes among the Kaibarttas: A case study in Barak Valley*, Assam. Ph.D. thesis submited to the Department of Anthropology, Dibrugarh University.

Aier, I.T.A. 1990. *The Religion of the Ao Nagas*. Jorhat: Assam Printing Works (Pvt.) Ltd.

Ajala, O.A. *et al*. 2005. Accessibility to Health Care Facilities: A Panacea for Sustainable Rural Development in Osun State, South Western Nigeria. *J. Hum Ecol.* 18 (2): 121-128.

Babu, K.S. 1998. Illness And Health Care in Madungula Mandal of Andhra Pradesh. *Man in India*. 78 (3&4): 255-268.

Babu, M.S. & P.D. Rao. 2006. Child Care among Racha Koyaks: A Tribal Group from Andhra Pradesh. *Man and Life*. Vol.32 (3-4):67-74.

Bairathi, S. 1991. *Tribal, Culture, Economy and Health* New Delhi: Rawat Publications.

Bareh, H. 1970. *Gazetteer of India*. Calcutta: Stress Sarawaty Press Ltd.

Barua, I. and A. Bharali. 2001. A Glimpse into Socio-Religious Life of the Deoris of Assam. *J. Hum. Ecol.* 12 (2): 87-94.

Barua, I. and R. Phukan. 1998. Socio-religious Aspects of Health Among Sonowal Kacharis. *The Eastern Anthropologist*. 51:4.

Barua, T. 1994. *Socio-cultural dimension of health practices among the Migrant Mundas : A case study in Assam Tea plantation*. Ph.D. thesis submitted to the Department of Anthropology, Dibrugarh University.

Bhadra, R.K. and J.B. Tirkey. 1997. Health Culture Practices in Rural Society: Case studies of Castes and Tribes of North Bengal. *Bulletin of Deptt. of Anthropology, Dibrugarh University, Dibrugarh*. Vol. XXV.

Bhagabati, A.C. 1991. Research Methods in Social Anthropology. *Assam Economic Journal, Department of Economics, Dibrugarh University, Assam, India*. Vol. VIII:89-94.

. The Tribe as a Social Formation: The case of the Tangsa of Arunachal Pradesh. *Bulletin of Deptt. of Anthropology, Dibrugarh University, Dibrugarh*. Vol. 16-17.

Bhagwat, S. and D. Chirmulay. 1997. Traditional Healing Practices in Rural Karnataka. *Man in India*. 77 (1):71-82.

Biswas, R.K., A.K. Kapoor. 2005. Health Seeking Behaviour among Saharia : A Primitive Tribe of Madhya Pradesh. *Indian Journal of Social Science Research*. Vol. 46 (3):249-260.

Bora, P. 2001. *Child Care and Development: A case study among the Mishings of Dibrugarh, Assam*. Ph.D. thesis submitted to the Department of Anthropology, Dibrugarh University.

Boruah, B.K. 1993. *Nagamese : The Language of Nagaland*. New Delhi: Mittal Publications.

Chaudhuri, B. (Ed.). 1986. *Tribal Health*. New Delhi: Inter-India Publications.

Chaudhury, R.H. 1982. *Social Aspects of Fertility with Special Reference to Developing Countries*. New Delhi: Vikas Publishing House Pvt. Ltd.

Chaudhuri, S.K. 2004. *Tribal Identity*. New Delhi: Rawat Publications.

Chutia, M. 1984. *Continuity and Change among the Chaudangs of Assam*. Ph.D. thesis submited to the Department of Anthropology, Dibrugarh University.

Coleman, J.W. and D.R. Cressey. 1987. *Social Problem*. New York: Harper & Row Publishers.

Dalal, A.K. and S. Ray (Ed). 2005. *Social Dimension of Health*. New Delhi: Rawat Publications.

Das, F.A. 1997. Study of Health Status: Physical Anthropological Perspective. *Bulletin of Deptt. of Anthropology, Dibrugarh University, Dibrugarh*. Vol.-XXV.

Das Gupta, P.K. 1984. *Life and Culture of Matrilineal Tribe of Meghalaya*. New Delhi: Inter-India Publications.

Das, I. 2003. Ethnomedicinal Practices among the Karbis of Goria Ghuli of Sonapur, Assam, with special reference to the Female Health Problems. *J. Hum. Ecol*. 14 (2): 119-124.

Devi, J. 2002. Property Rights and the Status of Women among the Rengma Tribe of Nagaland: A Case Study of Tseminyu Village. *Bulletin of Deptt. of Anthropology, Dibrugarh University, Dibrugarh*. Vol. 30.

Devi, T. 2004. "Relevance of Tribal Religion—An Overview", in *Undertaking Tribal Religion*. Edited by T. Mibang and S.K. Chaudhuri. New Delhi: Mittal Publications.

Doshi, S.L. and P.C. Jain. 2001. *Social Anthropology*. Jaipur and New Delhi: Rawat Publications.

Duarah, D.K. and S.D. Pathak. 1997. A Short Note on the Health Care Practices among the Nishis of Arunachal Pradesh. *Bulletin of Deptt. of Anthropology, Dibrugarh University, Dibrugarh*. Vol. XXV.

Dube, S.C. 1996. *Understanding Change; Anthropological and Sociological Perspectives*. New Delhi: Vikash Publishing House Pvt. Ltd.

Dutta, B.M. 2002. *Health status of the Tea labourers with speical reference to health seeking behaviour: A case study in Upper Assam*. Ph.D. thesis submitted to the Department of Anthropology, Dibrugarh University.

Dutta, P.C. 1990. *The Singphos*. Guwahati: Purbadesh Mudran, Assam.

Dwivedi, P. and A.N. Sharma. 2005. Utilization of Health and Family Welfare Services among the Baigas of Samnapur. *Man in India*. 85 (3&4):303-309.

Dzuvichu, K. 2005. Health Problems of the Aged among the Angami Nagas. *J. Hum. Ecol*. 17 (2): 101-107.

Edwin, R.A.S. and A. Johnson (Ed). 1932. *Encyclopaedia of Social Sciences*. Vol. IX-X. New York: The Macmillan Co.

Elwin, V. 1961. *Nagaland*. Calcutta: Stree Saraswaty Press Ltd.

—. 1969. *The Nagas in the Nineteenth Century*. London: Oxford University Press.

Firth, R. 1961. *Elements of Social Organisation*. London: Watts and Co.

Ghosh, B.B. 1982. *History of Nagaland*. New Delhi: S. Chand and Co. Ltd.

Goetz, P.W. (Ed).1768. *Encyclopaedia of Britannica*. Vol.26, Chicago:London.

Gope, T.K. 2004. *Social Environment and Health Care Practices: A Comparative Study among the Tribals in Tapan Block of Dakshin Dinajpur, West Bengal*. Ph.D. thesis submited in the Department of Sociology, North Bengal University.

Horam, M. 1975. *Naga Polity*. Delhi: B.R. Publishing Corporation.

—. 1977. *Social and Cultural Life of Nagas*. New Delhi: B.R. Publishing Corporation.

Hunter, D.E. and P. Whitten (Ed). 1776. *Encyclopedia of Anthropology*. New York: Harper and Row Publishers.

Jain, A.K. and A.N. Sharma. 2006. Feeding Practices, Child Immunization and Malnutrition Problems among the Traditional Prostitutes of Beria Caste of Sagar District, Madhya Pradesh. *Man and Life*. Vol.32 (3-4):61-66.

Jamir, N.T. and A. Lanunungsang (2005). *Naga Society and Culture*. Jorhat: Borkatoki and Co. Pvt. Ltd.

Jha, M. 1994. *An Introduction to Social Anthropology*. New Delhi: Vikas Publishing Hosue Pvt. Ltd.

Joshi, V. 1992. "Health, Disease and Social Structure: Ethnomedicine in a *Nagaland village"*, in *Nagaland: A Contemporary Ethnography*. Edited by S.M. Channa. New Delhi : Cosmo Publications.

Kannuri, N.K. 2005. "Koya perception of Health and Illness: An Ethnomedicinal Analysis", in *Social Dimension of Health*. Edited by A.K. Dalal and S. Ray. New Delhi: Rawat Publications.

Kanungo, J. & D.L. Mohanta. 2004. Reproductive and Child Health Care Status of Diffrent Social Groups of India: An Investigation into National Family Health Survey-II. *Man in India*. 84 (1&2):15-31.

Kar, R.K. 1993. Health Behaviour among the tribes of North-East India: A Profile. *Journal of Indian Anthropological Society*. 28 (2):156-164.

—. 1997. Anthropology and Health. *Bulletin of Deptt. of Anthropology, Dibrugarh University, Dibrugarh*. Vol.-XXV.

Kar, R.K. and J. Gogoi. 1995. "Health Culture and Tribal Life: A case study among the Noctes of Arunachal Pradesh", in *Indian Tribes, Health, Ecology and Social Structure*. Edited by R.C. Swarankar. Jaipur: Rupa Books Pvt. Ltd.

Kar, R.K. and T. Barua. 1997. Morbidity and Health Behaviour: A Case Study among the Migrant Munda Tea Labourers. *Bulletin of Deptt. of Anthropology, Dibrugarh University, Dibrugarh*. Vol. XXV.

Konwar, J.G. 2001. *Reproductive Health of Women: A case study in an Ahom village in Upper Assam*. Ph.D. thesis submitted to the Department of Anthropology, Dibrugarh University.

Kumar, M. and R. Kumar. 1987. "Environmental Impact of Slums on Health", in *Environmental Pollution and Health Hazards in India*. Edited by R. Kumar. New Delhi: Ashish Publishing House.

Kumar, R. (Ed). 2003. *Essays on Indian Culture*. New Delhi: Discovery Publishing House.

Lasuh, W. (Ed). 2002. *The Naga Chronicle*. New Delhi: Regency Publications.

Lynden, B. and M.P. Khonglah, 2004 : "Rural development an educational perspective", in *Dimension of Rural Development in North East India*. Edited by B. D. Roy and G. Das, New Delhi: Akansha Publishing House.

Maheo, L.M. 2004. *The Mao Naga Tribe of Manipur*. New Delhi: Mittal Publications.

Maiti, S. *et al*. 2005. Health Care and Health Among Tribal Women in Jharkhand: A Situational Analysis. *Stud. Tribes Tribals*. 3 (1):37-46.

Majumdar, D.N. 1933. Disease, death and divination in certain primitive societies in India. *Man in India*. 13:115-149.

Majumdar, D.N. and T.N. Madan. 1967. *An Introduction to Social Anthropology*. Bombay: Asia Publishing House.

Mandal, S.R. 1997. Social and Cultural Dimension of Mother and Child Health: Some Observations from A Muslim Village in West Bengal. Bulletin of Deptt. of Anthropology, *Dibrugarh University, Dibrugarh*. Vol.-XXV.

Medhi, B.K. and B. Paul. 2004. Health and Hygiene of the Nahs of Arunachal Pradesh. *Stud. Tribes Tribals*. 2 (1):23-27.

Medhi, B.K. and R. Hasan. 2003. Use of Plants in the Ethnomedical Practices of the Garos of Assam. *Man and Life*. Vol.29 (1-2):37-49.

Mehta, J.C. 1977. *Habitat, Human Settlements and Environmental Health*. Delhi: New Asian Publishers.

Mills, J.P. 1926. *The Ao Nagas*. London: Macmillon and Co. Limited.

Mohan, M. 1977. "Microbial Pollution and Public Health", in *Current Trends in Indian Environment*. Edited by D. Bandhu and K. Chauhan. Today and Tomorrow's Printers and Publishers.

Mojumder, A. 2006. Utilization of Health Care in North Bengal: A Study of Health Seeking Pattern in an Interdisciplinary Framework. *J. Soc. Sci*. 13 (1): 43-51.

Morris, B. 2006. *Religion and Anthropology; A Critical Introduction*. Cambridge University Press.

Murdock, G.P. 1965. *Social Structure*. London: The Macmillan Company.

Nagla, M. 2006. Culture and Health Care : An Interface. *Man in India*. 86 (1&2): 39-50.

Nanda, S. and R. Stephenson. 2001. Household Environment and Infant Mortality in India: A state level analysis with special focus to Orissa. *J. Hum. Ecol*. 12 (2): 81-86.

Pandey, G.D. *et al*. 2001. Socio-cultural Aspects and Health Care in Pando Tribe of Madhya Pradesh. *J. Hum. Ecol*. 12 (5): 391-394.

Pandey, P.L. *et al*. 2000. Some Aspects of Social Factors Affecting Fertility Behaviour of Gond Women. *Man in India*. 80 (3&4) : 251-258.

Patel, S. 1985. *Ecology, Ethnology and Nutrition*. Delhi: Mittal Publications.

Paul, S.K. 2006. "Health Care System Among The Tribals: The Shifting Paradigm Through Self Help Group", in *Health Problems and Health Care Systems Among The Tribes of India*. Abstract volume of National Workshop.

Pokarna, K.L. 1994. *Social Beliefs, Cultural Practices in Health and Disease*. New Delhi: Rawat Publications,

Prakash, N. 2001. Relevance of Social Science Concepts to Health System Management. *J. Soc. Sci.* 5 (1&2):133-137.

Prasad, K.R. and K. Nagraj. 2001. Socio-demographic correlates of Place of Delivery and Person conducting the Delivery in a Rural Community of Andhra Pradesh. *J. Hum. Ecol.* 12 (5): 357-362.

Rahman, A. 1998. *Household Environment and Health*. Delhi: B.R. Publushing Corporation.

Rajaratnam, A. *et al*. 1997. Maternal and Child Health Practices and Nutritional Status of Malto Tribals in Bihar. *Man in India*. 77 (1): 29-34.

Reddy, V.N.K. 1978. *Marriages in India*. Haryana: The Academic Press.

Rongmei, K.S. and S. Kapoor. 2005. Zeliangrong Today: A Naga Tribe of Manipur. *Stud. Tribes Tribals*. 3 (2):105-116.

Roy, A.D. 2002. A Social Profile of the Garo Hills District. *Man in India*. 82 (1&2): 165-176.

Roy, D. 1998. Educational situation in a Hill Village of West Bengal: A case study. *Man in India* 78 (3 & 4): 305 - 315.

Roy, R. *et al*. 1997. A study of Health Status of some Kharia and Mankhria Women from Orissa. *Bulletin of Deptt. of Anthropology, Dibrugarh University, Dibrugarh*. Vol.-XXV.

Saikia, J.K.K. 2003. "Religion: A Factor of Culture Change amongst Angamis in Nagaland", in *Tribes of North East*

India. Edited by Sarthak Sengupta. New Delhi: Gyan Publishing House.

Sangma, M.S. 1987. *History of American Baptist Mission in North East India*. Delhi: Mittal Publications.

Selvarajan, E. and R. Elango. 2004. *Rural Development Programmes and Externalities*. New Delhi: Serial Publications.

Sema, H. 1986. *Emergence of Nagaland*. New Delhi: Vikas Publishing House Pvt. Ltd.

Sen, S. 1987. *Tribes of Nagaland*. New Delhi: Mittal Publications.

Shameen, S. and T. Shameen. 2005. Traditional Health Care Practices of Munda Women: Continuity and Change. *Man and Life*. Vol. 31 (1-2):23-26.

Sharma, A. 2001. *Changing Modern Society*. New Delhi: Mittal Publications.

Sharma, A.K. 2005. "Perspectives on Health, Illness and Wellbeing: An Agenda for Future Research", in *Social Dimension of Health*. Edited by A.K. Dalal and S. Ray. New Delhi: Rawat Publications.

Sharma, C. and A.N.M. Irshad Ali. 2005. The Kaibartas: A Fishing Community of Assam, Their Society and Economy. *J. Hum. Ecol*. 17 (3): 205-209.

Sharma, P. 2002. Tai-Khamyang of Assam: Religious Life. *Bulletin of Deptt. of Anthropology, Dibrugarh University*. Vol. 30.

Shimmi, Y.L. Roland, 1988. *Comparative History of the Nagas, from ancient period till 1826*. New Delhi. Inter-India Publications.

Shimray, R.R. 1985. *Origin and Culture of Nagas*. New Delhi: Shimray Publications.

Singh, R.R. 1985. *The Mongsang Tribe of Manipur: A study on Changing Social Orientation of a small Tribal Group*. Ph.D. thesis submited to the Department of Anthropology, Dibrugarh University.

Singh, H.P. and M.C. Joshi.1990. "Shifting Cultivation in Nagaland", in *Shifting Cultivation in North East India*. Edited by D.N. Majumdar. New Delhi: Omsons Publications.

Singh, C. 2004. *Naga Politics, A Critical Account*. New Delhi: Mittal Publications.

Singh, Y.K. 2000. *Health Culture among the Mishings: A case study in Assam*. Ph.D. thesis submitted to the Department of Anthropology, Dibrugarh University.

Singh, P. 1972. *Nagaland*. New Delhi: National Book Trust.

Singh, K.S. (Ed). 1994. *Poeople of India Nagaland*. Vol. XXXIV.

Singh, K.R. 1987. *The Nagas of Nagaland*. New Delhi. Deep and Deep Publications.

Sinha, R., 1996: Equalisation of Educational Opportunities Scheduled Caste and Scheduled Tribe : Problems and Feature Strategies. *Man in India*. 76 (2):141-159.

Smith, W.C. 1857. *The Ao Naga Tribes of Assam*. Delhi: Gian Publications.

Spector, R.E. 1996. *Cultural Diversity in Health and Illness*. U.S.A.: Appleton and Lange Stanford, C.T.

Swarap, R. *etal*. (Ed). 1992. *Environmental Health, Education and Public Understanding; Encyclopaedia of Ecology, Environment and Pollution Control-2*. New Delhi: Mittal Publications.

Syamala, T.S. 2004. Do Health Worker Female and Traditional Birth Attendant Equipped to Provide Primary Health Care in Tribal Areas? Evidences from Tribal Andhra Pradesh. *Stud. Tribes Tribals*. 2 (2) : 119-124.

Tewari, V. K. 1991. "Healthy Housing: Urban India", in *Health Implications of Public Policy*. Edited by B. Ghosh. Bangolore: Indian Institute of Management.

Thakre, K. 1995. "The Bhills: Family, Marriage and Inheritance", in *Indian Tribes Health, Ecology and Social*

Structure. Edited by R.C. Swarankar. Jaipur: Rupa Books Pvt. Ltd.

Thangmi, 2002. *Ethnographic Study among the Thangal (Koirao) Tribe of Manipur*. Ph.D. Thesis submited to the Department of Anthropology, Manipur University.

Tiwari, P. and A.N. Sharma. 2001. An Assesment of Socio-Demographic Correlates Associated with Cases of Maternal Malaria. *J. Hum. Ecol*. 12 (5): 371-373.

Troisi, J. 1979. *Tribal Religion; Religious Beliefs and Practices among the Santals*. New Delhi: Manohar Publications.

Tyagi, D. 1997. Tribal Health in Anthropological Perspective. *Bulletin of Deptt. of Anthropology, Dibrugarh University, Dibrugarh*. Vol. XXV.

Vashum, R. 2000. *Nagas Right to Self Determination*. New Delhi. Mittal Publications.

Varma, G.R. *et al*. 2000. A study on knowledge of various family planning methods among rural population of Andhra Pradesh. *Man in India*. Vol. 80 (3 & 4): 331-336.

Verma, A. 2002. Antenatal Care and Birth Related Practices among the Baigas. *J. Hum. Ecol*. 13 (4): 257-261.

—. 2002. Socio-cultural correlates of Infant Mortality in a Primitive Tribe. *J.Hum. Ecol*. 13 (3): 203-207.

Vidyarthi, L.P. 1963. *The Maler : A Study of nature, man, spirit complex in a hill tribe of Bihar*. Calcutta: Book Land.

Vidyarthi, L.P. and B.K. Rai. 1976. *The Tribal Culture of India*. New Delhi: Concept Publishing Company.

Wells, A. 1970. *Social Institution*. London: Heinemann Educational Books Ltd.

Wells, P.S. 1980. *Culture Contact and Culture Change*. London: Cambridge University Press.

Westermarck, E. 1926. *A Short History of Marriage*. London: St. Martins Street, Macmillan and Co. Ltd.

Yadav, A. *et al*. 2001. Child Rearing Practices Among The Semi-Nomadic Lohar-Godiyas A Preliminary Observation. *Man in India*. 81 (3&4):391-395.

Yadav, A. and A.N. Sharma. 2002. Health Culture and Health Seeking Behaviour among the Semi-Nomadic Lohar-Gadiyas of Malthon Town of Sagar District, Madhya Pradesh. *J. Hum. Ecol*. 13 (6): 431-435.

Yonuo, A. 1974. *The Rising Nagas*. Delhi: Vivek Publishing House.

INDEX

Health Care Practices among the Ao Nagas

About the Author

Pranjal Boruah *(b. 1982)* in serving as an Assistant Professor in the Department of Anthropology, Dibru College, Dibrugarh, Assam. He did his Post Graduation in Social and Cultural Anthropology and PhD in 2008 from Dibrugarh University. He has to his credit serveral articles published in leading journals. Besides academic research, his area of interest is in social development and he is member of different professional bodies.